MANAGED BEHAVIORAL HEALTH SERVICES

MANAGED BEHAVIORAL HEALTH SERVICES

Perspectives and Practice

Edited by

SAUL FELDMAN

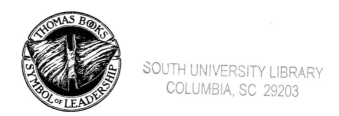

CHARLES C THOMAS • PUBLISHER, LTD.
Springfield • Illinois • U.S.A.

Published and Distributed Throughout the World by

CHARLES C THOMAS • PUBLISHER, LTD.
2600 South First Street
Springfield, Illinois 62704

©2003 by CHARLES C THOMAS • PUBLISHER, LTD.

ISBN 0-398-07348-1 (hard)
ISBN 0-398-07349-X (paper)

Library of Congress Catalog Card Number: 2002020459

With THOMAS BOOKS *careful attention is given to all details of manufacturing
and design. It is the Publisher's desire to present books that are satisfactory as to their
physical qualities and artistic possibilities and appropriate for their particular use.*
THOMAS BOOKS *will be true to those laws of quality that assure a good name
and good will.*

Printed in the United States of America
SM-R-3

Library of Congress Cataloging-in-Publication Data

Managed behavioral health services : perspectives and practice / edited by
Saul Feldman.
    p.   cm.
Includes bibliographical references and index.
ISBN 0-398-07348-1 (hard) -- ISBN 0-398-07349-X (pbk.)
1. Managed mental health care. I. Feldman, Saul.

RC480.5 .M3225 2002
362.2'0425--dc21
                                                                2002020459

CONTRIBUTORS

MICHAEL BENNETT, M.D.
    Associate Clinical Professor of Psychiatry
    Harvard Medical School

AUDREY BURNAM, PH.D.
    Senior Behavioral Scientist, RAND
    Director, RAND Center for Research
    on Alcohol, Drugs, and Mental Health

TAMARA CAGNEY, R.N., M.F.T., C.E.A.P.
    EAP professional

BRIAN J. CUFFEL, PH.D.
    Vice President, Research and Evaluation
    United Behavioral Health

NORMAN DANIELS, PH.D.
    Goldthwaite Professor
    Department of Philosophy
    Tufts University
    Professor of Medical Ethics
    Department of Social Medicine
    Tufts Medical School

RICHARD D. FLANAGAN, PH.D.
    Vice President
    Fort Hill Company
    Montchanin, Delaware

RICHARD G. FRANK, PH.D.
    Margaret T. Morris Professor of Health Economics
    Harvard Medical School

SHERRY A. GLIED, PH.D.
Associate Professor and Chair
Department of Health and Management
Mailman School of Public Health
Columbia University

MICHAEL A. HOGE, PH.D.
Associate Professor of Psychology (in Psychiatry)
Director, Managed Behavioral Healthcare
Yale University School of Medicine

JUDITH R. LAVE, PH.D.
Professor of Health Economics
University of Pittsburgh

WILLIAM MALONEY
Principal
William M. Mercer, Inc.

DANNA MAUCH, PH.D.
Former CEO, Magellan Public Solutions
Magellan Health Services, Inc.

SUSAN L. NEEDHAM, PH.D.
Chief Clinical Officer
Vice President, Product Development
Epotec, Inc.

JOAN M. PEARSON, PH.D.
Principal
Towers Perrin

JOHN PETRILA, J.D., LL.M.
Chair and Professor
Louis de la Parte Florida Mental Health Institute
University of South Florida

JAMES E. SABIN, M.D.
Clinical Professor of Psychiatry, Harvard Medical School
Director, Ethics Program, Harvard Pilgrim Health Care

SHARON A. SHUEMAN, PH.D.
Principal
Shueman Troy Associates

TOM TRABIN, PH.D., M.S.M.
Executive Director
Software and Technology Vendors' Association
Chair, Behavioral Informatics Tomorrow

WARWICK G. TROY, PH.D., M.P.H.
Principal
Shueman Troy Associates

Dr. Saul Feldman is the CEO of United Behavioral Health, a part of UnitedHealth Group and the executive editor of the journal *Administration and Policy in Mental Health*. He is a member of the Substance Abuse and Mental Health Service Administration's National Advisory Council, the Menninger Foundation's Board of Directors, and the MacArthur Foundation's Network on Mental Health Policy Research. Earlier, at the National Institute of Mental Health, he directed the national community mental health centers program and the Staff College. He is a past president of the American College of Mental Health Administration and a former adviser to the World Health and Pan American Health Organizations.

"The art of progress is to preserve order amid change and to preserve change amid order."

—Alfred North Whitehead

PREFACE

A decade ago, when the predecessor to this book was published, managed behavioral health organizations (MBHOs) were well into their adolescence–growing rapidly, unclear about their future, unsure about their identity, uneasy about their relationships, and, at least in their view, under-appreciated. Still growing, albeit much more slowly than in the past, MBHOs now dominate how behavioral health services are provided and paid for. They also have influenced behavioral health policy. Parity benefits, for example, would not likely have happened were it not for the well-documented, empirically based evidence that parity is affordable, but only under managed care.

The future of managed behavioral health is still unclear. To what extent, for example, is it likely to be a transitional object, less needed than in the past? Has it had an enduring and significant enough effect on the provider behavior that brought it about? Lest we forget, before the era of managed care, behavioral health services were too often characterized by long, expensive, and inappropriate, if not fraudulent, hospitalizations–particularly of children and adolescents. As a result of a lengthy investigation, "psychiatric hospitals and addiction centers paid over $500 million in Federal fines to settle charges of profiteering and diagnostic fraud in recruiting patients with generous mental health insurance" (Sharkey, 1999, p. 5). It was commonplace to use up limited substance abuse benefits on 28-day inpatient stays despite demonstrably less costly and more effective alternatives. As a result of all this and more, costs were escalating at a rate 20 to 30% higher than in general medical care, with no evidence of added value. If managed behavioral health were to disappear, would we return to what some would consider those "good old days?"

A decade ago, the cost of general health and behavioral health services was a major public concern, particularly its growing percentage of the gross national product. There were fearsome predictions of a linear progression that would, if nothing was done, severely damage the country's economy. The conventional wisdom was that health care costs were out of control, increasing much more rapidly then general inflation. Newspapers across the country spoke of behavioral health costs surging—even faster than other health care costs—and payers were especially troubled by the rise in hospitalization for adolescents with behavior problems and the like.

But there was something else going on, related to rising costs, but more subtle and at least as important. Whether it be in human services, foreign policy, the environment, or other major societal concerns, in order for change to occur, there must be real or fictional villains to blame, victims to pity, and potential saviors to root for. So it was with behavioral health (though *mental* health was the term more frequently used then). The designated villains were the private, for-profit psychiatric hospitals and the inpatient substance abuse facilities—blamed for profiteering, coerced admissions, bad or nonexistent care, and unnecessarily extended lengths of stay, terminated only when the benefits ran out. The victims were the patients, particularly but not exclusively children and adolescents; as reported by the media, they did not need to be hospitalized and were confined against their will, kept in the hospital too long, and psychologically damaged by the experience. To what extent these allegations were true—and to what extent they were hyperbole or a reflection of the media's hunger for tragic human interest stories—has never been clear, but it is likely that they are not entirely without foundation.

Clinicians were also vilified (albeit to a lesser extent) and were accused of seeing patients for too long, of not being able to demonstrate that the therapy was doing anybody any good, and of being indifferent to the societal consequences of the costs of their services. *Wave therapy*—an unkind but, unfortunately, not entirely inaccurate term—was used to describe the behavior of those psychiatrists who would walk through the hallway of a psychiatric hospital, wave to the patients in the rooms, and bill the insurer for each wave.

Managed care was then perceived as the savior, as the solution to the escalating cost problems, to the poor quality of care, to the absence of data, and to the lack of accountability by hospitals and clinicians. Like the HMOs before them, MBHOs, it was believed, would curtail unnecessary care and save money by providing the right services, at the right time, in the right place, at the right price.

Thus it was–a decade ago–that the villains, victims, and saviors were clearly identified and portrayed so convincingly that their images became fixed and part of the conventional wisdom. By the end of the 1990s, however, the first full decade of managed behavioral health, a profound change had taken place. At least in the perceptions of the public, the villains had traded places. Managed behavioral health was increasingly portrayed as the villain, whereas the providers, who a decade earlier had been portrayed as villains, came to be seen as victims. As before, patients remained the victims, but were now seen as being victimized by too little care rather than too much.

Who by now has not read or heard about needed services being denied? About clinicians not being allowed to care for their patients properly, being dictated to, if not exploited, by the MBHO? About so-called hard-hearted bureaucrats and insurance administrators making clinical decisions? And the list goes on. As with a decade ago, fiction and reality are interwoven, indistinguishable, but nonetheless persuasive.

The public's image of hospitals and clinicians was bad a decade ago; it is better now. The image of managed care was good then; it is worse now. Managed behavioral health–seen as the solution to the problems of a decade ago–is now, more frequently than in the past, portrayed as the problem. Fostered by the media, politicians, and special interest groups, simplistic generalizations abound as they did then. Then and now, the question should not be whether managed care, psychiatric hospitals, or clinicians, for that matter, are good *or* bad; they are, of course, good *and* bad, depending on what they do and how they do it. Differentiation is the key to understanding.

I leave it to those wiser and more courageous than I to predict who the next savior and what the next "solution" will be, how enduring, and how long it will be before the solution metamorphoses into the problem, at least in the mind of the public.

With time, MBHOs have become more sure about who they are, what they do, and why they do it. This heightened sense of security is, in good measure, engendered by their customers, who continue to see MBHOs as an important and permanent part of the behavioral health landscape. Employers, health plans, and other payers do not stop using MBHOs, although they may from time to time switch from one to another. Identity issues remain, although less so than in the past, as

MBHOs have added a number of services—disability, employee assistance, and others—and have broadened their scope, far beyond their traditional role.

Relationships with clinicians and facilities, however, remain far more problematic than those with customers. Managed health care therefore continues to be a leading topic of discussion in the professional media and wherever behavioral health practitioners gather. And the rhetoric, often negative and sometimes vitriolic, is only slightly less passionate now than a decade ago. Candidates for the presidency of the two major professional membership organizations (American Psychological and Psychiatric Associations), for example, apparently believe that they cannot possibly be elected without a strong and widely communicated position against managed behavioral health. It is ironic that those practitioners who are most critical of managed behavioral health did the most to bring it about in the first place. Had their behavior been different, so would the conditions under which they are now practicing; managed care would not have been needed.

Money, something that was in the past not discussed or argued about openly, remains an issue. Behavioral health practitioners tended to deny or at least not acknowledge their self-interest while actively pursuing it; they gave the impression that they viewed money "much like the Victorians viewed sex. It was seen as vulgar, as a sign of character defect, as something an upstanding professional would not be interested in" (Levinson & Klerman, 1972). Times have certainly changed. Whether or not related to the advent of managed behavioral health, financial self-interest is more overt than in the past. How much practitioners are paid and how promptly is not infrequently (or inappropriately) an important issue in their relations with MBHOs.

Provider concerns about managed behavioral health include the erosion of the professional prerogatives so highly valued by behavioral health professionals. These concerns are real and go to the heart of the major changes that MBHOs have brought about in the way that practitioners and hospitals do their work. The changes challenge what many behavioral health practitioners hold most dear and most zealously try to protect: their professional autonomy. The ability (or divine right) to be free of all controls over their behavior, to work in splendid isolation, is highly cherished by behavioral health professionals—particularly, but certainly not exclusively, by physicians. I have used the term "M.Deity" as a perhaps uncharitable description of this attitude in physicians; "Ph.Deity" is not far behind. This dimension—that is, the involvement (some would say intrusion) of MBHOs in clinical decisions that have historically been the almost exclusive domain of practitioners—has engendered the most opposition to, and most heated opinions about, managed behavioral health.

Other negative criticisms—not necessarily unrelated to money and power, but stated differently and in a more socially acceptable way—are about "quality of care" and "patient needs." To be sure, any time that a change of consequence to patient care takes place, its effects on quality must be addressed and closely examined. But not surprisingly, those who believe that their financial and power needs are threatened by change somehow seem always to see change as bad for the quality of care and the status quo as good, or at least better.

The effects of managed behavioral health are more clear now then they ever were. Access to outpatient care is up, inpatient care is down, costs are contained, utilization patterns have changed, community alternatives to hospitalization are more prominent, parity benefits have arrived, and employee assistance/work/life programs are now commonly part of the services that MBHOs provide. Nevertheless, still too "little is known about managed behavioral health's effect on treatment outcomes" (Feldman, Cuffel, & Hausman, 1999, p. 6). In an annotated bibliography listing 111 empirically based studies published between 1994 and 1998, only seven had to do with treatment outcomes. Moreover, those seven were all studies of the public sector even though over the past ten years, the amount of research done on managed behavioral health services has grown exponentially (Feldman et al., 1999). Most of the studies have focused on issues of cost and utilization, benefit design, and managed care in the public sector. So despite all the new research, conclusions about the effects of managed behavioral health on quality and outcomes are still indeterminate and very much in the eye of the beholder. Impassioned judgments on all sides continue to rely more heavily on anecdotal "evidence" than anything else.

It is clear that some of the processes used by some MBHOs do not reflect a sufficient understanding of the differences between control and accountability in their relationships with care providers. Control is undesirable; accountability is not. Accountability should be the essence of what good managed behavioral health is about–the accountability of providers and managers of care to each other, to the people they serve, to those who pay them, and to the public interest. Such accountability is not possible without data collection and analysis, and without appropriate processes to evaluate such factors as access, cost, and quality. None of this was possible in the days prior to the advent of managed behavioral health. It is much more possible now.

Accountability is also not possible without checks and balances, the constructive tension between care manager and practitioner when they interact around such issues as treatment planning and locus of care. This exchange between well-qualified professionals with somewhat different perspectives leads, in my judgment, to the best clinical decisions. But checks and balances work well only when the parties to the process are independent, neither being overly dominant. MBHOs must resist the temptation toward excessive control over practitioner behavior, however tempting with regard to efficiency and ease of operations that prospect may be. Failure to do so is to the detriment of patient care and practitioner autonomy.

MBHOs must also recognize that while they influence the nature of the interactions between practitioner and patient, quality of care is determined as it has always been, by what goes on in the consultation room between clinician and patient, in the hospital, and wherever else people who need help with behavioral problems are seen. Even with the best of intentions, practitioners who feel alienated from, and dictated to, by MBHOs are likely, unconsciously or not, to allow those feelings to affect their work with patients.

Care providers are not any less or more virtuous than care managers; opportunities for excessive self-interest are abundant and are available to both. Since the nature of behavioral health services allows care providers and managers a wide range of discretion, the opportunity to transform the public's needs into their own interests and the patient's problems into their own solutions is omnipresent for both. In such an environment, self-interest and sanctimony are not easily distinguished from altruism and devotion.

At its best, managed behavioral health can improve quality, reduce inappropriate utilization, control costs, and protect behavioral health benefits from being wasted on unnecessary care. But at its worst, it can deprive people of services they really need, truncate the role of behavioral health care providers, and damage the quality of the clinician-patient relationship that is so central to the success of the therapeutic process.

We have seen managed behavioral health at its best and at its worst. We have unfortunately not yet witnessed an appreciable enough increase in the ability of practitioners, payers, and society at large to tell the difference. Managed behavioral health continues to be a fact of life and may well be so for some time. There is no clear alternative, at least not yet, nor anytime soon. Done well, it can and does do good. It has the potential to do better still.

Saul Feldman
San Francisco, California
March 2002

REFERENCES

Feldman, S., Cuffel, B., & Hausman, J. (1999). *Administration and Policy in Mental Health, 27* (1)–(2), introduction.

Levinson, D. J., & Klerman, G. L. (1972, Winter). The clinician-executive revisited. *Administration in Mental Health,* pp. 64–67.

Sharkey, J. (1999, June 6). Mental illness hits the money trail. *New York Times,* p. 5.

INTRODUCTION

Much of what was published about managed behavioral health in its first decade is best described as opinion—often well expressed, but less well informed. This is not surprising, given the strong feelings that managed behavioral health evoked and the inevitable delay between the time that so profound a change begins, and informed analyses, published. In managed behavioral health's second decade, empirically based research has contributed greatly to what is known about its effects on such questions as access, utilization patterns, patient satisfaction, and economics. Strong opinions still abound, though tempered somewhat by data and also better founded than in the past.

This book is not free of opinion. But we have attempted (readers will judge how successfully) to keep the opinions as informed as possible. The chapters are based on the authors' personal experiences with managed behavioral health, what they know from the experiences of others, and the published literature. Where studies and data do exist, strong efforts have been made to incorporate them.

All the authors are experts in the particular areas of managed behavioral health about which they have written. Where the authors' proximity to, and personal experience with, managed behavioral health care might skew them one way or another, they and the editor have tried to be aware of it and mute the bias wherever possible.

The subjects included in the book are, in the editor's opinion, among the most important to its potential audiences: those involved in, or connected to, the managed behavioral health enterprise as payers, managers, providers, and health-benefit consultants; those who have a research or teaching interest in the subject; and decision makers in government and the private sector.

The choice of subjects in a multi-authored book is never easy, constrained by a number of factors, including the editor's judgment and the availability of willing and knowledgeable authors. The latter constraint was, in fact, not much of one at all. The subjects I had in mind and the people best able to write about them matched very well. If readers feel that either was not well chosen, it is clear where the fault lies.

ACKNOWLEDGMENTS

It would not have been possible to convey the breadth and complexity of managed behavioral health without the participation of contributors who, despite heavy commitments, were willing to lend their time and expertise to this project. I particularly appreciate their tolerance for so finicky an editor.

The editorial assistance of Stephen Scher and the persistence of my assistant Katie Egen made a book of what might otherwise have remained a work in process.

CONTENTS

MANAGED BEHAVIORAL HEALTH SERVICES

Chapter 1

CHOICES AND CHALLENGES

Saul Feldman

By any measure, managed behavioral health organizations (MBHOs) grew rapidly during the last two decades of the twentieth century, and the so-called carve-out now determines how over 100 million people in this country use their behavioral health benefits. The term *carve-out* came into common usage with the advent of MBHOs as a way to differentiate them from medical health organizations. The term is relatively new; the ideology, policy, and practice are not.

The opening of the first psychiatric hospital in America (Virginia Eastern Lunatic Asylum, 1773) was, in effect, the first behavioral health carve-out. It established a framework for the relationship between behavioral health and medical services that has endured for over two centuries. Since then, behavioral health services have for the most part remained organizationally separate from medical care. The reasons for this include: the discomfort, if not antipathy, with which "difficult and or unpleasant" patients with behavioral disorders were and are often viewed by physicians; powerful advocacy groups that value independence as a means of obtaining greater visibility and resources for behavioral health services; and the general perception by behavioral "healthers" that when their services are simply a unit within, and financially dependent on, a general health care organization, the services are more likely than not to be undervalued and underfunded. As Michael Bennett (1992, p. 79) has written,

Note: Portions of the discussion above previously appeared in the June 1998 Special Issue of the *American Journal of Managed Care* (pp. 5P59–5P67).

Forced to compete with the priorities of the general health care setting, and to operate within the value systems and models of care common to the medical setting, mental health often does not fare well. There is a tendency to underfund and to "medicalize": to rely excessively on active interventions and on techniques of diagnosis and treatment that emphasize the biological, sometimes at the expense of human service elements of care.

So the behavioral health carve-out involves new terminology but not a new practice—it is consistent with tradition and time-honored practice. What is new (about 20 years old) is the particular form that the carve-outs have taken—that is, as free-standing, predominately private, for-profit MBHOs that work with the already large, but still growing, number of employers, HMOs, insurers, and public sector agencies that have chosen to administer their behavioral health benefits differently from their medical.

CHARACTERISTICS

A typical MBHO contract with a customer is the outcome of a process that includes: a comprehensive response by the MBHO to a request for proposal; a presentation by the MBHO to the prospective purchaser (and frequently its health benefits consultant); and a negotiation process about rates, performance standards, reports, and implementation matters. A common part of the contract addresses performance standards—a major departure from unmanaged behavioral health services—that the MBHO is required to satisfy. The standards generally cover such things as telephone-response time, accuracy and timeliness of payments to providers, utilization targets, member satisfaction, access to services, and the like. Failure to meet any of these challenging standards requires the MBHO to return a portion of the fee it is paid.

MBHOs are generally paid in one of two ways: a flat fee per employee or per member for its services (generally referred to as "ASO," administrative services only); or a monthly per capita payment for each member or employee (under which the MBHO, like an HMO, is at financial risk for the cost of all the administrative and clinical services that it is required to provide). In general, MBHO contracts with HMOs include this capitated, "fully insured" type of payment; in effect, the HMO transfers to the MBHO its risk for the cost of behavioral health services received by its members. Most MBHO contracts with self-insured employers, however, are ASO; the employer retains the financial responsibility for the cost of the services, and benefits from whatever savings may come about from the management of the care.

It is not clear whether the way in which MBHOs are paid affects the process through which care is managed, the quality and the cost of care, or utilization patterns. In their study of the Massachusetts Medicaid MBHO, Frank and McGuire (1997) found, "In light of the contract's weak cost-savings incentives [for the MBHO], it may be surprising that so much was saved." In his study of an MBHO with both ASO and fully insured contracts, Sturm (1997) found no significant utilization differences when the care was managed by the same staff under the same clinical standards. These early findings suggest the need for further research on the relationship between how the MBHO is paid and how it performs.

Clinicians and facilities provide, under contract, the services for which the MBHO is responsible. These providers are "credentialed" and then, generally every two years, "recredentialed" in order to be certain that they continue to meet MBHO requirements such as licensure, ethical practice, and patient satisfaction. Most clinicians are paid in one of two ways—fee for service (the most common method) or capitated (typically a flat fee per member per month without regard to the amount of services they provide). This latter model puts clinicians at risk for the cost of the services that they provide to all those for whose care they are responsible. In effect, the less care they provide, the better off they are financially.

The fee-for-service model is dominant, but some clinicians and MBHOs prefer capitation. To the clinicians, capitation sounds attractive because it means payment in advance, greater autonomy, less accountability, and less interaction with the MBHO with regard to treatment plans, authorizations, and claims payments. But it may well raise difficult ethical and practice-management issues, particularly for clinicians who have had little experience with it and who are not skilled in time-limited, goal-focused treatment. For the MBHO, capitation saves time and money—less interaction with clinicians, less care management around patient needs, and fewer operational issues. But it also detracts from the "constructive tension" between the clinician and the MBHO.

Research is needed to help understand whether the financial incentives in the capitated model–for providers to do less–result in undertreatment. Prior to the advent of MBHOs, the unmanaged fee-for-service system, with its financial incentives for providers to do more, clearly resulted in overtreatment and cost inflation.

MBHOs have generally encouraged their network clinicians to form groups. As a result, group practice among behavioral health clinicians is more common than in the past. These groups, with or without "walls," are expected to engage in ongoing quality-assurance activities, to enhance access, and to handle the administrative arrangements such as billing more efficiently than individual practitioners. There is no evidence yet to suggest whether this is the case or what the effects of this shift to group practice have been on utilization patterns or on the cost and quality of care.

MBHOs cannot function properly without a technology that enables them to collect and use in their operations an extensive range of data, including: eligibility for services; utilization and costs; and referrals to, and extensive information about, providers (such as location, specialization, and performance). The requisite information about patients includes: presenting problems; diagnostic and treatment information; quality and outcomes of care; satisfaction; and the like. These data form the basis for assessing the MBHO's operations, as well as for extensive aggregate reports to its customers. The databases developed by MBHOs in the course of their work–data on the defined, circumscribed populations for whose care they are accountable–are an important resource for service researchers. Unfortunately, there has been too little use of the data that MBHOs acquire. As a result, research findings have had only a negligible effect on managed behavioral health services; "managed mental health organizations and services researchers are still strangers in a relationship that has never really been consummated" (Feldman, 1999, p. 49).

The data collected by the MBHOs should not go beyond what is required to assess whether treatment is proceeding appropriately, whether the patient is at risk, and what additional care may be required. Reports to employers or payers should be in aggregate only, with no patient-specific information. Whether the collection of this range of data by the MBHO threatens confidentiality has not yet been subject to sufficient analysis.

BEHAVIORAL HEALTH BENEFITS

Prior to the advent managed care, the traditional rigidity of insurers—exacerbated by their discomfort with what they considered to be the amorphous nature of behavioral health services and their distrust of behavioral health clinicians—caused benefits to be locked into impenetrable silos. As a result, treatment decisions were too often made based on what the benefit would allow; for example, care in the hospital even in those cases where less restrictive alternatives were likely to be more desirable and less costly. Managed care has changed all that. MBHOs can, and frequently do, move benefits and dollars across a wide range of services as patient needs suggest. Rigid benefit designs have all but disappeared as payers have discovered that in a well-managed system, they are not necessary and can even be counterproductive. Treatment patterns have changed as inpatient dollars are used to pay for other services that are less restrictive and expensive—for example, partial hospitalization and residential care. How these changes have affected patient care, who the major beneficiaries have been, and to what extent benefit flexibility under managed care, like the benefit silos it replaced, is simply a euphemism for a process that restricts care and saves money are questions that remain to be answered.

Another important byproduct of managed behavioral health care is benefit protection. Despite the move toward parity, behavioral health benefits remain far more limited than are those for general medical care. If the limited benefits are used up on expensive and unnecessary inpatient care, for example, and as is not infrequently the case, further treatment is required at a later time, there may be little or no benefit left to pay for it. The patient's options then are to forgo needed care, pay for it out of pocket, or seek it in the public sector—which was clearly the case with the traditional 28-day-stay model for substance abuse treatment. Since the alternatives to inpatient care generally cost only about 35% of a typical inpatient stay, a lot more of the benefit remains; if care is needed again, it is available.

SAFEGUARDS

But benefit flexibility can damage patient care as well, if it is used by the MBHO simply as a means to cut costs. So safeguards are needed and do exist, far beyond what is possible in unmanaged care. Most employers and health plans, for example, monitor the activities of the MBHO that they have selected. The processes that are used for such monitoring include the ongoing analysis of the extent to which performance standards are met, confidential employee-satisfaction surveys, and close attention to complaints from providers and patients who may be dissatisfied with their care. These and other issues are discussed regularly with the MBHO. Moreover, most MBHOs have highly visible complaint systems. Complaints are taken seriously, investigated, and reported to employers and health plans, many of which require the MBHO to do so. Negative "noise" will and has caused an MBHO to be fired. By contrast, one might ask: To whom do patients in an *unmanaged* system complain? And with what effect? How much leverage do they have?

Some employers use outside experts to review and evaluate the work of the MBHO. One method for doing so is the on-site audit that includes a review of records, quality standards, staff qualifications, and the care-management process. Another is the use of a panel of outside behavioral health clinicians to review the work done by the MBHO. (This is an irony of our times–behavioral health professionals as consultants to employers to monitor the work of managed behavioral health firms that monitor the work of behavioral health professionals.) Accreditation by such organizations as the Joint Commission on Accreditation of Healthcare Organizations, National Committee for Quality Assurance, and American Accreditation HealthCare Commission represents yet another safeguard.

Providers are not reluctant to report to employers–and directly to the MBHO–what they consider to be inappropriate practices. MBHOs also have an appeals process in place for providers who are unhappy about clinical issues. While these processes vary, they generally include review by top-level MBHO clinical staff if the issues are not resolved at a lower level. When disagreements occur, they are most often about the level and length of care, not about whether any care is needed. The professional associations actively encourage complaints about managed care from their members. As one example, for many years the American Psychiatric Association ran a prominent announcement on the front page of every issue of *Psychiatric News* that solicited complaints about MBHOs from psychiatrists. The American Psychological Association has been no less diligent.

Many employers, particularly large ones, select an MBHO based on the advice of outside consultants whose future business prospects are very much affected by their ability to help select the "right" MBHO and to help make certain that the one chosen does a good job. It is also clearly in the best interest of the MBHO to make good that choice, if it wants to be recommended by the consulting group to other prospective clients.

The values, standards, and professionalism of the clinicians in the MBHO's network—both the clinical-care managers employed by the MBHO and the clinicians with whom they interact and who actually provide the direct services—have a profound effect on the quality of the services provided in a managed behavioral health environment. The clinicians who provide care are not at all reticent to express their points of view about the care of particular patients for whom they are responsible—which is as it should be. These clinicians do not and should not passively accept the judgment of the MBHO when it conflicts with their own about what is best for patients. Since they are the clinicians who have the most direct contact with the patient, their opinions must have prime impact on the clinical decisions that are ultimately made.

The care managers employed by the MBHO are (or should be) well-trained clinicians who, while inevitably influenced by the organizational context in which they work, are unlikely to be co-opted by it. They have strong allegiances to the values and ethics of their professions. It has long been true that professionals tend to be more identified with, and loyal to, the standards of their professions and the associations to which they belong than to the organizations by which they are employed (Raelin, 1986). These allegiances and the professionalism of the care managers help neutralize what may be any undue influence on their behavior by the MBHO.

These safeguards do not guarantee that behavioral health care in a managed environment will be free of bad practice—and it is not. But no such safeguards—either in magnitude or kind—ever existed in unmanaged behavioral health care, where laissez faire prevailed, and protections against bad practice, where they existed at all, did so only at the extremes. The reluctance of health professionals, as well as the associations to which they belong, to identify and take action against unethical behavior or egregiously substandard practitioners is well documented. In managed behavioral health care, the safeguards against improper practice are far more extensive, better developed, and likely to be more effective. Determining just how well these safeguards work and how they can be improved are important areas for services research.

LIFE-CYCLE CHANGES

Organizations have life cycles—their own passages, or stages of development through which they go as they mature and grow. MBHOs are no exception. In the earlier stages of their lives, the late 1980s and early 1990s, they were busy creating a place in society, developing an identity, a service, a technology, and a market.

Like other organizations at this beginning stage, MBHOs were characterized by high innovation and clarity about their mission, but by uncertainty about the future and their place in it. In those early days, they were an amalgam of ambition, conviction, and anxiety about whether they would succeed and how.

Their policies and operations were likely to be flexible. Changes were made relatively easily; the leadership style tended to be informal and open; the organizational structures were flat; and egalitarianism characterized the relationships between staff at all levels. There was much emphasis on service, on mission, and on promoting themselves.

As MBHOs grew, made a place for themselves, and became more secure and successful, they gradually began to change, often without realizing it. They began to focus more on internal processes, and became more complex, more hierarchical, more dependent on written policies and rules. At this stage, it becomes easy to forget, without realizing or intending to, what the organization really is in business for—why it exists—and easy to let process triumph over purpose. In the "heady" pursuit of bigness, it is easy to forget, too, that size can be an enemy of responsive, humanistic health services if it is not recognized as a potential problem and if the organization does not undertake structural and other changes to deal with it.

Every human service organization, whether for-profit or not, has the exceedingly difficult task of balancing its service responsibilities, on the one hand, with its survival and its financial needs, on the other. There are no algorithms or decision pathways to help. It is a complex and delicate balance (service and quality are far less tangible than money), certainly for the leaders of MBHOs, who are, by virtue of what managed care organizations do, a step away, and sometimes too long a step, from where patients are being seen. So it is easy to forget how difficult it is to help people who have difficult problems, to forget what managed behavioral health should really be about, to forget why it exists, to forget what it feels like to be a patient. It seems to me that whether and to what extent this happens to a particular MBHO depends on the values and training of its leadership, the extent to which its customers are sensitive to these issues, and the influence of concerned staff and providers.

Many years ago, I was the director of a not-for-profit outpatient psychiatric clinic located on a busy street in New York City. The clinic's waiting room had large windows so that people walking by could easily look in. When I arrived in the morning, the window blinds would invariably be tightly closed and the waiting room unpleasantly dark, so I asked the receptionist to open them. She did so, and I went to my office. When I came out later in the day, the blinds were tightly shut, and once again, at my request, the receptionist opened them. This scenario went on far longer than it should have, until one day I decided (belatedly) to sit in the waiting room in order to observe first hand what was going on. I should have already known what I saw: patients in the waiting room were closing the blinds, worried about being seen by someone walking by who might recognize them.

This simple, but profound, experience was for me a reminder of the limits of authority (as the "boss," I couldn't get the blinds to stay open), a "wake-up call" that I should not have needed about the stigma associated with behavioral health services and about the importance of experiential learning. Notwithstanding good intentions, I had become insensitive to what it feels like to be a patient.

How well MBHOs reconcile their service and financial responsibilities, and how sensitive they are to the needs of patients, could well determine whether history will record them as anything more than a transitional object, as simply a temporary fix for the excesses of the past, a medicine with iatrogenic effects at least as bad as the illness it was intended to cure. That could well be the case if MBHOs fall victim to excesses of their own: too little care rather than too much, too few services rather than too many, too much control rather than too little. And there is little comfort in the knowledge that if this happens it would not be the first time, nor is it likely to be the last, that the solution to one set of social problems brings about others at least as difficult to resolve as the first.

PARITY

A decade ago, parity for behavioral health benefits was not unlike the quest for the Holy Grail—long sought after, highly desired, but no closer to being found despite years of trying. Nonetheless, parity has never been far from the top of the priority list for behavioral health advocates—citizen groups, professional associations, and government agencies. During the years that I was at the National Institute of Mental Health, parity was always a high priority. We worked hard to achieve it. The response from insurance carriers and many employers was always the same—it's too expensive, we are against mandates, and behavioral health is not a high priority.

Some 10 years ago, only 21% of the largest companies in America offered their employees behavioral health benefits as good as they had been 10 years before, and what had been generous outpatient benefits for federal employees had virtually disappeared because of high utilization and costs.

But then something changed. In 1996, the federal Mental Health Parity Act was enacted. Though limited in scope, the act was symbolically important. More than half the states have already followed suit with legislation that establishes parity for at least (in general) the major mental disorders. And in 1999, President Clinton issued a directive—a landmark in the history of behavioral health services in this country—granting full parity for all federal employees with respect both to mental health and substantive abuse treatment.

So why did this enormous change take place in the latter half of the 1990s? How did we achieve something that so many of us thought would never be possible? Did the traditional opponents of behavioral health parity change their minds, undergo some sort of ideological conversion? Did they lose their zeal? I think not. Credit certainly goes to the advocacy groups—despite the long odds against them, they never gave up—and to the state legislatures. The administration in Washington—particularly the Gores—was also a major factor.

But in my judgment, none of these factors would have made much difference if not supported by the analytic work done by respected economists in the field, using MBHO data. For what was really the first time, advocates had available the ammunition that they needed; that is, establishing parity for behavioral health benefits would not break the bank. Because of managed care, such benefits are affordable by any reasonable definition, but only so long as the care continues to be managed.

This is a singular contribution of MBHOs—one for which they have received too little recognition. It is also a reminder that enlightenment and enthusiasm are slender weapons without economics. This achievement presents an interesting conundrum to those providers who are, of course, among the major beneficiaries of parity but who are most critical of managed behavioral health. The object of their displeasure is, at the same time, the vehicle through which what they have long desired is being achieved—greater benefits for behavioral health services. They have greeted parity with enthusiasm; their silence about the contributions of managed care has been deafening.

Research is needed, and some is already under way, about the effects of behavioral health parity on access to care, on utilization, on quality and cost. Some critics are suggesting that even if managed behavioral health care played a role in bringing about parity, it will by its very nature obviate the positive benefits of parity by restricting access and limiting services.

THE CARVE-OUT

It seems to me that the term *carve-out*, which I referred to earlier, has a more negative connotation now than it did in the past; to its critics, it has become synonymous with the delivery of isolated, disconnected care. *Carved-out* care is juxtaposed to, and contrasted with, *integrated* care, suggesting that ipso facto there is a substantive and clear distinction between the two, and that the two are mutually exclusive. This is, to me, an example of crooked thinking, a faulty argument that confuses and prejudices a situation that demands precise expression and clarity of thought.

To behavioral health professionals, *integration* is an evocative and appealing word. It conjures up an image of harmonious race relations, of social justice, and, in behavioral health, of a well-adjusted person whose personality and behavior are said to be "integrated." To refer to something as *carved out* has, instead, a more dubious, separatist, even sinister ring, certainly much less appealing than *integrated,* at least superficially.

I referred earlier to the Virginia Eastern Lunatic Asylum, America's first psychiatric hospital, which predated the Declaration of Independence. Note that the asylum stood alone: it could have been, but was not, organized as a unit of a general hospital. Since then, outpatient psychiatric clinics, child guidance centers, and community mental health centers, as well as public and private hospitals, have developed in much the same way. The MBHO follows what has been a long tradition. While freestanding structures may be more prevalent in behavioral health care than in other fields of health care, the field of behavioral health care is not unique. Oncology, cardiology, and other medical specialty practitioner groups and hospitals exist in many parts of the country, separate from general medical care, and they are growing. Why are they not ordinarily referred to as "carve-outs?"

It is not clear what the effect of the managed behavioral health carve-out has been on the interaction between behavioral and general medical care. The relationship is certainly not what it should be. But there is no persuasive evidence that demonstrates why this is so and whether it is any worse than it used to be. Improving the relationship– and with it, the interaction of behavioral health and general medical care, as well as its practitioners–is a major piece of unfinished business for administrators, researchers, clinicians, and academic health centers. What has gotten much less attention than it deserves is the relationship between behavioral health and the other human services such as schools and social agencies, particularly for children. Behavioral health, managed or not, stands now as it always has and as it should, straddling the fence, with one leg in the human services and the other in general medical care–a challenging and sometimes painful position.

The goal, of course, is to help people whose problems go beyond the boundaries or expertise of any particular specialty. I believe it is useful here to differentiate a "vertical" organization, in which behavioral health would be a structurally integrated part of a larger health care organization, from a "virtual" organization, characterized by functional coordination and collaboration between independent organizations working together to help patients who need the services of them all. If, as I believe it should be, the objective is functional integration or coordinated care, then the relation between behavioral and general health care can take many forms. There is no inherent dichotomy between the so called "'integrated" and "carved-out" approaches; the behavioral carve-out is not synonymous with estrangement, nor should it be viewed as such.

But for behavioral health care, the integration issues go beyond those that have to do with medical care and the other human services. Too little attention is paid to the integration problems within the behavioral health field itself. Interdisciplinary rivalries, competing ideologies, and the discomfort between mental health and substance abuse are not unlike what characterizes a dysfunctional family. Despite some progress, we are still not doing a good enough job—for example, with the diagnosis and treatment of co-occurring disorders. There is now, however, a greater recognition of the problem and a higher priority for doing something about it.

TRAINING AND PRACTICE

New theories, changed social conditions, research findings, and the like should influence both the way that behavioral health professionals are trained and the way that they work. Managed behavioral health is one such change; new knowledge about evidence-based practice guidelines is another.

There remains much too large a gap between what is known and what is done. As *Mental Health: A Report of the Surgeon General* (Satcher, 1999, pp. 455–456) indicates:

> State-of-the-art treatments, refined through years of research, are not being translated into community settings. . . . A wide variety of community-based services are of proven value. . . . Yet a gap persists in the broad introduction and application of these advances in services delivery to local communities, and many people with mental illness are being denied the most up-to-date and advanced forms of treatment. New strategies must be devised to bridge the gap.

What is striking about this conclusion is that the gap persists despite the proliferation during the past 10 years of evidence-based practice guidelines that are intended as vehicles through which knowledge is translated into training and practice. Based upon research findings and the opinions of experts, the guidelines are designed to improve practice, standardize treatment for particular diagnoses, and reduce inappropriate variability in treatment. I suspect that of all the health care providers in this country, it would not be easy to find any who practice with more variability than those in behavioral health.

Where variability reflects provider bias or lack of knowledge rather than patient need, it results in services of questionable quality and in excessive costs. Unfortunately, evidence-based practice guidelines have helped very little. In addition to having only a negligible overall effect on how clinicians work with patients, they still seem to be unknown to many behavioral health professionals.

The recognition of the gap between knowledge and practice is not new, but efforts to bring about change have had little impact. In issuing a call to action, the American College of Mental Health Administration (2000, p. 43) notes:

> Considering the changes and challenges in health care, there was overwhelming consensus that not only are training and education problematic across disciplines, but training and education, both pre-professionally and for the existing workforce, are failing the field (and therefore the people we are supposed to serve) at all levels.

Alan Tasman, a former president of the American Psychiatric Association, has pointed out that the psychiatric profession is "training a generation that lacks even the most basic psychotherapeutic skills or framework for understanding mental functioning from a psychological perspective" (Drug focus shortchanges psychodynamics, 2000).

At United Behavioral Health our clinical care managers have compiled a list of "worst practices," those things that they and our psychiatric staff regularly encounter as they routinely interact with clinicians and facilities. These practices include: poorly prepared or—all too often—nonexistent treatment plans; children in outpatient therapy and or residential care with no involvement of the family in the treatment process; patients being seen in outpatient therapy over an extended period of time with a diagnosis of depression but with no psychiatric evaluation and no antidepressants even where there is a family history of depression; outpatient therapists treating patients with bipolar disorder but with no medical evaluation and no medication; absent or inadequate coordination between an outpatient therapist and a psychiatrist when a patient's care is split between the two; patients with a co-occurring disorder who are seen in outpatient therapy but with no chemical-dependency treatment; psychiatric hospitals that do not provide education programs for the families of patients hospitalized for major mental disorders, despite the proven efficacy of such family-education programs; the relative neglect of community alternatives to inpatient care; and the use of unproven or inappropriate interventions such as "holding therapy."

As with research findings about what works, and despite its dominance and durability, managed behavioral health care has had too little effect on what clinicians are taught. The resistance of faculty is key. According to Michael Hoge and colleagues, "[S]upervisors often present only negative views of managed care. . . . There are few faculty role models who have embraced the changing assumptions about practice patterns" (Hoge, Jacobs, & Belitsky, 2000, pp. 1001–1002). This neglect of the current and likely future behavioral health services environment, in which managed care will continue to be a major factor, cuts across all the behavioral health disciplines. Graduate training is not preparing students for the world in which they will be practicing. There is too little emphasis on such issues as treatment planning, community alternatives to inpatient care, brief goal-oriented treatment, group and family treatment, and co-occurring disorders. Yager, Dochery, and Tischler (1996) have described this state of affairs as "pedagogic malfeasance." It seems to me that disciplinary training–with its rigid requirements fostered by the major professional associations in concert with licensing bodies–is a major barrier to change. Of the many "sacred cows" in the behavioral health field, it is among the most sacred (and most self-serving). There may have been a time in the history of this country when it was necessary and important for psychiatrists, psychologists, psychiatric social workers, psychiatric nurses, and others to have their own schools or academic departments, their own professional associations, their own licensing or certification procedures, their own professional journals, and perhaps, above all, their own professional identities. But I believe that time has long passed.

Disciplinary training is wasteful, inefficient, and too expensive. It promotes unhealthy rivalry between professions (someone once said that if you asked a group of behavioral health professionals to form a firing squad, they would get into a circle), separates them by emphasizing their differences rather than their commonalties, and discourages interdisciplinary learning. Steven Hyman, a former director of the National Institute of Mental Health, has decried "the lack of exposure to behavioral science in psychiatry residential training." Moreover, "Many developing psychiatrists don't even know that relevant psychology journals exist" (Runck, 2000). There are, of course, some legitimate differences between the disciplines, but in the practice of psychotherapy, for example, most clinicians do pretty much the same thing. The differences that exist are based much more on the theories to which particular clinicians subscribe than on their disciplines. So why are they trained separately? And why do they continue to be taught so much that they use so little of? How much more of real value to patient care could be learned if the training content required by specific disciplines was replaced by a "disciplineless," evidence-based curriculum? Would it lessen the need for expensive and time-consuming postgraduate training institutes in which M.D.'s, Ph.D.'s, M.S.W.'s, and others try to make up for the deficiencies of their formal training?

What I believe we need instead of separate disciplines are "undisciplined" behavioral professionals (though some would say that they are already undisciplined enough), with degrees in behavioral health rather than in psychology, psychiatry, or the other disciplines. Students would pursue a graduate degree, preferably a doctorate in behavioral health, with an opportunity to specialize in such areas as children's services, geriatric care, addictionology, administration, and so on. They would have limited prescribing authority, consistent with their particular training in psychopharmacology and related subjects. This extension of prescribing authority would help to address what has become a major problem in this country (with no solution in sight): a severe shortage of, and inadequate access to, psychiatrists. Such training programs would, moreover, be unencumbered by the academic straitjackets all too common in the current, disciplinary training of behavioral health professionals.

The curriculum would focus on evidence-based treatment, and the content could range from biochemistry to community organization—whatever subject matters and teaching methods would help ensure that the graduates would be able to provide optimal patient care. The shape and substance of the training would reflect the needs of patients rather than the biases of faculty or the interests of specialized professional guilds. The time and money now wasted teaching things that practicing clinicians never really use again would be used much more effectively.

I realize that the sociology of professions is such that creating a new one and doing away with the old is a daunting task. But the effects of perpetuating a system that is failing–and that has been for some time–are deadly. Given how intractable and resistant to even modest change the current system has proven to be, the best we can hope for with it still in place is some tinkering at the margins, but no real improvement.

We need dramatic change, such as a rebirth of something like the Doctor of Mental Health program that was started at the University of California some 25 years ago. The program's creators "had the perhaps foolish, perhaps sober courage to dream that contrary to the lessons of human history a wholly new profession . . . could be conceived just by the compelling logic of its fit to the needs of the mentally and emotionally ill" (Wallerstein, 1991, preface). The five-year program combined three basic subject areas–biological, psychological, and social sciences–with a practicum experience and intensive clinical training, culminating in a professional degree analogous to those in law and medicine (as differentiated from a Ph.D.). Graduates were expected to be proficient in diagnosis, psychotherapy, and a specialty area such as behavioral health administration, psychological aspects of physical illness, or forensic psychiatry.

The program awarded its last D.M.H. degrees in 1986. Over its life, 75 people were graduated and went on to work in a variety of settings–HMOs, community mental health centers, public agencies. They were judged by those who supervised them as the best-trained behavioral health professionals with whom they had ever worked. Unfortunately, the program fell victim to budget cuts, strong opposition from the established behavioral health guilds (particularly psychiatry, since it was intended that the graduates would have limited prescribing authority), and rigid licensing requirements.

EXPANDED SERVICES

Employee assistance programs (EAPs) and, more belatedly, work/life services grew substantially in the 1990s and increasingly became part of what MBHOs provide. The marriage between managed behavioral health, work/life, and employee assistance programs is not yet entirely consummated because the parties to it come from different professional traditions and cultures that are not yet entirely compatible. Nonetheless, when melded together, the three types of program provide a range of services broader than what has been experienced ever before through a single plan or provider.

Work/life, an expression of some ambiguity, goes beyond the traditional EAP and is a response to corporate America's interest in enhancing employee performance and in *absence management* (a term that came into use in the 1990s). The latter refers to keeping employees on the job by helping them with everyday problems that would ordinarily either preoccupy them while working or cause them to take time off. The expression *concierge services*, which was formerly pretty much restricted to something provided by hotels, is often used as an overall descriptor of what work/life programs do. The range of services appears almost unlimited. I know, for example, of a recent instance where a work/life program proposal to a prospective customer was rejected because it didn't include pet services—it does so now.

These programs have substantially expanded the boundaries of managed behavioral health, as has the Internet, which is already demonstrating its enormous capacity. For people seeking help, the Internet has the potential to transform and enhance their access to information, to treatment, and to sources of help beyond what has been possible in the past, and to do so quickly and easily. For providers, the Internet can mean enhanced access to clinical information (for example, practice guidelines), to patient referrals, to a new way of doing therapy, and to greater efficiency, particularly in how clinicians relate to MBHOs.

In a sense, the Internet represents a "catch up" for the behavioral health field. For far too long, we were spectators watching the self-help movement develop around us, but not with us. The past decade has seen an explosion of self-help material, much of it related to behavioral health. One can walk into any bookstore and literally see shelves of books and CDs on parenting, marital issues, self-esteem, and the list goes on. The Internet gives us an opportunity to catch up—and far more quickly than anyone thought possible just a few years ago. And MBHOs are embracing it rapidly—I hope not too much so.

I am concerned about the growth of counseling and therapy over the Internet–not only by MBHOs, but also by clinicians in private practice. I worry that the rate at which it may grow will exceed our ability to handle it wisely and well. Nonverbal communication, how a patient looks and acts, posture, facial expressions, and the like have been important in face-to-face therapy. What, if any, are the surrogates for these factors in therapy over the Internet? What are the other differences? Is special training needed for clinicians? Who will do the training? What will they teach? Who will fund and do the research that will help evaluate the effects of this Internet therapy? These and other questions abound. The answers are obviously not yet known, but we must begin working toward them.

One of the things that we need to understand better is whether and to what extent Internet-based services will add to, or substitute for, more traditional and more expensive services. The Internet has great potential for bringing behavioral health services to people who, because of geography or personal inclination, would not ordinarily take advantage of opportunities for face-to-face help. But is there a danger that the Internet will be used inappropriately–by clinicians and by MBHOs as a substitute way of providing care to people who really should be seen in person? The Internet is, after all, less costly and more convenient.

There are, of course, other troubling Internet issues to worry about, not the least of which is confidentiality. Despite assurances to the contrary, I believe that there is a legitimate concern about security, more so in behavioral health than in medical care, given the sensitivity of the problems with which we deal. Unresolved questions about confidentiality may be one of the primary reasons why Internet use so far–by those who have access to it as managed behavioral health members–is still quite low.

CONCLUSION

I have tried in this chapter to discuss what I believe to be some of the important things that have happened in and around managed behavioral health: the major characteristics and growth of the carve-out; its life cycle and effect on benefits; integration issues; parity; the gap between knowledge, training, and practice; EAPs and work/life services; and the Internet. Other topics were possible and perhaps preferable. Those I selected come from my now nearly 15 years of experience as a managed behavioral health executive, leavened by my prior incarnations while in government at the National Institute of Mental Health and also by my earlier work in outpatient psychiatric clinics.

It is far easier to discuss what *has* happened than what *will*, to reflect rather than predict. In that spirit, it is not at all clear to me what MBHOs will be like in the future, or even whether they will continue to exist. Managed behavioral health care came along at a time when it was needed; it has brought about major changes in the behavioral health landscape. But the conditions that bred and sustained it are no longer what they were: public alarm at cost increases, with slight accountability and no discernible added value; a surplus of inpatient beds; insufficient attention to effective alternatives to inpatient care; and reduced behavioral health benefits as a means to control costs. Now there is at least a partial mental health parity benefit (in most of the states), a full parity benefit for federal employees, far greater use of outpatient services than 10 years ago, enhanced continuity of care, and a range and depth of data that, more than ever before, may help us determine what all of this means. To what extent these developments are attributable to managed care, I leave to the judgment of behavioral health historians.

REFERENCES

American College of Mental Health Administration. (2000). Sounding a call to action. *Behavioral Healthcare Tomorrow, 9* (3), 43–44.

Bennett, M. J. (1992). Managed mental health in health maintenance organizations. In Feldman, S. (Ed.), *Managed Mental Health Services* (pp. 61–82). Springfield, IL: Charles C Thomas.

Drug focus shortchanges psychodynamics, Tasman says. (2000, July 7). *Psychiatric News, 35*. Available at <http://www.psych.org/pnews/00-07-07/drugfocus. html>.

Feldman, S. (1999). Strangers in the night: Research and managed mental health-care. *Health Affairs, 18* (5), 48–51.

Frank, R. G., & McGuire, T. G. (1997). Savings from a Medicaid carve-out for mental health and substance abuse services in Massachusetts. *Psychiatric Services, 48,* 1147–1152.

Hoge, M. A., Jacobs, S. C., & Belitsky, R. (2000). Psychiatric residency training, managed care and contemporary clinical practice. *Psychiatric Services, 51,* 1001–1005.

Raelin, J. (1986). *The Clash of Cultures.* Boston, MA: Harvard Business School Press.

Runck, B. (2000, August 4). Behavioral science too often ignored, says NIMH head. *Psychiatric News, 35.* Available at <http://www.psych.org/pnews/00-08-04/behavioral.html>.

Satcher, D. (1999). *Mental health: A report of the surgeon general.* Rockville, MD: National Institute of Mental Health.

Sturm, F. (1997). How expensive is unlimited mental health care coverage under managed care? *Journal of the American Medical Association, 278,* 1533–1537.

Wallerstein, R. (Ed.). (1991). *The Doctorate in Mental Health: An Experiment in Mental Health Professional Education.* Laham, MD: University Press of America.

Yager, J., Dochery, J., & Tischler, G. (1996, Fall). Training psychiatric residents for managed care: Fundamental values and proficiencies and an outline for a model curriculum. *American Association of Directors of Psychiatric Residency Training Newsletter,* pp. 3–6.

Chapter 2

EFFECT ON CLINICAL PRACTICE

Audrey Burnam

The rapid emergence and dominance of managed care approaches to the delivery of behavioral health services since their advent in the late 1980s is breathtaking. Even more remarkable is the rise of the managed behavioral health organization (MBHO) as the leading provider of these services. In less than two decades, the concept of managed behavioral health care has been embraced with such vigor that it now affects just about every aspect of how behavioral health services are organized, financed, and delivered in both the private and public sectors. These changes would, in turn, be expected to have a significant impact on the patterns of service utilization, on the quality of care provided, and on the clinical workforce and its practice style. Although research assessing these changes is still sparse, and the time lag for producing relevant research is frustratingly slow relative to the pace of industry change, there is now a suitable body of empirical literature—albeit incomplete and weak in some places—that can be consulted to evaluate how well managed care is working in the behavioral health arena.

This chapter reviews the available literature on those changes in specialty behavioral health service delivery that appear to be linked with the rapid emergence of managed behavioral health care. It examines evidence on patterns of service use, quality of care, and changes in the ways that behavioral health specialists run their businesses and provide clinical care. Note the intentional use of the phrase "appear to be linked," rather than the more decisive "caused by," since it is difficult to discern, even in the best of studies, either the degree to which these various changes are directly attributable to the diverse array of structures and processes that are encompassed in the term "managed care," or the degree to which they result from overall market and social shifts that are not specific to managed care technologies. Legislation to achieve parity of behavioral health insurance benefits is also discussed in this chapter because cost containment under managed care has clearly created a context in which parity policies can be embraced.

BEFORE MANAGED CARE

In order to provide some understanding of the context and intended consequences of the managed care revolution in behavioral health, we begin by briefly summarizing key features of the behavioral health care delivery system in the United States prior to the advent of managed behavioral health care (see Edmunds et al., 1997; Gerstein & Harwood, 1990; Institute of Medicine, 1996; Mechanic, 1999).

1960s to 1970s: The Community Mental Health Movement

The modern behavioral health delivery system was sharply influenced by the community mental health movement that began in the early 1960s. This movement shifted the treatment of mentally ill patients from state-directed psychiatric hospitals to outpatient and partial-hospitalization programs that emphasized new psychopharmacologic treatments and a variety of counseling, rehabilitative, and supportive services. The result was a dramatic decline in the number of public mental hospital beds—from 560,000 in 1955, to only 77,000 in 1995 (Bachrach, 1996). By the 1980s, both the uninsured poor and patients with severe mental illness received services largely from community-based facilities funded with direct federal and state dollars. These community-based models of care emphasized a continuum of services, including outreach, case management, outpatient care, and inpatient alternatives such as partial and day hospitalization. Long-term psychiatric hospitalization was considered appropriate for only a few of the most severely impaired psychiatric patients. Although the early community mental health centers increased access to mental health clinic services, they were also criticized for their failure to serve adequately the most severely mentally ill.

Through an infusion of categorically distinct public funding in the 1970s, a separate substance abuse treatment system also emerged. This system initially focused on treatment of alcoholism and heroin addiction and consisted largely of freestanding facilities offering outpatient and residential treatment programs. Models of care included methadone maintenance for heroin addicts and a diverse array of non-drug programs that often embraced the notion of rehabilitation within a self-policing and supportive community of peers. Programs tended to require relatively long-term participation; many members of the counseling staff in these substance abuse treatment facilities had personal addiction experience but little formal professional training.

1970s to 1980s: Expansion of Insurance Benefits

Also during the 1970s and early 1980s, private insurance benefits for mental health and substance abuse treatment began to expand under state mandates requiring employer-based plans to offer coverage for mental health and substance abuse treatment. Traditional indemnity insurance for behavioral disorders greatly expanded during this period, but these benefits were more heavily restricted than general medical care benefits—through the application of lower hospital-day and outpatient-visit limits, annual and lifetime dollar limits, and high copayments. In addition, because of skepticism regarding the value of "talk" therapies, traditional indemnity benefits tended to provide for relatively generous inpatient stays (for example, 30 days), but quite limited outpatient benefits, and seldom reimbursed intermediate alternatives to inpatient care (Freeman & Trabin, 1994). Medicaid insurance (public insurance for poor families with children and the disabled) also expanded and included state options to reimburse a wide range of rehabilitative and supportive services for the seriously mentally ill. By federal regulation, however, Medicaid could reimburse inpatient psychiatric care only when provided in general medical hospitals.

In response to the expansion of public and private fee-for-service insurance benefits, private specialty facilities grew during the late 1970s and 1980s. Admissions to private inpatient psychiatric treatment facilities, as well as to psychiatric inpatient units in general hospitals, dramatically increased during this period. Between 1972 and 1992, the number of private psychiatric hospitals grew from 150 to 475, and non-federal general hospitals with separate psychiatric services increased from 797 to 1,616 (Manderscheid & Sonnenschein, 1996). This same general period was also one of rapid expansion of inpatient care for children (Burns, 1991) and of inpatient chemical-dependency programs for alcohol and drug addiction (for those with private insurance) (Frank, Salkever, & Sharfstein, 1991; McKusick et al., 1998).

The Gap between Publicly and Privately Financed Behavioral Health Care

The 1970s and 1980s, then, gave us reverse trends in increasingly distinctive public and private sector markets. The directly funded public mental health system, which served the poor and most people with serious mental illness, had shifted dramatically from nearly exclusive reliance on psychiatric inpatient care to a continuum of community-based services. It retained only a modest capacity to treat patients in state psychiatric hospitals. The directly funded public substance-abuse treatment system developed largely outside of hospitals and medical models, and spawned, instead, many specialized treatment facilities. Medicaid beneficiaries generally received their services with the uninsured poor within the directly managed public systems (few private providers were attracted to the low reimbursement rates for mental health care, and Medicaid benefits for substance abuse treatment were limited), but these beneficiaries also had much greater access than the uninsured poor to Medicaid-reimbursed inpatient psychiatric care within general hospitals, including hospital-based detoxification from alcohol and drug addiction.

Privately insured people received a very different type of care. Traditional fee-for-service indemnity insurance expanded benefits for mental health and substance abuse treatment, and fueled a reverse trend toward hospitalization for a wide range of psychiatric and substance abuse problems. This trend included a surge in inpatient treatment of children and adolescents. Private insurance also increased access to outpatient treatment with highly credentialed behavioral health specialists (largely psychiatrists and Ph.D. psychologists)–but only for a limited number of visits.

The irony of these distinctive markets and reverse trends is that by the 1980s, the United States was treating the sickest patients (those with serious mental disabilities, as well as chronic alcoholics and hard-core drug addicts) in systems that emphasized outpatient care and relied heavily on paraprofessional and peer-counseling staff. At the same time, the employed and their dependents (generally with less severe problems) with private health insurance were being treated in a system that relied heavily on professional staff and hospital-based care.

Late 1980s: The Rise of Managed Care

By the mid-1980s, both public and private payers were concerned about the costs of behavioral health care. For public payers, the directly funded service system was capped, so to speak, by federal grants and by state and local budget allotments. The costs of the Medicaid fee-for-service insurance program, however, were not so easily contained. Medicaid mental health and substance abuse treatment costs escalated at an annual rate of 8.8% between 1986 and 1996, greatly outpacing general inflation (McKusick et al., 1998). This increase was of concern not only to the federal government, but to many states, which pay on average half the costs of this federal entitlement program. At the same time, employers–the major private payers–became increasingly concerned about the rising cost of health insurance premiums: a leading culprit was the rapidly increasing expense of private mental health and substance abuse benefits (Frank et al., 1991).

Managed behavioral health care emerged in the late 1980s in response to employer concerns about these escalating costs. Some analysts, such as Freeman and Trabin (1994), suggest that the conceptual roots of managed behavioral health care are found in two earlier developments. One was the community mental health movement that, in its emphasis on community-based rather than hospital care, embodied cost-effectiveness principles (Feldman, 1994). This movement not only led to a complete restructuring of the public system of care, but generated many of the initial leaders of managed behavioral health care. The other development leading to managed behavioral health care was the rise of Employee Assistance Programs (EAPs), which began as early as the 1950s and 1960s as employer-sponsored services designed to provide advice, counseling, and treatment referral for substance abuse problems in the workplace. EAPs gradually evolved to address a broader scope of behavioral health issues in the workplace and to manage the use of behavioral health specialty services.

The growth of the managed behavioral health care industry over the past decade has been phenomenal. Findlay (1999) recently reported that approximately 78% of Americans who have health insurance, either private or public, are presently enrolled in some kind of managed behavioral health plan. This is more than a doubling of enrollment in managed behavioral health care since 1993. The early managed care model of the full-service health maintenance organization (HMO) that provided both behavioral health care and general medical services hardly exists today. HMOs now overwhelmingly "carve out" behavioral health services; that is, either the employer or the HMO separately contracts with an MBHO to cover mental health and substance abuse insurance benefits. A 1997 survey of MBHOs and HMOs showed that nearly 90% of participants were enrolled in a specialty managed behavioral health plan, while the remainder received behavioral health care directly from an HMO (Oss, Drissel, & Clary, 1997). Many MBHOs were spawned in the late 1980s and early 1990s, and fierce competition has rocked the industry. Through a rapid succession of mergers and acquisitions, three private, for-profit MBHOs currently have more than half of the market share, and only 10 organizations control 80% of the market (Oss et al.).

The public Medicaid market has also made significant shifts toward managed care—following, and in many ways also modeling, the approaches developed in the private sector. Under pressure to control the escalating costs of their Medicaid fee-for-service insurance programs, states used opportunities provided through federal waivers to restructure their Medicaid programs. Many states developed capitated contracts (in which a fixed fee is provided for each beneficiary) with private managed care organizations to provide health services to their Medicaid populations. Broad reforms undertaken by a few states greatly expanded Medicaid insurance eligibility to include all the poor; they financed their new state insurance systems with blended Medicaid dollars and directly managed federal and local dollars. The federal Substance Abuse and Mental Health Services Agency tracked public managed care in 1998 and reported that 47 states had implemented 97 managed behavioral health programs. A little more than half of these programs were specialty behavioral health carve-outs, and the remainder were general medical plans that included some mental health or substance abuse services (Substance Abuse and Mental Health Services Administration, 1998).

While states are adopting some aspects of employer-based managed care models, they are also creating distinctive approaches that take into account not only the unique features of an enrollee population that is disproportionately chronically ill, but the existence of a specialized set of public safety-net providers that have traditionally served this population. In state plans, acute-care service benefits are often distinguished from long-term-care service benefits: acute-care benefits are provided as part of the main medical managed care plan, with long-term-care benefits covered by a specialty behavioral health carve-out plan. Half of the states with carve-out programs have contracted their management to either public agencies or public/private partnerships. Although the majority of the programs tracked in 1998 reported that they covered mental health services, substance abuse services were only seldom included; if included, they were integrated either with the main medical plans or with mental health services in a behavioral health plan.

While low-income women and children who compose most of the Medicaid population typically receive limited behavioral health benefits as part of a Medicaid managed care plan, states have increasingly extended more comprehensive managed behavioral health care to those with serious mental disorders (Bazelon Center for Mental Health Law, 2000). Of the 31 states that have adopted managed care models for the seriously mentally ill, all but 2 use specialized behavioral health carve-outs. Most (21) are statewide managed care programs, while the remainder have been implemented in specific counties, regions, or smaller pilot areas.

PATTERNS OF SERVICE USE

Both the private and the Medicaid fee-for-service insurance environments offered incentives that favored lengthy, expensive hospital stays. The resulting escalation of costs for behavioral health care set the stage for payers to turn to managed behavioral health care. We might expect, then, that managed care strategies to contain costs would focus on reducing inpatient care and substituting lower-cost outpatient and intermediate services. The evidence supports this expectation with respect to inpatient care and the more flexible use of benefits to provide intermediate services, but the story with outpatient services is more complex. The consequences of cost containment are reviewed below, looking first at Medicaid managed care programs and then at employer-based health plans.

The Public Sector: Impact of State-Initiated Reforms

The public behavioral health system varies greatly across states in per capita spending and in the ways that care is organized and delivered. To these state-run systems falls the responsibility of caring for most of the chronically and seriously mentally ill. This mandate has long been challenging in view of the complex needs of such patients, coupled with constrained resources and fragmented funding streams. And concerns about this vulnerable group have been heightened with the penetration of managed care models into the public sector. Many states have, indeed, moved cautiously into managed care demonstrations; it has been feared that managed care approaches, successful in the private sector, may undermine gains made in community-based models of care that emphasize supportive and rehabilitative services for the seriously mentally ill. For example, some states have left the disabled population in the traditional fee-for-service system when introducing a managed Medicaid program, or have set up special behavioral carve-outs for the seriously mentally ill that leave in place traditional safety-net providers, such as community mental health centers. Because of special concerns about the seriously mentally ill, many evaluations of managed care in the public sector have focused on this population.

The Massachusetts and Utah Experience

Two key evaluations conducted in Massachusetts and Utah show that Medicaid reforms implementing managed behavioral health carve-out plans have reduced the use of inpatient hospital care. Both states had managed care demonstrations that included both welfare families (AFDC) and the disabled (SSI) Medicaid populations. The evaluators of these demonstration programs examined the impact on utilization among all eligible Medicaid beneficiaries. Both evaluations reported large reductions in inpatient hospital costs in the first year. Utah's program involved capitated contracts with community mental health centers. In the first year of the program, hospital admission rates were 17% lower than expected, which was disproportionately due to drops in rates for the AFDC population (Christianson et al., 1995). In Massachusetts, where a private managed behavioral health company was contracted to provide services (and also carried financial risk up to a limit), hospital admissions dropped by 7%, and the length of hospital stays was shortened by 12% (Dickey, 1997).

Shifts in outpatient care were less apparent in these demonstrations. The Massachusetts evaluation found a slight decline (3%) in outpatient utilization relative to what would be expected in the absence of managed care, but overall outpatient use continued to increase (Dickey, 1997). No changes in outpatient behavioral health visits were found in the Utah evaluation (Christianson et al., 1995).

A related study of the impact of a capitated managed behavioral health program in an unidentified U. S. city examined the initial level of care assigned by a case manager to adult intakes during the first $2^{1}/_{2}$ years of the program (Thompson, Burns, Goldman, & Smith, 1992). The study documented that inpatient assignment dropped by nearly a half while initial assignment to outpatient care increased, a pattern that was consistent across all clinical categories.

The Colorado and Minnesota Experience

Evaluations of managed Medicaid programs in Colorado and Minnesota focused on samples of adults known to have serious mental illness prior to the implementation of managed care. For this subgroup of Medicaid enrollees, the reported changes in utilization of services in the first year were relatively modest. In Colorado, a carvedout, capitated Medicaid behavioral health program was provided by different managed care contractors in two regions: in one region the state contracted with community mental health services that both managed and delivered services, and in another region the contract was held by a partnership between a private managed care organization and community mental health centers. The Colorado evaluation found only a small and insignificant reduction in the probability of inpatient admissions in the two managed care regions relative to a fee-for-service area. In contrast, hospital costs among users were significantly reduced in the managed care sites, reflecting shortened lengths of stay. Use of any outpatient care among this sample declined more in managed care sites than in the fee-for-service site; however, outpatient costs among users did not (Bloom et al., 1998).

An early capitated Medicaid program in Minnesota provided behavioral health benefits as part of an integrated health plan, delivered by one of seven local HMOs (Christianson & Gray, 1994). An evaluation of the program found little difference in the use of services, either inpatient or outpatient, between the capitated plan and fee-for-service care among a sample of adults with serious mental illness.

State Programs Targeting the Severely Mentally Ill

Some states have implemented targeted capitated programs, which are designed specifically to provide care for the most severely mentally ill or high-cost behavioral health service users in their public systems; community-based provider organizations assume the risk for a relatively small group of high-risk enrollees. These programs, evaluated in New York, Oregon, and California, reduced the number of days of inpatient hospitalization and increased the use of community-based clinical and rehabilitation services (Chandler, Hu, Meisel, McGowen, & Madison, 1997; McFarland et al., 1995; Reed, Hennessy, Mitchell, & Babigian, 1994). Unlike programs for the broader Medicaid population, these targeted programs did not appear to decrease costs for this selected and very sick group of patients. The programs did, however, appear to increase use of a range of case-management, clinical, and rehabilitative services that is more consistent with comprehensive community-based models of care for the severely and persistently mentally ill (see also Kapur, Young, Murata, Sullivan, & Koegel, 1999).

Behavioral Health Services for Children

Stroul and colleagues (1998) broadly surveyed managed behavioral health services for Medicaid children. After conducting visits to programs in 10 states, these investigators concluded on the basis of site reports that the managed care programs in 7 states improved access to home- and community-based services for children; those in 6 states improved the availability of case management; and the programs in all 10 states made it more difficult to get hospital care. They note a trend in all states toward briefer, more problem-focused treatment approaches.

An evaluation of a North Carolina Medicaid behavioral health carve-out for youth by Burns and colleagues (1999) analyzed claims data that demonstrated similar shifts in care. In North Carolina, the Medicaid behavioral health carve-out program was managed by local mental health authorities in 10 of 40 mental health areas. In the first two years of the program, the local authorities were at full risk only for inpatient care, while in the next two years of the demonstration, they were at full risk for both inpatient and outpatient care. Inpatient care declined dramatically over the four years of the study. Residential alternatives to hospital care, as well as outpatient, case-management, and wrap-around services, greatly increased in the first two years of the demonstration, and slightly declined or leveled off in the next two. Overall, more youth were served at greater intensity in the managed care program areas than in the traditional fee-for-service Medicaid areas. While total costs in both fee-for-service and managed care areas increased over the four years of the demonstration, costs in the last two years of the managed care program declined slightly, whereas costs in the fee-for-service areas continued to climb.

Managed Substance-Abuse Treatment Programs

There has been little study of the impact of managed care on sub-stance abuse treatment in the public sector, probably because Medicaid funds are not directed to this specialized area as much as they are to general behavioral health care. When substance abuse ben-efits are included in a state's managed Medicaid program, they are often restricted to the traditional Medicaid-eligible population, who account for a relatively small share of the state's public expenditures for substance abuse treatment.

The few evaluations of Medicaid reforms aimed at substance abuse treatment services consistently find large drops in inpatient treatment and increased use of detoxification services. In the Massachusetts Medicaid demonstration, Callahan and colleagues (1995) reviewed the first year of the program, which included managed benefits for substance abuse, as well as for mental health. They found that costs for substance abuse treatment declined by 48%, while costs for mental health treatment dropped by only 19%. The evaluation team reported a large drop in inpatient hospitalizations for substance abuse and increased use of freestanding detoxification services, acute residential treatment, and methadone treatment.

In Minnesota, Finch and coworkers (1992) reported declines in both inpatient admissions and outpatient visits under managed care for seriously mentally ill Medicaid enrollees with a prior history of substance abuse treatment. The study cited earlier by Thompson and colleagues (1992) of managed behavioral health care in an unidentified city noted a similar trend. In reviewing the level of care assigned by a case manager to adult behavioral health intakes with a substance abuse diagnosis, the evaluators found that admission to inpatient hospitalization was dramatically reduced over time, replaced largely by assignment to detoxification services.

Summary

Management of Medicaid benefits has been consistently associated with large declines in inpatient care leading to large cost reductions for the broad Medicaid population, at least in the first year or two following transition from a fee-for-service model. There is little evidence of expansion of outpatient services to counter declines in inpatient care. For Medicaid children in managed care programs, however, alternatives to hospitalization, such as residential care and intensive community-based services, appear to have expanded to substitute for declining inpatient care. And with Medicaid substance abuse treatment services, there is some evidence that managed care replaced inpatient care with freestanding detoxification services.

In evaluations of targeted programs that capitate care only for the most vulnerable and highest-cost patients–those with severe and persistent illness–managed behavioral health care has not had a dramatic impact on the cost of their care. Cost reductions, if any, were modest. These programs, however, appear to have achieved some success in shifting care from hospital inpatient units to a wide range of clinical, supportive, and rehabilitative services delivered in community-based programs.

The Private Sector:
Impact of Changes on Employer-Based Health Plans

Early studies of managed health care in employer-based health plans focused on outpatient behavioral health services because inpatient care was rarely used. One of those studies, the Health Insurance Experiment conducted by RAND in the mid-1970s, showed that behavioral health expenditures for outpatient care were nearly three times lower for enrollees assigned to a prepaid HMO than for those assigned to a fee-for-service medical insurance plan (Manning et al., 1989). Although enrollees in the prepaid plan were more likely to use any behavioral health outpatient care, those who used the services averaged one-third the visits of those in fee-for-service care; they were also more likely to receive their care from a primary care provider or a psychiatric social worker than from a psychiatrist or psychologist (Wells, Manning, & Benjamin, 1986). Another early study done in the late 1970s examined the costs of outpatient care for Washington state employees who selected from a choice of medical plans, including an HMO, an independent practice association (IPA), and a fee-for-service indemnity plan (Diehr, Williams, Martin, & Price, 1984). The costs were much higher in the fee-for-service plan than for the IPA and HMO. The managed care plan enrollees were more likely to use any behavioral health care than enrollees in the fee-for-service plan, but their average number of visits was much lower.

The Behavioral Carve-Out

It is not surprising that the growth and dominance of the behavioral carve-out industry during the 1990s has attracted the attention of a number of recent studies. They chiefly examined the changes in costs and utilization of services when large employers began to contract for mental health and substance abuse services with a carved-out MBHO. For example, Sturm and colleagues (1998) looked at these changes for the state of Ohio employee program. They found that the switch to a behavioral carve-out from a traditional fee-for-service plan was associated with a large initial drop in both inpatient days and outpatient visits that then continued to decline slightly over the seven years of managed care that were examined. Over the entire period, annual inpatient days dropped by an order of magnitude (from 204 to

20 per 1,000 enrollees), and outpatient visits dropped by half (from 1,060 to 476 per 1,000 enrollees). The carve-out also provided inter-mediate services that were not covered under the fee-for-service plan, including group residential treatment (utilized at 10 days per year per 1,000 enrollees) and intensive outpatient care (utilized at 34 days per year per 1,000 enrollees).

Other researchers carried out a similar analysis for the state of Massachusetts employee program (Huskamp, 1998; Ma & McGuire, 1998; Merrick, 1998). Their evaluations found large declines in costs of hospital care that were due both to a shift from inpatient hospital-ization to less intensive partial hospitalization, and to reductions in length of stay. Ma and McGuire also reported large reductions in out-patient care, including declines in the rate of use of any outpatient care (drops of 25% and 33% for mental health and substance abuse care, respectively) and in the number of outpatient visits per user (declines of 25% and 17% for mental health and substance abuse visits, respec-tively).

Goldman and colleagues (1998) looked at the changes in behav-ioral health care for a large U.S. employer that switched benefits from a fee-for-service plan to a managed behavioral carve-out. They found that access to behavioral health care improved, as indicated by an increased probability that enrollees would use any behavioral health services. Furthermore, the probability of an inpatient admission dropped by 40%; the average length of hospital stay for behavioral health care shortened; and the average number of outpatient visits declined. New intermediate services were included in the carve-out plan (including residential care and day treatment), but they account-ed for a relatively small proportion of costs (11%) in 1996.

A study of Alcan Aluminum's switch from an unmanaged indem-nity behavioral benefit to a behavioral carve-out found that access to any behavioral health care increased over time (from 4.1% to 6.1%), while costs decreased by about 70% (Cuffel, Goldman, & Schlesinger, 1999). A unique feature of this study was that it examined general medical costs among enrollees to see if changes in behavioral health care use affected those costs. No shifts in costs to the medical plan were detected; in fact, there was a small decrease in medical care costs among users of behavioral health care under the carve-out.

A study of another large company revealed that substituting a carved-out behavioral health plan for another form of managed care–

a preferred provider organization (PPO)–had little impact (Grazier, Eselius, Hu, Shore, & G'sell, 1999). Inpatient care was already very low under the PPO and did not change with the switch to a carved-out behavioral health plan. Access to outpatient services did increase somewhat, and overall costs were lower, but the intensity of outpatient care was similar before and after the change.

In the single study of employer-based care that focused specifically on care for substance abuse, Stein and colleagues (1999) found that a behavioral carve-out had a major impact on substance abuse services for a large Midwestern employer whose behavioral health benefits were originally covered under 23 different HMOs. The number of inpatient days and outpatient visits for substance use disorders sharply decreased under the carve-out, and the use of intermediate services (residential treatment, recovery homes, partial hospitalization, day treatment, and intensive outpatient) increased.

Summary

Because of the dominance of managed behavioral carve-out plans in the private sector, studies conducted in the 1990s focused on assessing their impact on employer-based health care. The results demonstrate that carved-out managed behavioral health care reduces both inpatient and outpatient service utilization relative to traditional fee-for-service plans. Little difference in utilization was found, however, in the one study that compared a company's switch from a PPO to a behavioral carve-out. Behavioral carve-outs also seem to have little impact on access to behavioral health services, that is, on the proportion of enrollees using any behavioral health services: at times access appeared to be greater, and at other times poorer, with the carve-out. There is also, however, a consistent pattern of evidence showing that carve-outs, by taking advantage of benefit flexibility, increase the use of intermediate behavioral health services, such as nonhospital residential treatment, partial and day treatment, and intensive outpatient treatment. This shift in care may be substituting for inpatient hospital care.

Discussion: Service Use under Managed Care Programs

The clearest consequence of managed behavioral health care is that it has shifted patterns of service utilization. These shifts are clearly responsive to pressures from payers to control costs. Managed care has consistently driven down the use of costly inpatient care and has often reduced total outpatient visits, most typically by reducing the average number of visits per outpatient user and by either maintaining or reducing access to care.

Managed care has the potential to provide more flexibility of behavioral health benefits than traditional indemnity insurance, and this flexibility appears to be used in a way that is generally consistent with goals of efficiency—substituting lower-cost services for higher-cost ones when there is no apparent loss in value. The evidence suggests that managed behavioral health care has broadened services in employer-based health plans beyond traditional inpatient and outpatient care to include a variety of intermediate services, such as partial hospitalization, day hospitalization, residential treatment, and intensive outpatient treatment, all of which may be substituting to some extent for costlier inpatient care. These changes in utilization patterns and the substitution of lower-cost services have clearly contributed to the financial savings seen under managed behavioral health care compared to traditional fee-for-service indemnity insurance.

There are exceptions to the pattern of cost containment achieved through shifts in service utilization. For managed care programs that have targeted populations with high need for intensive services, such as the severely mentally ill and Medicaid children, reductions in inpatient care have been achieved, but the substitution of highly expanded community-based services has tended to increase overall costs of care. Managed care in these instances has principally been a tool for implementing service models that value community- over hospital-based settings, and that can provide more flexible services geared to the specific needs of the client.

OUTCOMES AND QUALITY

It is clear that by reducing the utilization of services, managed behavioral health care has succeeded in containing and even reducing costs. But what impact have these changes had on the quality of the care received? It is easy to speculate that quality suffers, which is a view held by many in the behavioral health specialty professions and by the public. That negative image, however, is not backed to date with strong evidence showing that declines in quality of clinical care or patient outcomes necessarily follow from managed behavioral health care.

At this still early stage of managed care, the evidence about its impact on the quality of care is sparse. Part of the problem is that ferreting out data on this issue is more challenging than finding information on costs. Some insight, however, is provided by the five studies discussed below; they compared outcomes under managed care with fee-for-service plans using reasonably well controlled designs. These studies most often showed no detectable differences across plan types, although they did find some evidence that managed care has a detrimental effect on outcomes for selected measures.

Public Sector Outcomes

Publicly funded Medicaid demonstration evaluations conducted in Minnesota and Colorado, which followed samples of adults with serious mental illness, found that managed care had little impact on outcomes (Bloom et al., 1998; Lurie, Moscovice, Finch, Christianson, & Popkin, 1992). In Utah, a sample of adults with schizophrenia was followed for four years after implementation of a capitated carve-out plan for the Medicaid population, and the patient outcomes were compared with those of another group receiving care in a traditional Utah Medicaid program (Manning et al., 1999). Although patients in both groups showed improvements in their mental health status over time, those in the carve-out plan had significantly smaller improvements by the last two years of the study, especially for those who were most severely ill at the study's outset.

Outcomes in Employer-Based Health Plans

Relatively little work has been reported on behavioral health outcomes under managed care for employed populations, and what is available is now highly dated. The RAND Health Insurance Experiment conducted in the 1970s found no differences in behavioral health outcomes between enrollees in an HMO and those receiving fee-for-service care (Wells, Manning, & Valdez, 1990). The Medical Outcomes Study conducted in the 1980s compared outcomes for a sample of patients with depression who were receiving care from behavioral health specialists and general medical providers under pre-paid versus fee-for-service arrangements (Rogers, Wells, Meredith, Sturm, & Burnam, 1993). Differences across plans were found only for psychiatrists' patients, who were also on average the sickest patients: the prepaid patients, but not the fee-for-service patients, declined on a measure of role and physical functioning over two years. The authors suggest that this difference may be explained by the prepaid patients having received less intense care than the fee-for-service ones; for example, the latter had fewer behavioral health visits and were less likely to be using antidepressant medications over time. No differences were found between the two patient groups, however, for measures of depressive symptoms.

While no recent behavioral health outcomes studies of privately insured populations have been published, one recent report by Gresenz and Sturm (1999) suggests that patients with severe mental illnesses may be more dissatisfied with the care they receive under managed behavioral health plans. The patients in this study included those with schizophrenia and bipolar affective disorder, as well as those with substance abuse problems, and they were more likely to disenroll from carved-out behavioral health plans.

Examining the Data

There are two ways to view the null findings reported so far in the outcome studies. We could surmise that the reductions in the intensity of behavioral health services delivered under managed behavioral health care are sensible–that this insurance approach has eliminated care having very little or no expected benefit. It is also possible, however, that the reason that these studies generally fail to establish differences in quality of care is that *measures of outcomes* among enrollees are not very sensitive to the *quality of care* provided. Outcomes, for example, are a function of many individual characteristics of patients that are outside the control of the plan or the provider. They include such factors as the initial severity of the illness, other co-morbidity and lifestyle factors, and the individual's willingness to seek care and follow a provider's advice. In fact, these characteristics may drive the variations in outcomes and swamp any effects attributable to plans.

Process of Care

Process measures—that is, measures of the care actually delivered by providers to patients—may be more sensitive measures of quality of care because these are measures that providers and plans can affect more directly. In order for process measures to be convincing indicators of quality, however, they must reflect clinical procedures or services that have demonstrated efficacy. While the empirical literature is far from complete, the evidence now supports practice guidelines for treatments of schizophrenia, depression, alcoholism, and other mental and substance use disorders, and provides the basis for examining a variety of process-of-care measures as indicators of quality of care.

Few researchers have used process-of-care measures to evaluate managed behavioral health care's impact on quality. One notable exception is the work by Popkin and colleagues (1998), who abstracted medical records of patients with schizophrenia in an evaluation of a Medicaid reform in Utah. They then compared 19 process-of-care measures before and after the initiation of a capitated managed behavioral health plan. The authors found that after managed care, there was a reduction in the percentage of patients with psychotherapy visits and crisis visits, and an increase in the percentage having a case manager. These shifts from traditional therapeutic encounters do not have clear implications for quality of care, because there is little empirical evidence that psychotherapy is effective for persons with schizophrenia, and the reduction in crisis visits could be a reflection either of better clinical management or of greater barriers to this mode of care. Two other process measures did suggest declines in quality, however: there was an increase in the percentage of patients who terminated treatment or who were lost to follow-up, and an increase in the percentage of patients prescribed antipsychotic medications at suboptimal dosage levels.

Opposite results were found in an analysis of an employer-insured population. Merrick (1998, 1999) used claims data for Massachusetts state employees to examine a single quality-of-care indicator—the probability of an outpatient follow-up within a month after discharge from inpatient hospital care for major depression. She found higher rates of outpatient follow-up (at both 15 and 30 days postdischarge) after the initiation of a managed behavioral carve-out than before the carve-out—when employees received their behavioral health care through fee-for-service indemnity plans or a PPO. These results suggest an improvement in the continuity of care for patients hospitalized with depression under managed behavioral health care.

Although no studies have compared processes of care for substance abuse treatment across plan types, the study by Thompson and colleagues (1992) is relevant. In examining utilization of services after the implementation of a managed behavioral carve-out, this study found that hospitalizations for substance abuse were being replaced by detoxification services. This finding suggests a decline in quality of care under the carve-out, since detoxification in the absence of substance abuse rehabilitation services has no demonstrated lasting benefit for patients.

Discussion

Evaluating the quality of care that patients receive under managed behavioral health plans is not easy. The few studies that have addressed this issue so far have only scratched the surface in finding answers. Measures of outcomes may be crude indicators, at best, of quality of care; given the importance of individual-level prognostic factors, which are outside the control of the provider, the differences in the quality of clinical care may have to be quite large in order to be detectable in observational studies of outcomes. Measures of the process of clinical care are more direct and therefore a more sensitive yardstick for evaluating quality of care, but only rarely have evaluations directly examined that process. When they did, the findings were equivocal. In the two studies discussed above, one found some indications of poorer quality treatment for schizophrenia under a managed Medicaid plan, while the other found better post-hospital follow-up with depressed patients after the switch to a managed behavioral carve-out under an employer-based plan. Although these two studies do not begin to allow us to make any generalizations about the impact of managed behavioral health care on quality of care, they do suggest that the story may be complicated and depend on the particular features of a managed care plan and its enrollees.

Some critics have warned that we should not overestimate the impact that managed care organizational and financing changes, in themselves, can have on provider practice, and that altering provider behavior to improve quality of care is extremely difficult (Bazelon Center for Mental Health Law, 2000). Within any particular managed care environment, focused and well-conceived efforts to influence provider behavior are probably required in order to improve the quality of clinical practice. We would speculate, however, that organizational and financing changes might more easily result in declines in quality of care, particularly when access to care is impeded.

Much more work is needed to assess the impact of managed care on the quality of care; further evaluation of processes of care known to influence patient outcomes seems the most promising route. Not only will process measures be more direct and sensitive to variations in quality of care than outcome measures, but they provide more information about how to improve the quality of care.

CLINICAL PRACTICE

The clinical workforce has been buffeted by major changes in the health care industry, as evidenced by the general uproar from behavioral health specialists, and their struggles are evident from even a cursory reading of the trade press. Managed care has influenced their job markets, income, clinical autonomy, and organizational and clinical roles. The managed care era clearly challenges the behavioral health professions to forge new roles, to regain or redefine the boundaries of clinical autonomy in making decisions, and to mitigate the ethical and legal problems that they confront. Changing trends in clinical treatments, such as reliance on briefer psychotherapeutic approaches and rapid adoption of new psychopharmacologic treatments, have likely been accelerated by managed care. In this section, we present evidence of managed behavioral health care's influence on clinical practice.

Changes in the Workforce

Scheffler and colleagues (1998) document significant shifts in the disciplinary make-up of the specialty behavioral health provider workforce between 1989 and 1995. While the number of clinically trained social workers, advance practice nurses, and other master's-level clinicians nearly doubled, the ranks of clinical and counseling psychologists grew at a smaller rate (24%), and the number of practicing psychiatrists remained steady. Estimates of the number of practicing behavioral health workers in 1995 included 33,000 psychiatrists, 70,000 licensed psychologists, 125,000 licensed clinical social workers, and 7,000 clinical nurse specialists with behavioral health specialties.

One explanation offered for these workforce changes is the use of a broader array of providers in managed care environments than in traditional fee-for-service plans, where specialty behavioral health treatments were typically reimbursed only if provided by a psychiatrist or Ph.D.-level psychologist. Thus, managed care organizations may be reducing costs and be benefiting from economies of scale by triaging severely ill patients to higher-paid psychiatrists and psychologists, and by referring less severely ill patients to master's-level clinicians.

Most practicing psychiatrists and psychologists report that they are in managed care provider panels, though many of their patients have other sources of financing. Psychiatrists surveyed in 1997 (Zarin, West, Pincus, & Tanelian, 1999) said that, on average, 36% of their patients were in managed care plans, 30% were in nonmanaged public plans, and 29% were in nonmanaged private plans. Among practicing clinical psychologists surveyed in 1996, 84% reported that they were in managed care provider panels, with about half of their services to patients provided under some form of managed care (Murphy, DeBernardo, & Shoemaker, 1998). Social workers are increasingly branching beyond traditional public-agency roles to work as behavioral health clinicians in private-practice settings, where they are participating in managed care networks (Gibelman & Schervish, 1996).

Relatively little is known about how managed care has changed the organization of clinical practice, although a trend away from solo practice and toward group practice has been noted. While early staff-model HMOs were characterized by in-house programs that valued collaboration among multidisciplinary staff, the recent dominance of open panels of specialty providers in managed behavioral health networks can accommodate traditional solo practice and may have dampened the trend toward multidisciplinary group practice (Bennett, 1992). Some studies indicate that behavioral health providers are more likely to work as part of a multidisciplinary team in managed care networks (Domino, Salkever, Zarin, & Pincus, 1998), but this difference has not yet been well documented. Although psychiatrists may be following the general trend among physicians to move from solo to group practices in which they are less likely to share ownership (Simon & Born, 1996), clinical psychologists still predominantly work as solo practitioners (Phelps, Eisman, & Kohout, 1998).

Changes in Income and Staffing

Data on income for specialty behavioral health workers are readily available and suggest a leveling (and perhaps even a recent decline in real dollars) in the earnings of psychiatrists and psychologists since 1990 (Scheffler et al., 1998; Simon & Born, 1996; Williams, Wicherski, & Kohout, 1998). The earnings of master's-level behavioral health clinicians, however—consistent with a growing demand for these practitioners—appear to have significantly increased throughout the 1990s (Scheffler et al.).

The leveling of private-practice incomes for psychiatrists and psychologists may reflect the bargaining power of managed care plans, which typically negotiate lower-than-customary fee schedules for network providers and risk-based contracts with large provider groups. Income declines may also reflect a reduced market demand for behavioral health specialists in response to the tighter controls over utilization of behavioral health services that were introduced by managed care. Scheffler and Ivey (1998), for example, examined staffing patterns for two full-service HMOs in 1995 and reported that the number of behavioral health specialists per 100,000 enrollees was much lower than would be expected in view of the staffing rates for the states in which the HMOs were located. Relatively low staffing rates were apparent for psychiatrists (4–5 per 100,000 enrollees), psychologists (2 per 100,000 enrollees), and clinical social workers (8–14 per 100,000 enrollees). Furthermore, both HMOs decreased their behavioral health specialty staffing rates between 1992 and 1995. Other studies examining psychiatrist staffing in HMO environments have reported similar findings—low rates of psychiatrists to enrollees compared to a fee-for-service environment (Dial, Bergsten, Haviland, & Pincus, 1998). But these HMO data are not likely to reflect the provider staffing in behavioral carve-out plans that are the dominant form of managed care today. A description of all participating providers in the network of one large behavioral carve-out revealed a staffing mix that was proportionately higher in psychologists than what was found in HMOs: 20% psychiatrists, 36% psychologists, and 19% social workers (Scheffler & Ivey), though this comparison is limited by absence of information on how many full-time equivalents are represented in the network.

Challenges to Clinical Autonomy

Managed care not only influences the organization and income of behavioral health specialty practice, but generally entails external oversight of clinical decisions made by practitioners. Such oversight is widely viewed by practitioners as intrusive, burdensome, and an impediment to the provision of good clinical care. Psychologists surveyed about managed care changes convey concerns that utilization-management requirements have increased the administrative burden on clinical practices and have had a negative impact on quality of care (Murphy et al., 1998). Most psychologists in the survey reported increased paperwork and phone contacts associated with utilization review. About half said that managed care had a negative impact on the quality of the care that they provided, and posed ethical dilemmas not addressed by their professional code. Although a survey of physicians conducted by Donelan and colleagues (1997) was not directed specifically at psychiatrists, it did find that many physicians are unhappy with changes in the health care system. Those practicing in high HMO-penetration states were more likely to report problems in their practices, including pressure to see more patients and limitations on prescribing drugs, ordering tests, and making referrals. Zarin and colleagues (1999), who surveyed psychiatrists in the American Psychiatric Association practice research network, reported that 42% of patients enrolled in managed care plans had a change in treatment due to their plans' financial or resource constraints, compared to 30% of patients in nonmanaged plans. Physician members of the American Society of Addiction Medicine were surveyed in 1998 by Galanter and colleagues (1999). The majority of respondents reported that managed care had a negative impact on the quality of care for substance use disorders and on their ethical practice of medicine, and that it added to their workload. Similarly, a survey of outpatient substance abuse treatment units (Alexander & Lemak, 1997a, 1997b) found that administrative burden increased as a function of greater utilization-management requirements, and that facility directors viewed many of these oversight mechanisms negatively. Interestingly, this survey also asked directors about aspects of treatment that might be positively affected by managed care. They viewed managed care to be associated with an absence of limits on the number of outpatient sessions and with plan requirements to follow up with clients after discharge (Alexander & Lemak, 1997b).

Changing Clinical Technologies

Psychotherapy

Historically, approaches derived from psychoanalytic and related dynamic theories have dominated the practice of psychotherapy, particularly within psychiatry, but also within clinical psychology and social work. Individual psychotherapy delivered by a highly trained specialist over a sustained course of visits is the preferred mode of delivering these treatments. While psychoanalysis has had its ups and downs in popularity, never has it been more threatened than by managed behavioral health care. Weissberg (1994, p. 180), for example, bemoans the influence of managed care on dynamic psychotherapy, blames unchecked managed care operations for dramatic drops in new psychoanalytic trainees, and expresses concern that managed care will "legislate or administer an effective treatment modality out of existence." Reimbursement for any mental health therapy has long been limited in traditional fee-for-service indemnity plans by outpatient benefit limits and copayments, making long-term psychotherapy affordable only for those who had unusually generous plans or could pay the added out-of-pocket expenses. MBHOs, however, have generally adopted policies that specifically exclude psychoanalytic approaches—by excluding practitioners from provider panels and denying or limiting reimbursement for these treatment approaches (Barron & Sands, 1996). Leading psychiatrists tend to agree that psychoanalysis has become an even greater luxury, limited to those who can afford to pay (Detre & McDonald, 1997; Olfson & Weissman, 1997; Sharfstein, 1997).

Managed care leaders see the exclusion of long-term psychotherapeutic treatments as justified by principles of effectiveness and efficiency (Bartlett, 1994), and have embraced, instead, brief-psychotherapy approaches rooted in theories from behavioral and cognitive psychology (Hoyt, 1994). These approaches are time-limited and focus on the alleviation of specific problems or symptoms, rather than on underlying psychodynamic causes. Cummings (1996) argues that success as a psychotherapist in the managed care era requires a fundamental shift in values from those of a traditional "dyadic" model of psychotherapy that depends on establishing a sustained relationship between therapist and patient, to a "catalyst" model where brief treatments are provided intermittently by the therapist as a catalyst to patient change. While brief psychotherapeutic approaches are not new in clinical psychology (see Bloom, 1992), most clinical psychologists, even recent graduates, have little or no training in these approaches (Cummings). Managed care leaders have cause for concern that clinical training is not keeping pace with changes in practice (Feldman, 1994). Psychotherapists appear to be responding to managed care pressures by learning on the job (Hoyt). And yet there are fears that many psychotherapists may simply be using abbreviated versions of traditional approaches and are delivering individually oriented psychodynamic therapy in fewer visits and with little benefit (Bennett, 1992).

Pharmacology

Increasing reliance on psychopharmacology in the treatment of behavioral disorders, heralding what some call "an era of psychopharmacological revolution" (Joseph, 1997, p. 21), is a trend that has paralleled the growth of managed care. An analysis of national data by Pincus and colleagues (1998) showed that between 1985 and 1994, visits to psychiatrists in which psychotropic medication was prescribed nearly doubled; this increase was largely due to growing use of a new class of antidepressant drugs—selective serotonin reuptake inhibitors (SSRIs)—first introduced in 1988. Medication is now the most common treatment provided by psychiatrists to their patients. In a 1997 survey, for example, psychiatrists reported prescribing psychotherapeutic medications to 90% of their patients, whereas two decades earlier, nonanalyst psychiatrists in private practice prescribed medication to less than one-third of their patients (Pincus et al., 1999). The increased reliance on psychopharmacologic treatments certainly reflects influences beyond managed care, including important gains in knowledge of molecular biology and the development of new, effective psychopharmacologic agents. Beyond these factors, however, managed care has likely encouraged the diffusion and use of drug treatments in the care for behavioral health problems. Managed behavioral health care has been particularly receptive to psychopharmacologic treatments because they are consistent with the goal of efficiency and are demonstrably effective (Joseph, 1997). Furthermore, psychiatric drug therapy, like brief problem-oriented psychotherapy, is consistent with the symptom-focused approach to treatment favored by managed behavioral health care.

Clinical Roles

The roles of psychiatrists appear to have shifted quite dramatically with the growth of managed care. Many of these changes undoubtedly reflect a broader shift in psychiatry from psychodynamically based paradigms to a more biological, evidence-based understanding of behavioral health problems and technologies. Psychiatrists are prescribing more medications; they are now far less likely to deliver any form of psychotherapy; and most of their patients have a severe psychiatric disorder (Pincus et al., 1999). In 1997, for example, psychiatrists provided psychotherapy to less than half of their patients (43%) even though many (38%) were receiving services—most often, individual psychotherapy—from other behavioral health providers. Psychiatrists have differentiated themselves from other behavioral health clinicians by retaining unique roles in managing psychotherapeutic medications, and in evaluating and supervising the care of patients with severe or medically complex illnesses (Olfson & Weissman, 1997; Sharfstein, 1997). Psychiatrists have been among the key leaders and innovators building and shaping the managed behavioral health care industry. Yet some psychiatrists caution that psychiatric training falls short in sufficiently preparing psychiatrists for new roles in the managed care era. Meyer and McLaughlin (1998) identify service areas in which psychiatric training needs to be improved, including brief psychotherapies, alternatives to inpatient treatment, the integration of psychopharmacology and psychotherapy, and the treatment of patients with co-occurring mental illness and addictive disorders.

Unlike psychiatrists, clinical psychologists as a profession have generally not led efforts to redefine their roles or their specific clinical niche in the managed care environment (Bobbitt, Marques, & Trout, 1998), and clinical training has not shifted to smooth the way for the next generation's entry into managed care networks (Cummings, 1996). In 1996, only 5% of psychologists reported that they did any psychoanalysis, but most reported providing individual therapy (94%), marital therapy (88%), family therapy (72%), and psychological testing (71%) (Murphy et al., 1998). It is clear, however, that psychologists have experienced pressures from managed care to modify their traditional practices. A majority of psychologists surveyed in 1996 reported that they experienced reimbursement problems for marital therapy and psychological testing, and nearly half experienced reimbursement problems for family therapy (Murphy et al.). Although the professional association of psychologists has focused its efforts on actively resisting managed care, Cummings (1996) describes a groundswell of changes among clinical psychologists as they adapt their practices in order to participate and thrive in managed care networks. He includes among these changes a "stampede" to join with other behavioral health specialties in multimodal group practices and a "rush" to acquire new skills in brief therapeutic techniques. Cummings foresees that market pressures may ultimately force Ph.D.-level psychologists out of business or into clinical research or supervisory roles, while a rapidly expanding workforce of master's-level psychologists takes their place as the dominant providers of psychotherapy.

Discussion

The changing professional workforce and patterns of clinical care raise new issues for the clinical professions about their differentiation from, and relationship to, each other. Psychiatrists and clinical psychologists have developed more distinctive roles relative to each other and are forging new roles relative to the burgeoning workforce of master's-level clinicians. Models of multispecialty team care have emerged. Yet there is still much debate within the professions over different visions of their future in the managed care era. New practitioners are often not well prepared for the changing clinical-practice landscape because clinical training has not kept pace with market changes.

And dissatisfactions about managed care abound among clinicians, who largely still work in traditional private practice settings. In particular, the demise of long-term psychodynamic therapy for all but the wealthy does not rest easily on exceedingly well trained professionals convinced of the value of this approach and experienced in its practice.

Managed care presents serious challenges to the behavioral health professions, but it may also stimulate evaluation of, and improvements in, clinical care—if clinical training, provider organizations, and managed care technologies are turned to this goal. As Bartlett (1994, p. 33) notes, "What was originally perceived as an assault on the practice of the behavioral health professions may well be a major force in the demonstration of their value . . . and expand access to appropriate and affordable care."

PARITY OF BEHAVIORAL HEALTH BENEFITS

A significant policy effect of the containment of behavioral health care costs under managed care has been legislative action to provide parity of behavioral health insurance benefits. In employer-based insurance plans, limits on behavioral health coverage have generally been much more restrictive than those for general medical care. In 1997, for example, three-fourths of employers who offered behavioral health benefits imposed more limits on behavioral health coverage than on general medical coverage; typical annual restrictions were 30 days or $5,000 for inpatient care, and 24 days or $2,000 for outpatient visits (Buck, Teich, Umland, & Stein, 1999). A key lobbying issue for behavioral health advocates has been the promotion of behavioral health parity legislation, at both federal and state levels, that would eliminate differential restrictions and thereby increase nominal behavioral health benefits. Until recently, opponents successfully argued that behavioral health parity would result in excessive increases in health care premiums and be too costly for employers. Predictions of high increases in costs were from earlier data, when most employer-based behavioral health benefits were in traditional fee-for-service indemnity plans, but had not taken into account the sweeping transition to managed behavioral health care.

In recent years, parity legislation has been enormously successful, which is due, at least in part, to revised projections of the costs of implementing the law under managed behavioral health care. These projections showed little increase in costs (for example, Sturm, 1997). In 1996, a Federal Mental Health Parity Act was passed; this act prevents employers from imposing different annual or lifetime dollar limits for mental health coverage than they do for general medical coverage. By 2000, 44 states had passed their own legislation, and 31 of these states imposed further requirements on employers than those imposed by the federal law. Despite this success, however, parity regulations are limited in scope. The federal legislation exempts small employers, and it allows other differential limits, such as limits on inpatient days and outpatient visits, and higher deductibles and copayments. And state laws do not affect self-insured employers (including many large employers), which are exempt under the federal Employee Retirement Income Security Act of 1977. Even with parity legislation, the most recent available data suggest that, overall, limits imposed on behavioral health insurance coverage offered by employers have become more restrictive over the past decade (Hay Group, 1998). Those who have most to lose under continuing benefit restrictions in the managed care era are those with severe mental disorders and children with serious emotional problems (Peele, Lave, & Xu, 1999).

The debate on behavioral health parity, along with advocacy on behalf of those with serious mental illness, thus continues. As more experience is gained with expanded benefits under managed care, further strengthening of parity legislation at state and federal levels seems likely, with recent parity legislation in California—as well as for all federal employees (under President Clinton's executive order)—leading the way. Although experience under managed behavioral health carve-outs paved the way for parity legislation, it is likely that the tough parity mandates in California and also for federal employees will, in turn, shift the remaining fee-for-service mental health benefits into managed care plans in order to contain costs.

FURTHER QUESTIONS

Cost-containment mechanisms of some sort are now inevitable, and a rational management of behavioral health resources is, at least in theory, much more preferable to arbitrary benefit limits that adversely affect the sickest people. To date, much of the research accumulated about managed care has been directed at comparing a managed care plan with a traditional fee-for-service plan. But with traditional fee-for-service mental health benefits fast becoming a thing of the past, new areas of inquiry need to be addressed. Much variability exists both across the organizations that manage behavioral health care and in the specific arrangements of these organizations with payers and providers. There are good reasons to expect that these variations have implications for access to, and quality of, care, and they may explain some of the differences in results across studies. Yet there has been no systematic description of the ways that managed care organizations differ, and very little comparison across organizations or features of managed care. Such studies are needed to inform the future evolution of managed behavioral health care.

We know much less about the impact of managed care on treatment for substance abuse problems than for mental health problems. This is an important gap in knowledge both in public systems of care and in employer-based health plans. Underdetection and undertreatment are of particular concern with respect to substance abuse, since persons with such problems may not be highly motivated to seek care. But the personal and social costs of not treating substance abuse are high. Demonstrated.standards of care are less well developed for substance use disorders than for many mental disorders, and there is little consensus regarding essential provider skills and credentials, or differentiation of roles among diverse professional and nonprofessional practitioners. It would not be surprising if managed care tools discouraged adequate treatment of substance abusers, yet the managed care revolution also provides an unparalleled opportunity to develop demonstrable standards of care for substance abuse, and to usher in wide-scale improvements in the quality of substance abuse treatment.

Finally, we must find approaches for evaluating at what point the costs of behavioral health care are driven too low, with widespread underservice the inevitable result. Behavioral health services are particularly vulnerable to skimping because they have historically been viewed as more discretionary by payers and health plans. What should we make of steeper declines between 1988 and 1997 in employer-based costs of behavioral health care relative to general health care (Hay Group, 1998)? Or of the report that utilization management of hospital stays has reduced length of stay much more for behavioral disorders than for other medical conditions (Wickizer & Lessler, 1998)? Or of states with highly publicized failures of Medicaid behavioral health reforms when they attempted to reduce historical spending levels while expanding service benefits to new populations (Chang et al., 1998)? In some circumstances, behavioral services may be bearing too much of the brunt of health care cost-containment efforts. Future policy and evaluation issues in managed behavioral health care must include the development of information and systems to better monitor access to, and quality of, behavioral health services.

REFERENCES

Alexander, J. A., & Lemak, C. H. (1997a). The effects of managed care on administrative burden in outpatient substance abuse treatment facilities. *Medical Care, 35,* 1060–1068.

Alexander, J. A., & Lemak, C. H. (1997b). Managed care penetration in outpatient substance abuse treatment units. *Medical Care Research and Review, 54,* 490–507.

Alliance for Health Reform. (1999). *Managed care and vulnerable Americans: Mental health care coverage* (Issue Brief No. 98–01). Washington, DC: Author.

Bachrach, L. L. (1996). The state of the state mental health in 1996. *Psychiatric Services, 47,* 1071–1078.

Barron, J. W., & Sands, H. (1996). *Impact on managed care on psychodynamic treatment.* Madison: Connecticut International Universities Press.

Bartlett, J. (1994). The emergence of managed care and its impact on psychiatry. *New Directions for Mental Health Services, 63,* 25–35.

Bazelon Center for Mental Health Law. (2000). *Effective public management of mental health care: Views from states on Medicaid reforms that enhance service integration and accountability.* New York: Milbank Memorial Fund.

Bennett, M. J. (1992). Managed mental health in health maintenance organizations. In S. Feldman (Ed.), *Managed mental health services* (pp. 61–82). Springfield, IL: Charles C Thomas.

Bloom, B. L. (1992). *Planned short-term psychotherapy: A clinical handbook.* Boston: Allyn and Bacon.

Bloom, J. R., Hu, T., Wallace, N., Cuffel, B., Hausman, J., & Scheffler, R. (1998). Mental health costs and outcomes under alternative capitation systems in Colorado: Early results. *Journal of Mental Health Policy and Economics, 1* (1), 3–13.

Bobbitt, B. L., Marques, C. C., & Trout, D. L. (1998). Managed behavioral health care: Current status, recent trends, and the role of psychology. *Clinical Psychology: Science and Practice, 5,* 53–66.

Buck, J. A., Teich, J. L., Umland, B., & Stein, M. (1999). Behavioral health benefits in employer-sponsored health plans, 1997. *Health Affairs, 18* (2), 67–78.

Burns, B. J. (1991). Mental health service use by adolescents in the 1970s and 1980s. *Journal of the American Academy of Child and Adolescent Psychiatry, 30* (1), 144–150.

Burns, B. J., Teagle, S. A., Schwartz, M., Angold, A., & Holtzman, A. (1999). Managed behavioral health care: A Medicaid carve-out for youth. *Health Affairs, 18* (5), 214–225.

Callahan J. J., Shepard, D. S., Beinecke, R. H., Larson, M. J., & Cavanaugh, D. (1995). Mental health/substance abuse treatment in managed care: The Massachusetts Medicaid experience. *Health Affairs, 14* (3), 173–184.

Chang, C. F., Kiser, L. J., Bailey, J. E., Martins, M., Gibson, W. C., Schaberg, K. A., Mirvis D. M., & Applegate, W. B. (1998). Tennessee's failed managed care program for mental health and substance abuse services. *Journal of the American Medical Association, 279,* 864–869.

Chandler, D., Hu, T., Meisel, J., McGowen, M., & Madison, K. (1997). Mental health costs, other public costs, and family burden among mental health clients in capitated integrated service agencies. *The Journal of Mental Health Administration, 24* (2), 178–188.

Christianson, J. B., & Gray, D. Z. (1994). What CMHCs can learn from two states' efforts to capitate Medicaid benefits. *Hospital and Community Psychiatry, 45,* 777–781.

Christianson, J. B., Manning, W., Lurie, N., Stoner, T. J., Gray, D. Z., Popkin, M., & Marriott, S. (1995). Utah's prepaid mental health plan: The first year. *Health Affairs, 14* (3), 160–172.

Cuffel, B. J., Goldman, W., & Schlesinger, H. (1999). Does managing behavioral health care services increase the cost of providing medical care? *Journal of Behavioral Health Services & Research, 26,* 372–380.

Cummings, N. A. (1996). The resocialization of behavioral healthcare practice. In N. A. Cummings, M. S. Pallack, & J. L. Cummings (Eds.), *Surviving the demise of solo practice: Mental health practitioners prospering in the era of managed care* (pp. 3–9). Madison, CT: Psychosocial Press.

Detre, T., & McDonald, M. C. (1997). Managed care and the future of psychiatry. *Archives of General Psychiatry, 54,* 201–213.

Dial, T. H., Bergsten, C., Haviland, M. G., & Pincus, H. A. (1998). Psychiatrist and nonphysician mental health provider staffing levels in health maintenance organizations. *American Journal of Psychiatry, 155,* 405–408.

Dickey, B. (1997). Assessing cost and utilization in managed mental health care in the United States. *Health Policy, 41* (Suppl.), S163–S175.

Diehr, P., Williams, S. J., Martin, D. P., & Price, K. (1984). Ambulatory mental health services utilization in three provider plans. *Medical Care, 22* (1), 1–13.

Domino, M. E., Salkever, D. S., Zarin, D. A., & Pincus, H. A. (1998). The impact of managed care on psychiatry. *Administration and Policy in Mental Health, 26* (2), 149–157.

Donelan, K., Blendon, R. J., Lundberg, G. D., Calkins, D. R., Newhouse, J. P., Leape, L. L., Remler, D. K., & Taylor, H. (1997). The new medical marketplace: Physicians' views. *Health Affairs, 16* (5), 139–148.

Edmunds, M., Frank, R., Hogan, M., McCarty, D., Robinson-Beale, R., & Weisner, C. (Eds.). (1997). *Managing managed care–Quality improvement in behavioral health.* Washington, DC: National Academy Press.

Feldman, S. (1994). Managed mental health–Community mental health revisited? *Managed Care Quarterly, 2* (2), 13–18.

Finch, M., Lurie, N., Christianson, J., & Moscovice, I. (1992). The treatment of alcohol and drug abuse among mentally ill Medicaid enrollees: The utilization of services in prepaid versus fee-for-service care. In R. Frank & W. Manning (Eds.), *Economics and mental health* (pp. 292–306). Baltimore: Johns Hopkins University Press.

Findlay, S. (1999). Managed behavioral health care in 1999: An industry at a crossroads. *Health Affairs, 18* (5), 116–124.

Frank, R. G., Salkever, D. S., & Sharfstein, S. S. (1991). A new look at rising mental health insurance costs. *Health Affairs, 10* (2), 116–123.

Freeman, M. A., & Trabin, T. (1994). *Managed behavioral healthcare: History, models, key issues, and future course.* Washington, DC: Center for Substance Abuse Treatment and Managed Behavioral Health Care.

Galanter, M., Keller, D. S., Dermatis, H., & Egelko, S. (1999). *The impact of managed care on addiction treatment: A problem in need of solution* (American Society of Addiction Medicine Report). Available at <http://www.asam.org/ppol/managedcare.htm>.

Gerstein, D. R., & Harwood, H. J. (Eds.). (1990). *Treating drug problems* (Vol. 1). Washington, DC: National Academy Press.

Gibelman, M., & Schervish, P. H. (1996). The private practice of social work: Current trends and projected scenarios in a managed care environment. *Clinical Social Work Journal, 24,* 323–338.

Goldman, W., McCulloch, J., & Sturm, R. (1998). Costs and use of mental health services before and after managed care. *Health Affairs, 17* (2), 40–51.

Grazier, K. L., Eselius, L. L., Hu, T., Shore, K. K., & G'Sell, W. A. (1999). Effects of a mental health carve-out on use, costs, and payers: A four-year study. *Journal of Behavioral Health Services & Research, 26* (4), 381–389.

Gresenz, C. R., & Sturm, R. (1999). Who leaves managed behavioral health care? *The Journal of Behavioral Health Services & Research, 26,* 390–399.

Hay Group. (1998). *Health care plan design and cost trends–1988 through 1997* (News release prepared for the National Association of Psychiatric Health Services, Association of Behavioral Group Practices, and National Alliance for the Mentally Ill). Available at <http://www.naphs.org/News/hay99/hay99toc.html>.

Hoyt, M. F. (1994). Characteristics of psychotherapy under managed behavioral healthcare. *Behavioral Healthcare Tomorrow, 3* (5), 59–62.

Huskamp, H. A. (1998). How a managed behavioral health care carve-out plan affected spending for episodes of treatment. *Psychiatric Services, 49,* 1559–1562.

Institute of Medicine. (1996). *Pathways of Addiction.* Washington, DC: National Academy Press.

Joseph, S. (1997). *Symptom-focused psychiatric drug therapy for managed care.* Binghamton, NY: Haworth Medical Press.

Kapur, K., Young, A. S., Murata, D., Sullivan, G., & Koegel, P. (1999). The economic impact of capitated care for high utilizers of public mental health services: The Los Angeles PARTNERS Program experience. *Journal of Behavioral Health Services & Research, 26,* 416–429.

Lurie, N., Moscovice, I. S., Finch, M., Christianson, J. B., & Popkin, M. K. (1992). Does capitation affect the health of the chronically mentally ill? Results from a randomized trial. *Journal of the American Medical Association, 267,* 3300–3304.

Ma, C. A., & McGuire, T. G. (1998). Costs and incentives in a behavioral health carve-out. *Health Affairs, 17* (2), 53–69.

Manderscheid, R. W., & Sonnenschein, M. A. (Eds.). (1996). *Mental health United States, 1996* (DHHS Publication No. SMA 96-3098). Washington, DC: Government Printing Office.

Manning, W. G., Liu, C., Stoner, T. J., Gray, D. Z., Lurie, N., Popkin, M., & Christianson, J. B. (1999). Outcomes for Medicaid beneficiaries with schizophrenia under a prepaid mental health carve-out. *Journal of Behavioral Health Services & Research, 26,* 442–450.

Manning, W. G., Wells, K. B., Buchanan, J. L., Keeler, E. B., Valdez, R. B., & Newhouse, J. P. (1989). *Effects of mental health insurance: Evidence from The Health Insurance Experiment* (RAND R-3815-NIMH/HCFA). Santa Monica, CA: RAND.

McKusick, D., Mark, T. L., King, E., Harwood, R., Buck, J. A., Dilonardo, J., & Genuardi, J. S. (1998). Spending for mental health and substance abuse treatment, 1996. *Health Affairs, 17* (3), 147–157.

McFarland, B. H., Bigelow, D. A., Smith, J. C., Hornbrook, M. C., Mofidi, A., & Payton, P. (1995). A capitated payment system for involuntary mental health clients. *Health Affairs, 14* (3), 185–196.

Mechanic, D. (1999). *Mental health and social policy: The emergence of managed care* (4th ed.). Boston: Allyn and Bacon.

Merrick, E. L. (1998). Treatment of major depression before and after implementation of a behavioral health carve-out plan. *Psychiatric Services, 49,* 1563–1567.

Merrick, E. L. (1999). Effects of a behavioral health carve-out on inpatient-related quality indicators for major depression treatment. *Medical Care, 37,* 1023–1033.

Meyer, R. E., & McLaughlin, C. J. (1998). The educational missions of academic psychiatry. In R. E. Meyer & C. J. McLaughlin (Eds.), *Between Mind, Brain, and Managed Care* (pp. 49–76). Washington, DC: American Psychiatric Press.

Murphy, M. J., DeBernardo, C. R., & Shoemaker, W. E. (1998). Impact of managed care on independent practice and professional ethics: A survey of independent practitioners. *Professional Psychology: Research and Practice, 29* (1), 43–51.

Olfson, M., & Weissman, M. M. (1997). Essential roles for psychiatry in the era of managed care. *Archives of General Psychiatry, 54,* 206–208.

Oss, M. E., Drissel, A. B., & Clary J. (1997). *Managed behavioral health market share in the United States, 1997–1998.* Gettysburg, PA: Behavioral Health Industry News.

Peele, P. B., Lave, J. R., & Xu, Y. (1999). Benefit limits in managed behavioral health care: Do they matter? *Journal of Behavioral Health Services & Research, 26,* 430–441.

Phelps, R., Eisman, E. J., & Kohout, J. (1998). Psychological practice and managed care: Results of the CAPP practitioner survey. *Professional Psychology: Research and Practice, 29* (1), 31–36.

Pincus, H. A., Tanielian, T. L., Marcus, S. C., Olfson, M., Zarin, D. A., Thompson, J., & Zito, J. M. (1998). Prescribing trends in psychotropic medications: Primary care, psychiatry, and other medical specialties. *Journal of the American Medical Association, 279,* 526–531.

Pincus, H. A., Zarin, D. A., Tanielian, T. L., Johnson, J. L., West, J. C., Pettit, A. R., Marcus, S. C., Kessler, R. C., & McIntyre, J. S. (1999). Psychiatric patients and treatments in 1997: Findings from the American Psychiatric Practice Research Network. *Archives of General Psychiatry, 56,* 441–449.

Popkin, M. K., Lurie, N., Manning, W., Harman, J., Callies, A., Gray, D., & Christianson, J. (1998). Changes in the process of care for Medicaid patients with schizophrenia in Utah's prepaid mental health plan. *Psychiatric Services, 49,* 518–523.

Reed, S. K., Hennessy, K. D., Mitchell, O. S., & Babigian, H. M. (1994). A mental health capitation program: II. Cost-benefit analysis. *Hospital and Community Psychiatry, 45,* 1097–1103.

Rogers, W. H., Wells, K. B., Meredith, L. S., Sturm, R., Burnam, M. A. (1993). Outcomes for adult outpatients with depression under prepaid of fee-for-service financing. *Archives of General Psychiatry, 50,* 517–525.

Scheffler, R. M., & Ivey, S. L. (1998). Mental health staffing in managed care organizations: A case study. *Psychiatric Services, 49,* 1303–1308.

Scheffler, R. M., Ivey, S. L., & Garrett, A. B. (1998). Changing supply and earning patterns of the mental health workforce. *Administration and Policy in Mental Health, 26* (3), 85–99.

Sharfstein, S. S. (1997). Essential roles for psychiatry in the era of managed care. *Archives of General Psychiatry, 54,* 212–213.

Simon, C. J., & Born, P. H. (1996). Physician earnings in a changing managed care environment. *Health Affairs, 15* (3), 124–133.

Stein, B., Reardon, E., & Sturm, R. (1999). Substance abuse service utilization under managed care: HMOs versus carve-out plans. *Journal of Behavioral Health Services & Research, 26,* 451–456.

Stroul, B. A., Pires, S. A., Armstrong, M. I., & Meyers, J. C. (1998). The impact of managed care on mental health services for children and their families. *Future of Children, 8* (2), 119–133.

Sturm, R. (1997). How expensive is unlimited mental health care coverage under managed care? *Journal of the American Medical Association, 278,* 1533–1537.

Sturm, R., Goldman, W., & McCulloch, J. (1998). Mental health and substance abuse parity: A case study of Ohio's state employee program. *Journal of Mental Health Policy and Economics, 1,* 129–134.

Substance Abuse and Mental Health Services Administration. (1998). *Managed Care Tracking System: State profiles on public sector managed behavioral health care and other reforms.* Rockville, MD: National Clearinghouse for Alcohol and Drug Information.

Thompson, J. W., Burns, B. J., Goldman, H. H., & Smith, J. (1992). Initial level of care and clinical status in a managed mental health program. *Hospital and Community Psychiatry, 43,* 599–603.

Weissberg, J. H. (1994). Reflections on managed care, health reform, and the survival of dynamic psychotherapy. *Psychoanalysis of Psychotherapy, 11,* 177–180.

Wells, K. B., Manning, W. G., & Benjamin, B. (1986). Use of outpatient mental health services in HMO and fee-for-service plans: Results from a randomized controlled trial. *Health Services Research, 21,* 453–474.

Wells, K. B., Manning, W. G., & Valdez, R. B. (1990). The effects of a prepaid group practice on mental health outcomes. *Health Services Research, 25,* 615–625.

Wickizer, T. M., & Lessler, D. (1998). Effects of utilization management on patterns of hospital care among privately insured adult patients. *Medical Care, 36,* 1545–1554.

Williams, S., Wicherski, M., & Kohout, J. (1998). *Salaries in Psychology 1997: Report of the 1997 APA Salary Survey* (Research Office, American Psychological Association). Available at <http://research.apa.org/97salary/homepage.html>.

Zarin, D. A., West, J. C., Pincus, H. A., & Tanielian, T. L. (1999). Characteristics of health plans that treat psychiatric patients. *Health Affairs, 18* (5), 226–236.

Chapter 3

CLINICAL-RISK MANAGEMENT

Michael Bennett

The essence of managing medical care, including behavioral health care, is appraising and managing risk. With the evolution of organized, managed systems of health service delivery over the past decade or more, the concept of financial-risk management is generally appreciated as the driving force behind both the changing configurations of health care delivery systems and the continuous reshaping of the landscape of ownership and owner behavior. Clinical risk, which underlies financial risk, is a less appreciated and understood variable. As used in this chapter, clinical-risk management refers to the policies and procedures that organizations managing health care use to protect themselves against the impact of adverse incidents while providing optimal care to the populations they serve. Managed care organizations have developed and systematized such mechanisms and processes to varying degrees.

The profound changes in health care delivery over the past 20 years were driven initially by concerns about cost containment, primarily on the part of payers. With the failure of the Clinton initiative to reform health care at the national level, ongoing reconfiguration has incorporated many of the considerations that drove that initiative: the need to increase access, to improve quality, and to broaden the population whose care is managed. With increased concern about the underserved, there has also been a shift in focus from individual insurees to populations, and from fee-for-service to prospective forms of reimbursement, in which the needs of a population may be anticipated and planned for. These trends, along with improving methods of monitoring clinical activities and outcomes, have increased financial risk by forcing organizations that manage health care to meet expanding expectations while continuing to conserve costs. The problem is exacerbated by advances in technology, costly new medications and procedures, and higher levels of patient awareness of treatment options, especially through the Internet and the mass media. In this environment, organizations that provide the best *value*–which may be understood as the best outcomes relative to cost–are likely to succeed. Shrinking profit margins place an increasing burden on such organizations to define "good enough" care and to calculate and manage the risks that such a concept entails.

The management of behavioral health care poses special problems with respect to providing value to enrollees and also to the purchasers of health insurance, who make the actual decisions about coverage. The boundaries of behavioral health care are vague, and concepts such as medical necessity may be difficult to define (Bennett, 1996; Sabin & Daniels, 1994). Procedures such as psychotherapy lack agreed-upon definitions; the roles of providers overlap; and each new edition of the Diagnostic and Statistical Manual of Mental Disorders, upon which most practitioners base their diagnoses, becomes more broadly inclusive. Clinicians compete with each other and vie for ascendancy in an already saturated market and in an environment that promises more work for less pay (Bennett, 1994). As in the case of general health care, organizations that represent clinicians maintain an attitude toward managed care–the assortment of structural and process controls that define organized systems of health care delivery–that borders on the paranoid. Gamesmanship, challenges to authority, and threats of litigation–by both sides–confound the problems. Perhaps as a measure of their initial success in reducing costs, the agents of managed care have provoked a backlash not only among clinicians, but also among patients and the organizations that represent their interests. The public clamors for reform, and there are calls both for improved redress in areas of disagreement between clinicians and care managers, and, more generally, for a general softening of management-imposed constraints on the autonomy of providers and patients alike. Legislation and litigation, as well as efforts to invoke the protections of the Employee Retirement Income Security Act (Sederer & Bennett, 1996; Appelbaum, 1993), increase the element of legal and therefore financial risk for organizations that contract to manage care. Such risks have reshaped the landscape, leaving fewer organizations managing care for larger populations in an increasingly regulated and monitored environment. It appears that everyone is inspecting everyone else's work.

Managed behavioral health care may be understood as a reform phenomenon spurred by the excesses in cost in the unregulated environment of the 1970s and early 1980s (Bennett, 1992). The growth of managed systems has reawakened the god of regulation–ironically, with the blessing and cooperation of behavioral health care providers, who are usually opposed to regulation in any form. This surprising trend is common to health care providers generally. With the proliferation of regulatory bodies and mechanisms (for example, the National Committee for Quality Assurance and the Joint Commission on Accreditation of Healthcare Organizations), the cost of managing care has increased and even driven some organizations out of the business. Consolidation has led to fewer players that are increasingly pressed to turn a profit (or its not-for-profit equivalent) in an increasingly scrutinized and monitored environment. Since the core activity is the provision of health care services, organizational risk ultimately boils down to clinical risk: the way services are either provided or not provided to individual patients. Thus, appraisal and management of clinical risk are critical to the well-being of all managed systems. In a larger sense, managing clinical risk is a guiding principle for the calibration of a delivery system–more specifically, in making decisions about service intensity, level and duration of care, need for aftercare, and degree and nature of outreach and oversight. These principles can be best demonstrated by describing one organization's approach to clinical-risk management over a three-year period.

In the remainder of this chapter, I will describe a series of strategies for managing clinical risk–focusing on lethality–within a large, for-profit managed behavioral health organization (MBHO). These initiatives evolved over the course a three-year period under the direction of a psychiatrist (the author), whose job initially was to review all member deaths in order to assess the potential for liability. As a product of these reviews, the perceived potential for quality improvement led to the creation of a program for clinical-risk management, at the core of which was a committee comprising attorneys, quality-improvement (QI) and provider-relations managers, and clinicians. This committee was responsible to and closely linked to the corporate QI body. I will describe the program in more detail, focusing on its key features:

1. the process for auditing all patient deaths and certain other serious adverse incidents
2. findings from the audits, and the programmatic implications of those findings
3. direct effects of audit findings on organizational policies and procedures
4. secondary or indirect effects on organizational philosophy and culture

I will also describe the problems associated with such a program and suggest how they may be addressed in the current environment. Finally, I will present a broad vision of clinical-risk management as it pertains to new and emerging configurations of managed care, and suggest how the concept may be expanded beyond inspection and integrated into the organizational culture.

MANAGED CARE AND MANAGED RISK

There are three reasons why the managed behavioral health care environment is particularly well suited to the challenge of managing clinical risk. First, given the most common contemporary configuration for managing behavioral health care–a for-profit MBHO, which is a business entity that is structurally and operationally independent (that is, "carved out") of the general medical setting–the culture is likely to be a variant of that found in all business enterprises. Such a culture includes continuous attention to risk in the form of liability, with clinical liability being the equivalent of product liability. Second, managed systems require collection and monitoring of data as a precondition of fulfilling the contractual obligation to a payer. Regulatory requirements, as well as payers' performance expectations, increasingly demand both clinical and demographic information, including data on outcome, member and patient satisfaction, and the like. Adverse incidents must be monitored, and policies must be in effect to demonstrate attention to the quality of care rendered. When problems in care are identified (especially those relating to adverse incidents), it is expected that corrective steps will be taken and documented. Risk management is a close corollary of quality improvement, which is a mandated core concept required for success. Third, the successful MBHO must operate with some collective notion of acceptable risk in mind–a consequence of providing care that aims to be optimal but not necessarily state-of-the-art.

Because of these and other considerations, which will become apparent in the discussion to follow, managed behavioral health care offers an opportunity to develop strategies for managing clinical risk that may be relatively difficult to achieve in more loosely managed (or unmanaged) systems. The degree to which MBHOs have, in fact, developed such strategies remains unclear.

Audits of Adverse Incidents

The author's organization, like many other such organizations, had long had in place a process for auditing certain serious adverse incidents, most commonly those involving the death of a member. Driven by legal concerns, such audits included chart reviews, teleconferences involving clinical and care-management participants, and a report that was directed toward a staff attorney whose job it was to assess the potential for liability. Because of concerns about discoverability (that is, discovery of the evaluation by litigants who might use such information to support law suits), reports had historically been filed away and therefore not used in any systematic manner to improve systems or to educate providers or staff. The method used to conduct such reviews was variable, largely dependent on the person who conducted the review–a senior clinical manager.

Beginning in 1995, certain changes were made. The process was standardized, and a flow chart was developed to assign responsibility for its various stages. Incident reports, which alerted the organization that a serious event had taken place, were to be accompanied both by a narrative describing what was known about the event and by a standardized database providing demographic and clinical information to the attorney, who would, in turn, use a screening device developed by the Risk Management Committee to determine whether the incident met the threshold for a corporate audit. This threshold was based mainly on the seriousness of the event and its potential for liability. All member deaths and certain other serious occurrences met this threshold, while lesser incidents were handled through other channels.

When an event met the threshold, the attorney requested a corporate audit, which then set in motion a series of steps to acquire the necessary documentation and to schedule and conduct a 90-minute teleconference with the clinical and care-management participants. Following the teleconference, a report was prepared for the attorney.

Audit Findings and Implications

Since mortality audits may identify significant flaws requiring correction, such audits have been found in other settings to be an excellent vehicle for promoting quality improvement (Kinzie et al., 1992). Based upon the audits that we conducted in late 1994 and early 1995, assumptions were made about the most important and recurrent systems and clinical issues in the care of these high-risk patients. Six parameters of care were identified as indicators of possible gaps either in the provision of care or in the system for overseeing care. Auditors were asked to assess these parameters from a systemic perspective in order to inform QI staff regarding necessary improvements in systems, staff training, and oversight of providers. Cumulative data (in which individual cases could not be identified—a protection against possible discovery in litigation) would be shared periodically with staff in local programs. In additional, each auditor was asked to assess the quality of the audit itself so that necessary changes and improvements could be made.

In 1995, the first annual report was prepared for senior management. It detailed the changes that had been made, described the major findings in cases reviewed over the year, and made a series of recommendations. All suggestions were approved. The most significant findings were:

> 1–6. Auditors had identified repeated problems in six areas of care: (1) inadequate medical care or oversight; (2) lack of necessary outreach by providers; (3) insufficient involvement of families in treatment; (4) incomplete treatment plans; (5) inadequate communication among providers treating the same patient; and (6) failure on the part of providers to obtain past histories and records of their patients. The most common event audited was suicide, most commonly by the use of a gun (almost 50% of all cases).

7. Providers rarely offered services to survivors, and care managers often failed to make contact with survivors and to offer care as needed. There also appeared to be a general conviction–despite the lack of any supporting evidence–that such contact might increase the risk of lawsuits.
8. There was no standardized instrument in place for gauging clinical risk, and there was great variability among care managers and their psychiatric backups about how to evaluate and monitor this dimension of assessment.
9. Although a framework for managing high-risk cases was in place in many parts of the system, it was not well correlated with any system for monitoring lethality. The "high-risk patient" was not consistently defined.

The report's recommendations, which were based on the above findings, constituted the first components of a clinical-risk management program, from which other initiatives evolved. The goal of the program was to improve the quality of care for patients with evidence of lethality (predominantly suicidal potential) rather than to prevent suicides per se. This strategy was based on the assumption that patients who commit suicide are among the most difficult patients treated, and that the system therefore ought to be working at its very best in providing their care. The occurrence of a suicide in a system designed to promote healing should raise questions about whether or not the system has functioned optimally. Any gaps found would presumably indicate similar gaps in the care of other, less severely ill patients. Addressing identified gaps ought therefore to lead to a general improvement in the care of all patients treated in the system. Theoretically, at least, some future suicides might also be prevented.

The following recommendations were made to senior management. First, auditors should begin to assess systematically the six parameters of care noted previously and also three others (which appeared less consistently problematic): assessment and diagnosis; adequacy of documentation; and adequacy of services offered to survivors (Figure 1). Second, a policy and a procedure should be developed for routinely offering services to survivors of deceased members–and in a manner that does not expose the organization or its clinicians to increased legal risk. Third, because of the common use of guns in suicide, and because of the strong association between suicide and affective disorders, a protocol should be developed and promulgated that

Figure 1

QUALITY OF CARE ASSESSMENT

*to be completed by auditor following audit
and returned with report to corporate counsel*

Patient (initials only)..............................Nature of incident..

Auditor...Area...............................Region............................

Date of incident.....................................Date of audit ....

Rate the quality of care provided in this case from 1 to 5 for each of the following nine parameters, where 1=excellent, 2=good, 3=average, 4=poor, and 5=unacceptable (See Key)

parameter	rating				
assessment/diagnosis/characterization of problem	1	2	3	4	5
quality of treatment plan/treatment	1	2	3	4	5
documentation/adequacy of records	1	2	3	4	5
medical oversight/quality of medical care provided	1	2	3	4	5
adequacy of followup/outreach	1	2	3	4	5
coordination/communication among treaters	1	2	3	4	5
adequacy of case management/MBC oversight	1	2	3	4	5
adequacy of family/significant other involvement	1	2	3	4	5
attention to needs of survivor(s)	1	2	3	4	5
other (specify)	1	2	3	4	5

....

Key: 1 **Excellent:** *optimal practice; exceeds both MBC and community standards*
      2 **Good:** *more than meets MBC and community standards*
      3 **Average:** *meets MBC and community standards, but barely*
      4 **Poor:** *fails to meet MBC and community standards*
      5 **Unacceptable:** *calls for corrective action*

DO NOT COPY OR FAX, OR DISCUSS FINDINGS REPORTED ON THIS FORM

would restrict access to guns for any patient in treatment for any form of affective disorder while treatment was in progress. Fourth, the procedures for assessing and documenting risk status should be updated and standardized, and procedures should be developed for identifying and closely following high-risk patients, especially those with demonstrated or suspected lethality. Finally, the education of providers and staff about assessing and monitoring lethality should be made a high priority, and new methods should be found to address this need.

Since this particular MBHO was an organization structured as discrete business units spread across the country, it was necessary to find a means to educate staff and providers as close to their practice sites as feasible. (The audit conference could be used for such a purpose, but only with respect to the clinicians and staff involved in each given case.) Beginning in the fall of 1995, evaluations of performance were shared with staff of local programs. These evaluations, which were based on the auditors' assessments, presented data on local performance and compared it to the organization's overall experience in all units for the same time frame. In addition to presenting comments about the care rendered by clinicians, the reports provided cumulative critiques of the MBHO unit's patterns of intake, risk assessment, referral, and oversight, and identified quality concerns that were to be further investigated by local management through QI channels. No identifiable case was described, a precaution that was necessary in order to protect confidentiality. There was little response to the red flags raised by such reports, however, until the National Committee for Quality Assurance (NCQA) issued its new requirements two years later. In general, the efforts of the clinical-risk management program gained impetus as payers and regulatory bodies increased their demands that MBHOs demonstrate functional QI programs and initiatives.

In addition to the reports, education of clinicians under the clinical-risk management program took three forms. The first teaching initiative comprised a set of best-practice guidelines for assessing and managing the suicidal patient (Bennett, 1996). These guidelines were developed with the active input of staff, providers, and national experts, and were then offered to network physicians. Placing minimal emphasis on demographic variables, the guidelines stressed the problems associated with managing the care of suicidal patients, and then recommended methods to address those problems. The strong association between suicide and psychic anxiety was noted (Fawcett, Clark,

& Busch, 1993), as was the importance of safety planning. Contracts for safety, which had been noted to be in place in at least 15% of cases of completed suicides, were discouraged in the absence of a complete assessment, and the effective monitoring, of risk factors. This advice is consistent with observations in the literature about how risky the common practice of safety contracts may be (Simon, 1991). These guidelines were distributed to over 3,000 network clinicians who requested them after they were made available free of charge, and were widely disseminated among organizational staff. In a second teaching initiative, a series of teleconferences were scheduled in order to describe the guidelines in detail to staff, and to answer questions about how best to use them. This initiative complemented the training sessions on risk management that had already been in place for new staff.

In order to support the use of the best-practice guidelines, new tools were developed for schematizing them. In response to the observation that many clinicians had no systematic approach to assessing and monitoring lethality, and were apt to limit their exploration of suicidal potential to the presence or absence of lethal ideation, a flow chart (Figure 2) was created to provide a model for exploring acknowledged ideation. Based on information gleaned from the audits, two sets of risk factors indicating the *imminence* and *severity* of the suicidal risk associated with suicidal ideation were compiled (Figure 3). The degree of risk was assumed to be quantifiable (though actual suicide might not be predictable) in this manner. Patients might be characterized as high in both parameters, low in both, or high in one but not the other (Figure 4), placing them in one of three categories: high, moderate, and low risk. Case scenarios were developed to illustrate how strategies for *containment* and *safety planning*–which often are confused with each other but should be considered as separate elements of a treatment plan–might vary depending on this type of schematized appraisal (Figure 5). These instruments, while having limited predictive value, were useful heuristically; the aim was not to prevent suicide, but to assess and manage risk, a more achievable objective.

Revision of the organization's utilization-management (UM) guidelines took place in 1996, offering another opportunity to shape the organization's approach to risk management. Unlike its predecessors, this version of the UM guidelines included many of the general risk-management imperatives described above, as well as specific recom-

Figure 2

EVALUATION OF SUICIDAL IDEATION

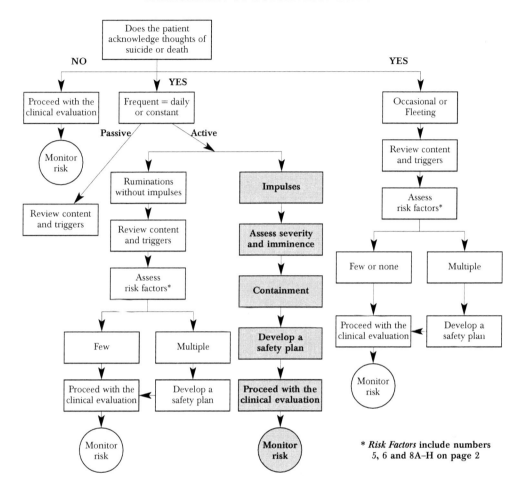

* *Risk Factors* include numbers 5, 6 and 8A–H on page 2

Figure 3

ASSESSING THE IMMINENCE AND SEVERITY OF SUICIDAL IMPULSES

Indicator of Imminence	*Indicator of Severity*

Indicator of Imminence

1. A specific plan
2. Intent to act on the plan
3. Specificity of means
4. Availability of the chosen means
5. Defensive breakdown, as indicated by:
   a. a high level of psychic anxiety*
   b. a report of global insomnia
6. Diminished barriers, as indicated by:
   a. evidence of impulsivity and/or recent life-threatening behavior
   b. ego syntonicity of suicidal option
   c. substance-induced disinhibition
   d. rejection of assistance
   e. rehearsal or preparation for death

* *psychic anxiety* refers to a state of emotional turmoil or agitation, with or without somatic anxiety symptoms.

Indicator of Severity

7. High lethal potential of planned means
8. The presence of one or more of the following *risk factors*:
   a. patient meets DSM IV criteria for depressive disorder (any subtype), schizophrenia (any subtype), substance abuse/dependence or BPD
   b. dual or multiple diagnoses**
   c. history of MH or SUDS hospitalization during the last year
   d. history of previous suicide attempt(s)
   e. access to guns
   f. family history of suicide (inquire about date and note proximity to current date)
   g. recent or impending loss
   h. social isolation

** comorbid mental health, substance-related and/or severe medical disorders

When suicidal impulses are present, the degree of lethality is a product of their imminence and severity, two overlapping but separable parameters of risk. While the *risk factors* listed in 8a–h should be appraised for any patient, they are likely to be most significant for patients with acknowledged suicidal impulses. For such patients, a careful review of both *imminence* and *severity* indicators should precede decisions about containment and safety planning, as elaborated on page 3. Depending on the presumptive degree of lethality, as evaluated by the presence of both imminence and severity indicators, the following steps should be considered:

. . . .

High: **A medical emergency calling for immediate *structural containment***

Moderate: **Consider alternative forms of containment, followed by a safety plan**

Low: **Containment may not be necessary, but safety planning should be a component of the treatment plan. Risk should be considered low but present, and an effort made to understand the "why now?" of the expressed lethality as well as the patient's agendas.**

Figure 4

THE FOUR QUADRANTS OF LETHAL RISK

SEVERITY

IMMINENCE

High imminence/ low severity:	*High imminence/high severity:*
Example: the patient who frequently acts self-destructively when stressed and may do so manipulatively. Acts may be of limited lethality, but may have the potential to escalate. Chronic risk. Suggests character pathology.	Example: the severely depressed patient, with any category of this disorder, including adjustment disorders; the patient with severe psychic anxiety; depression associated with schizophrenia. Acute risk: this is a medical emergency.

Degree of risk: moderate
Strategy: non-structural containment
      safety planning
      why now?
	Degree of risk: high
	Strategy: immediate structural
	      containment (usually
	      requiring a hospital)

Low imminence/low severity:	*Low imminence/ high severity:*
Example: the patient who is responding to an acute stressor or who is attempting to convey something to another person using this evocative device. May be acute or chronic, if pattern becomes established. Common in adolescents.	Example: Chronic depression with persistent lethality but no acute regression; chronic alcoholism associated with social isolation and depression; schizophrenia in the early stages, following hospitalization. May be acute or chronic risk.

Degree of risk: low
Strategy: why now?
      perform risk assessment
      safety planning as needed
	Degree of risk: moderate
	Strategy: non-structural containment
	      safety planning
	      why now?

Figure 5

CONTAINMENT AND SAFETY PLANNING

CONTAINMENT: This term refers to a variety of options for protecting the patient at acute risk for harming self or others; these may be employed selectively, tailored to the degree and nature of risk. The level of achievable safety and security is one of the structural elements that MBC uses in defining levels/sites of care.

HIGH RISK: The patient with suicidal impulses of high severity and high imminence requires immediate ***physical or structural*** containment, usually in a hospital, where appropriate security measures may be instituted, followed by comprehensive assessment and treatment planning. A safety plan should then become part of the treatment plan.

MODERATE RISK: When suicidal risk is rated as moderate, other containment options should also be considered during a level of care assessment; these include: ***psychosocial*** (engagement of collaterals; consideration of higher intensity and/or frequency of services; stabilization of associated situational factors; clarification of the proximal event(s) leading to the acutely lethal state ("why now") and empathic linkage with the patient's pain in response to them); ***chemical*** (use of medication appropriate to the diagnosis; immediate treatment of states of agitation; elimination of possible disinhibiting substances); and ***strategic*** (limiting access to suicidal means, especially firearms; taking steps to modify a pathogenic environment). In all instances, safety planning should be instituted in order to ensure continuing management of risk, which should then be carefully monitored.

LOW RISK: For patients in the low risk category, immediate containment may not be necessary, but factors contributing to lethality should be carefully assessed, with particular emphasis on the "why now" and a safety plan should be developed as part of the overall plan of treatment. Inpatient care may be contraindicated in some instances of low risk.

SAFETY PLANNING: The key element in a safety plan is its continuity over time. Suicidal risk tends to wax and wane and must be continuingly monitored in the patient with demonstrated lethality. Elements of a safety plan include:

1. Assurance that the patient is competent to participate in such planning: ie., understands the risks of failing to keep treaters and collaterals informed about his/her risk status
2. Coordination/communication among treaters and with significant others
3. Alliance with the patient through a mutually developed plan of treatment*
4. Continuation of the key elements of containment instituted at the point of entry
5. Provision for emergency contact and intensification of services as needed
6. Anticipation of possible destabilizing events and agreement on how to deal with them
7. Continuing monitoring of lethality through careful, repeated assessments

* *No harm* contracts may be useful only when such alliance exists, and ***should never be used in lieu of safety plans.*** Such contracts, verbal or written, run the risk of conveying to the patient that the therapist does not want to hear about lethality and/or wishes to protect himself/herself legally from actions of the patient.

mendations for assessing and managing lethality. This tool and the guidance it provides on assessing and monitoring risk will be described in some detail below as one of the direct effects that audit findings had on program development, clinical philosophy, policies, and procedures.

Direct (Primary) Effects of Audit Findings

One of the major functions of any MBHO is determining whether patients meet criteria for a given service intensity or level of care. This process, leading to authorization for reimbursement, may involve either case managers alone or—when a redirection (that is, a modification of a service request made by a patient or clinician) or a denial of such authorization occurs—both case managers and psychiatrists. The tool that particular MBHOs use to systematize this process is a set of UM guidelines that the MBHO has either developed itself or drawn from an external source. Modification and updating of these guidelines takes place periodically.

In 1996, when the author's company decided to rewrite its UM guidelines, the author was asked to cochair the process—thus providing an opportunity to include parameters of care management that reflected what had been learned from audits. Recommendations were made for family involvement at all levels of care, especially for young patients; for lethality assessments that included risk factors concerning severity and imminence; for routine assessment of substance use for all patients entering treatment; for medical clearance and involvement of all active clinicians (including outpatient therapists and primary care physicians) when patients were treated at higher levels of care; and for safety planning as a component of discharge plans when patients with demonstrated lethality moved from higher to lower levels of care (that is, when discharged from a hospital to partial inpatient, residential, intensive outpatient, or outpatient care).

The new UM guidelines sought to promote focused interventions associated with longitudinal treatment planning, including rehabilitative services for patients requiring them. The first section of the guidelines was a model for treatment planning, which included the core elements of risk appraisal. The guidelines, designed for the use of staff relating to network providers, were introduced through telephonic training of all company case managers and psychiatrists. The expectation was that these clinical managers would, in turn, then orient their local network clinicians. Risk management was conceived very broadly to apply not only to the management of lethality, but also to the general challenge of ensuring adequate aftercare, preventing recurrence, and ensuring that dual and multiple diagnosis is considered for all patients. The aim was to encourage focused care that would be efficient, effective, and safe.

In considering the direct effects of audit findings on organizational policies and procedures, as well as on clinical philosophy, some brief vignettes will serve to illustrate the types of issues identified. Although this material is drawn from audits, no identifiable case will be used, because of confidentiality concerns. The quality indicators noted were the ones most commonly observed to be problematic.

Gaps in Medical Care or Medical Oversight

> *Case 1:* The patient was a 71-year-old widow with a long history of alcohol abuse and depression. She was admitted to a free-standing psychiatric facility for detoxification and for treatment of a recurrence of her depression, which was associated with suicidal impulses. A known diabetic, she was treated with insulin and other appropriate medications. A blood sugar of 40 mg/dL was noted by the nursing staff, but there was no documentation that this finding was reported to the covering physician or that it was treated. The patient was subsequently discovered unresponsive and was transferred to a medical facility, where she received further, appropriate treatment related to her diabetes.

> *Case 2:* The patient was a 59-year-old divorced auto mechanic with a history of depression and of multiple hospitalizations for alcohol and benzodiazepine detoxifications. His psychiatrist maintained him on a regimen of bupropion, diazepam, and zolpidem, with only fair control of his depression. The patient had occasionally been hospitalized acutely suicidal. No change was made in his medications over a two-year period, and there was no indication that substance abuse treatment was ever considered or discussed.

These cases illustrate two frequently encountered problems: inadequate screening for, or treatment of, coexisting medical and substance use disorders in patients being treated for depression or other mental disorders, and overreliance on benzodiazepines over long periods of time, even in circumstances where a pattern of abuse of substances is known to exist.

Mental health clinicians often fail to evaluate and arrange treatment for substance use disorders. Many studies of suicide highlight the importance of substance abuse, either on a long-standing basis or at the point of the suicide, as an important factor (Marzuk & Mann, 1988; Murphy, 1988; Weiss & Stephens, 1992). This connection was borne out in the audits; approximately half of all completed suicides in our sample were associated with substance abuse in some form. As is indicated in Figure 3, substance use may contribute to both imminence and severity of lethality. MBHOs, through their case managers, are in a position to raise consciousness about this problem, and in some instances care managers may facilitate the linkage between addiction-treatment professionals and the mental health clinician treating the patient.

The patient's medical status is of particular concern in a MBHO carve-out because of the gap created between behavioral health and medical care. Behavioral health clinicians often do not maintain contact with primary care and other medical caregivers, and therefore fail to collaborate with them. Efforts had periodically been made in the author's MBHO to ensure coordination between primary care and behavioral health clinicians by requiring that the reports of behavioral health evaluators be routinely sent to medical caregivers. Providers cooperated with this requirement only some of the time. This practice was considerably strengthened when client organizations more uniformly began to require it, and has recently has been standardized in conformance with NCQA requirements.

With high-risk patients, in particular, coordination of care is essential lest one provider assume that all communications received are also being received by other, concurrent clinicians. It is well known in this context that most patients who suicide have reported their lethality to someone, but not necessarily to a behavioral health care provider; many such patients have seen nonpsychiatric physicians and may have made allusions or direct threats shortly before their deaths (Bharucha & Satlin, 1997). In addition, patients may be receiving conflicting advice, counseling, or psychotherapy from multiple sources or may be receiving medications from more than one clinician. Finally, the contribution of physical illnesses, especially when associated with persistent pain, has long been recognized as a potential contributor to lethality (Bharucha & Satlin). The new audit process at the author's MBHO underscored the importance of these issues and raised consciousness among case managers and psychiatric staff about ensuring such collaboration.

In response to gaps in medical care or in oversight of care, the author's MBHO examined and improved its psychiatric staffing, and backup services were made more readily available to case managers. In addition, since case managers often complained that they found it difficult to question a network psychiatrist's treatment–especially where medication was concerned–the MBHO's own psychiatrist began, when indicated, to intervene consultatively more frequently with treating clinicians.

The prescribing of benzodiazepines presents two major problems. First, it has been noted that physicians, including psychiatrists, often prescribe this class of drugs for patients suffering from depression, and may do so in the absence of an antidepressant (Oquendo, Malone, Ellis, Sackeim, & Mann, 1999). Although the short-term use of a benzodiazepine may be warranted for patients who are depressed and have symptoms of anxiety, many of the antidepressants may be sufficient alone after the medication begins to exert its full effects. It is noteworthy in this context that certain forms of anxiety, characterized by Fawcett and colleagues (1993) as *psychic anxiety*, may be strongly associated with completed suicides. In contrast to *somatic anxiety*, which is characterized by prominent physical symptoms (shortness of breath, tremor, muscle tightness, and so on), psychic anxiety is characterized by a sense of impending doom and may signal a sense of loss of control. Although this type of anxiety should be vigorously treated, it may be a symptom of depression (so-called agitated depressions) and may respond in time to the antidepressant alone. Clinicians should be wary of limiting their treatment of anxiety to those patients who qualify for a concurrent diagnosis of anxiety disorder, which may not include the patient with such agitation; anxiety disorders themselves have also been noted to be associated with lethality (Cox, Direnfeld, Swinson, & Norton, 1994). Partly as a result of the changes brought about by the audit process, the organization's case managers and their backup psychiatrists have been trained to identify those patients who are placed on benzodiazepines for extended periods of time, and to raise questions about the need for such medication. The concern is less about addiction, which is probably rare with this class of drugs, than about the possibility that the treatment is inadequate or that the diagnosis has been incorrect.

A second, larger problem with prescribing benzodiazepines, as exemplified in the second case, is the use of these medications in the care of patients with known addictive disorders. Not only are such patients at risk for inappropriate utilization of potentially addictive medications, but the use of antianxiety medication may mask withdrawal symptoms and complicate the recovery process. Of course, in many cases the patient is actively abusing substances and is not in effective recovery, an even more ominous concern.

It should also be noted that it became obvious through the auditing process that clinicians would sometimes persist in their treatment strategies despite the lack of progress. As an example, a psychiatrist might use a low dose of an antidepressant over long periods of time in the absence of clinical improvement. Suggestions for reevaluation, alternative strategies, or consultation might be made in such cases. The rapid evolution of psychopharmacology places a demand on the busy practitioner to keep up, but not all do. Studies of depression and of the suicidal patient have repeatedly indicated the inadequacy of treatment, even by psychiatrists (Keller et al., 1986; Oquendo et al., 1999). Telephonic review with an informed, psychopharmacologically sophisticated psychiatric colleague, when presented in a respectful manner, was usually found to be welcome and valuable.

Lack of Necessary Outreach by Providers

Case: The patient was a 65-year-old business executive who presented with symptoms of depression related to the impending breakup of his marriage. He was being treated by both a psychiatrist and a psychotherapist. The latter met with the couple and learned that the husband had been abusive, but there was no documented plan to deal with this problem or to communicate this information to the psychiatrist. Similarly, the psychiatrist learned of a threatened suicide, but the record failed to document that this information was shared with the psychotherapist or that it was explored with the patient. The patient was placed on fluoxetine and trazodone, and given a 3-week supply of each medication. As the marriage continued to deteriorate, the patient reported to his psychotherapist that he had followed his wife one evening, suspecting that she was seeing another man. There was no documented evaluation of this behavior or possible lethality. When the patient dropped out of treatment, there was no documented outreach on the part of either clinician.

This case demonstrated multiple problems. First, there was no systematic approach on the part of either clinician to the assessment and monitoring of lethality, or to safety planning in the face of worrisome reports from the patient. Second, no communication took place between the clinicians. Third, large doses of medication were dispensed to a potentially suicidal patient without any provision for guaranteeing safety. Finally, the patient was allowed to drop out of treatment without any subsequent attempt at outreach by either provider—despite evidence that the patient was a potential risk to himself and possibly to his wife.

The weakest part of any MBHO oversight system is its management of outpatient treatment. Since clinicians will not usually report their contacts with the patient until it is time for reauthorization of benefits, there is no opportunity to identify high-risk patients who may require close case management. When patients have been hospitalized, discharge planning will usually address such matters, and case management may then be tighter. In the case of outpatient treatment, however, the MBHO may be required—sometimes by law—to authorize a specified number of visits and may be barred from obtaining any clinical information other than diagnosis and demographics. Risk assessment at the point of entry into the system is impossible under such circumstances. Consequently, because of the difficulty of working with a large network of clinicians in solo practice—who may not have well-developed methods of risk assessment and may not communicate with other clinicians—many MBHOs favor working with group practices, where such collaboration is easier and where policies and procedures are in place for dealing with missed appointments (through routine outreach). In the particular case presented above, these practices would have been important elements in the patient's care (although there is no guarantee that the outcome would have been different).

Insufficient Involvement of Families in Treatment

> *Case:* The patient was a 45-year-old unemployed beautician with a history of 30 hospitalizations over a 20-year period for depression and alcohol abuse. Her diagnosis was bipolar disorder. Though she did well when maintained on valproate, her usual pattern was to stop her medication, to drink, and to become symptomatic, often suicidal. She had a large, supportive family, but they were not involved with her caregivers and were not asked to participate in her care. Despite her pattern of alcohol abuse, she was not treated for this disorder. Reports of cocaine use were not explored. During the last two years of her life, during which she was hospitalized eight times, the patient reported "family problems" and, on one occasion, reported having assaulted family members. This report was not explored. Her suicidality markedly increased for reasons that never became clear, and multiple attempts took place before the actual suicide.

This case again demonstrates ineffective care, with regard both to the management of her substance abuse and the failure to clarify the reasons for the change in the nature of the patient's illness (including an increased level of lethality). Though her family was repeatedly characterized as "supportive," they were never enlisted in her care. The patient, in that sense, was treated out of context. This lack of context became particularly important when her behavior toward the family apparently changed, which suggested that psychosocial stressors may have been contributing to the decline. Although this patient's pattern was well established, and she was clearly difficult to treat, her providers failed to take note of her longitudinal course and of the changes that were taking place. As is often the case in this era of descriptive psychiatry, it appears that the disorder, rather than the patient, was being treated.

Failure to Diagnose, Leading to an Inadequate Treatment Plan

> *Case:* The patient was a 31-year-old bookkeeper who presented for relationship problems and was followed over a period of several months by a psychotherapist, who saw her both alone and jointly with her lover. At her second visit, she reported a recent auto accident, but the possibility of a subintentional suicide at-

tempt was not considered. When the patient reported "vegetative degeneration," it was learned that she had become anorectic and was losing weight, sleeping poorly, unable to concentrate, anhedonic, anergic, and indecisive. Concluding that she was depressed, her therapist recommended that she contact her primary care physician in order to discuss the possible use of medication. The patient did not do so, and the matter was dropped. Relaxation exercises were prescribed and psychotherapy continued, but the record did not document either a psychiatric referral or any exploration of her reluctance to use medication.

Although this patient was observed to be depressed, the record did not indicate a formal lethality assessment, a mental status exam, or an attempt to address her resistance to the use of medication. These lapses are not uncommon among nonmedical clinicians, who may be reluctant to refer because they are concerned that the patient will leave their care, because they have no working collaboration with a trusted psychiatrist, or because they are themselves resistant to the use of drugs. Problems such as those noted for the patient above may be difficult to identify and address when the patient is seen only on an outpatient basis. Close oversight is less and less common for these patients, however; most MBHOs have come to the conclusion that outpatient case management for routine referrals is not cost-effective. The major method of control is the use of a network of clinicians who practice in patterns acceptable to the MBHO and who are known to meet acceptable standards of practice. MBHOs that are exploring contracts with group practices based on prospective reimbursement may delegate all care, including case management, to such entities, with the understanding that the group practice will assume both clinical and fiscal accountability—in which case the job of the MBHO becomes collective monitoring of quality.

Indirect (Secondary) Effects of Audit Findings

One feature of MBHOs that is central to their prosperity is the ability to adapt to a constantly changing environment. Those unfamiliar with the culture of these organizations often attribute an ideological basis to their activities, but nothing could be farther from the truth. MBHOs are highly pragmatic and plastic, taking the form required at the time, and often taking a variety of forms to suit different clients.

Because of this organizational characteristic, it is difficult to trace the evolution of any single feature, such as a risk-management program; policies and procedures are written and rewritten in response to a host of factors operative at any given time, rather than as part of a planned strategy of development. Nevertheless, it appears that the audit process and the associated quality reviews did make inroads into the organizational culture of the author's MBHO and left their mark in a few specific ways:

1. *The importance of clinician documentation.* Behavioral health clinicians were found in the audit process to document poorly. Deficits were also found in the MBHO's own accounts of case management. Improvements in both of these areas became an organizational priority that was reinforced by burgeoning regulatory requirements and supported by the improvement in internal information systems. As part of such documentation, standardized risk-assessment tools were developed, though these were tailored to the requirements of certain client organizations. For example, the requirements of a Medicaid contractor might be quite different from those of a national corporate account. Both types of clients, however, are requiring increased levels of documentation of MBHO activity, particularly in cases that have a potential for liability.

2. *High-risk case management.* Most MBHOs have some system in place for identifying patients whose course should be monitored over time. This approach is sharply at variance with MBHOs' historical emphasis on acute-care episodes—one of the major criticisms leveled at such organizations. It was largely the assumption of responsibility for more severely disturbed populations, in which persistent and recurrent mental disorders are relatively common, that produced this shift in emphasis. In the case of the particular MBHO described in this chapter, the risk-management program, with its identification of failed treatment as a common precursor to completed suicide, also contributed to this shift in perspective. More generally, it is in the interest of MBHOs to maintain high-risk patients in treatment and potentially prevent the type of regression that precedes hospitalization, rather than to give undue emphasis to crisis intervention that treats returning patients as though they were new to the system.

An additional reason to develop a tracking program for high-risk cases is that MBHOs (and their client organizations) are extremely concerned about disaffected patients who become publicly visible and create what is termed "noise." Efforts to identify patients who may be at risk for future hospitalization–and for future appeals and complaints–may be every bit as important to MBHOs' risk-management programs as is the identification of lethal patients.

In addition to case management, the high-risk tracking programs that were developed in the author's MBHO featured interdisciplinary planning conferences focusing on patients displaying patterns either of nonalliance with treatment (often called "noncompliant") or of repeated use of costly resources (often called "recidivist"). It is noteworthy that the terms used to describe such patients reflect the ambivalence felt toward them in all systems of care. This ambivalence may blunt the concern of caregivers, as well as that of the overseers of care, and may be reflected in the provision of a secondary diagnosis of personality disorder–which does nothing to mitigate risk.

3. *Provider credentialing/recredentialing.* It is required of MBHOs that they credential and recredential network providers, usually at two-year intervals. Risk management enters into the process at the outset by identifying clinicians having open or ongoing legal issues, which then must be clarified in order to reassure an MBHO that no increased liability will be assumed by placing in the network a clinician whose quality or safety of care is in question. As for clinicians already within the network, having an audit process in place makes it possible to identify those clinicians (and also facilities) whose practice is suspect based on an adverse incident of sufficient magnitude to warrant a corporate audit. In order to preserve the nondiscoverability of the audit itself, action is rarely taken to discipline or remove a clinician or a facility based solely on audit findings. The practice is to submit a recommendation to the clinical managers of the program with which the clinician or institution involved in the case was associated, and to suggest that the local medical or clinical director conduct an audit of a sample of the clinician's or institution's other cases with features similar to the case already examined through the corporate audit. The aim is to correct any

found deficits. Criteria were developed by the author's organization to allow for consistency in record review and to permit an informed decision about what, if any, action should be taken. The willingness of a provider or facility to correct identified gaps in practice might then be used as a requirement for continuing network participation.

Throughout the process of clinician review, efforts are made to adopt an attitude of responsible quality improvement. Thus, the primary concern–beginning with feedback during the audit–is the continuing education of the clinician and of the MBHO staff, with the goal of improving performance rather than weeding out problem clinicians. The exception is the case in which the audit demonstrates a clear danger to other patients, which requires more immediate action.

4. *Dual diagnosis.* The audit process reinforced other messages coming from QI programs, client input, and an increasingly publicized emphasis on dual and multiple diagnosis within the professional community. Routine assessment of substance-use patterns for all patients who presented with mental disorders, and the reverse, became standard for case managers and supervising physicians. With its emphasis on rapid stabilization at high service-intensity sites (that is, ones providing inpatient, partial inpatient, or residential services), the MBHO favors early intervention in a case that is not going well. The finding that over half of all completed suicides were associated with substance abuse reinforced such practices.

5. *Sensitivity to the needs of survivors.* The procedure of routinely offering services to survivors of a patient death has become a standard one. Case managers and the patient's clinicians may also be considered survivors. Since many clinicians have no formal method of reviewing and processing their responses to such a traumatic event, their involvement in the entire audit and review process may help them with this task. Addressing the needs of survivors to a suicide is likely to represent not only humane care, but good risk management; it carries the potential to preserve the remaining alliance and may lessen survivors' desire to find a scapegoat.

6. *Awareness of gun ownership/access as a key variable.* Through both the gun protocol and the emphasis in teaching sessions–the

importance of gun ownership/access has been underscored. Including gun ownership as a factor in risk assessment has become part of the organizational culture.

RISK MANAGEMENT: PROBLEMS AND PROSPECTS

The experiences described above may be of value to those attempting to introduce a risk-management program into an MBHO. Certain types of problems should be anticipated, however. Clinicians are often advised not to participate in the audit process because of the legal risks involved. (Although attempts can be made to minimize such risks, they remain present.) For example, efforts to enlist the support of the Psychiatrists' Purchasing Group, the major organization that provides malpractice coverage for psychiatrists, proved unsuccessful in that the organization's attorneys believed that they could not advise their clients to participate in such reviews. The difficulty of engaging psychiatrists was in sharp contrast to the ease of obtaining cooperation from the network's nonphysician clinicians. Perhaps psychiatrists' fear of lawsuits is too great to overcome this reluctance, even though the audit process may be helpful in directing their attention to gaps in practice that need to be addressed. The approach we took was to insist, at a minimum, that psychiatrists provide their records. If no records were provided, disciplinary action would follow. Not only is such cooperation part of the network-membership contract, but the absence of a record suggests that no record exists, which is a violation of standard practice. It was our experience that the average quality of records was appallingly poor for all categories of clinicians. We have tried to address this issue, thus far unsuccessfully, through the professional organizations. Other means must be found to deal with this issue (see below).

A second problem is the difficulty of standardizing practice in a system that is so strongly tailored to the needs and preferences of particular client organizations. This problem can be addressed by establishing minimal standards that can then be varied as clients require—for example, with regard to the development and use of risk-management instruments.

A third issue, already referred to in some of the cases, is the difficulty of conducting risk assessment for outpatients when the MBHO may have no contact with them until an adverse incident occurs. This situation is in flux, but the trend is toward selective contracting, with delegation of responsibility for quality and risk management to provider groups engaged in some form of risk-sharing arrangement– which creates an oversight role for the manager of care. The role of the MBHO then becomes one of ensuring accountability rather than that of attempting to micromanage patient care. The precise terms of accountability should be determined only if and when a client contract specifies that risk assessment and monitoring are required. The MBHO can then set standards for how these goals should be achieved–for example, through establishing: minimum requirements for risk-assessment tools; standards for lethality monitoring; and best-practice guidelines for the risks associated with specific disorders (such as eating disorders, substance abuse, schizophrenia, borderline personality disorder, and depression) or populations (adolescents, the elderly, patients with persistent and recurrent mental disorders).

A fourth set of problems concerns documentation–which appears to be related, in turn, to the failure of many practicing clinicians to develop appropriate methods to record their activities. In our experience, this inadequacy appeared to be most common in individual, office-based practices–which presents yet another reason to prefer group practices that have the necessary administrative supports.

A final problem concerns the state of clinicians' current knowledge and the resulting risks associated with clinicians' failure to keep up-to-date. Despite its initial promise, organized continuing education must be regarded as a failure in this respect. With the great changes that have taken place in behavioral health care over the past few years, however, continued learning has become even more crucial. Nonetheless, it was a repeated finding that clinicians, including psychiatrists, often fell back on what they knew how to do and, when clinical progress was not evident, tended to do more of the same rather than something different. Many clinicians appeared unprepared to work in the managed environment, which requires a fundamental shift to the needs of a population and to the use of evidence-based treatment strategies aimed to promote a specific desired outcome in the briefest possible time. The goals of managed care are primarily related to restoration of functional integrity rather than cure–a frame of reference alien to many practitioners. We found, for example, that many psychiatrists were unfamiliar with substance-use disorders and how to assess and manage them, often had limited knowledge of the various strategies for augmenting medications when necessary, and often did not have clear strategies for dealing with resistant or nonallied patients. Although case managers may be helpful in some cases, limitations in skill or knowledge remain a great problem. A wealth of knowledge is available on the Internet (as well as elsewhere), but many of the clinicians, in our experience, were not prepared to take advantage of it and, more generally, appeared to be poorly educated to function in the current, managed environment. Weeding out such clinicians may become a central task for managers of care, since professional organizations may not be willing to acknowledge or address such problems.

It was our experience that some clinicians respond well to pointing out the need to update their knowledge. For example, the development of a best-practices document on assessing and managing the suicidal patient met with enthusiasm, and many network clinicians requested copies. The best chance for necessary learning may lie in the threat of competition for a declining number of available positions for clinicians within the group practices that will come to dominate the practice environment. Dual requirements for adult learning will be present (Budman & Armstrong, 1993): active learning, and learning in the context of the clinician's own practice. Ultimately, well-trained (or retrained) clinicians who approach the care of each patient with thoughtfulness and clarity, and who document their process of making decisions, are the best risk managers.

Other Aspects of Clinical-Risk Management

The risk-management program described above was but a beginning. Movement from inspection to forethought and planning—and transforming the culture into one that is attuned to clinical risk as a key driving force in clinical decision making—is a much broader task. One limitation we encountered was the structure within which we operated. The clinicians were not at risk and often saw their primary obligation as treating each particular patient rather than as addressing the needs of the population as a whole. Clinicians were reimbursed on a fee-for-service basis, creating perverse incentives to keep the patient coming, to resist referral to a potential competitor, and to offer only those services that they felt competent to provide. There was no reward for providing outreach, dealing with corollaries (except in office visits that were billable), communicating with other clinicians providing treatment, or finding new and more efficient ways to manage complex patients. These issues all have great relevance for the internalization of risk management as a principle that guides practice.

Despite these limitations, clinicians are likely to practice certain forms of risk management both to protect themselves from liability and to meet legal requirements. For example, most clinicians have some idea that they are required to report certain types of abuse, warn potential victims, address questions of competence with regard to motor vehicle operation, and the like. Clinicians also are taught to recognize the need to maintain reasonable boundaries with their patients, and to understand the risks of not doing so. Commitment laws, which vary from state to state, become relevant for some clinicians but are poorly understood by most. Finally, though the matter came up infrequently in the MBHO experience described, there is the matter of assessing and managing the assaultive or dangerous patient. In our experience, most clinicians (aside from emergency room staff) deal with this matter by avoiding it if at all possible.

For certain routine aspects of risk management, the periodic training and the continuing education currently practiced by most clinicians—who attend a few conferences, read a bit, and take an occasional course—may be useful. In this context, it would be helpful to ensure a familiarity with Simon's (1992, pp. 125–153) strategies for assessing dangerousness and with various protocols for managing the suicidal patient. If the clinician is to go beyond this limited approach, however, certain contextual factors are important. Since these factors appear to coincide with the direction in which managed behavioral health care is moving, it may be useful to enumerate them:

1. *The clinician should be placed at risk financially for the population served.* One of the more contentious questions in health care concerns the impact of placing clinicians at financial risk for the cost of care delivered to the populations they serve. This question is of great importance, given the likely proliferation of risk-sharing contracts and the likely growth of physician service networks and other such vehicles to manage them.While some may argue that financial risk encourages venality and leads to undertreatment, combining it with mechanisms to monitor the health status of insurees, as well as their satisfaction with the

care they receive, appears to offer protection against such consequences, while underscoring the principle of accountability.

In the presence of mechanisms to monitor the quality of care, risk sharing challenges the clinician to manage care in a manner that balances "doing good" with "doing well"; that is, to arrive at a treatment plan that is optimal, safe, efficient, effective, and characterized by neither undertreatment nor overtreatment. It is in the clinician's interest to quickly identify and address clinical impasses, and to collaborate with any and all who can help maximize outcome: for example, to speak with clinicians treating the same patient, involve the family, obtain old records in order to clarify diagnosis, or seek appropriate consultation when the patient fails to improve on an initial regimen. Parsimony of intervention and the use of the lowest service intensity for the shortest time that will produce the necessary outcome become internalized, guiding principles (within the constraint of patient safety). Managing financial risk may therefore lead the clinician to a more enlightened management of clinical risk.

2. *The clinician should work collaboratively with other clinicians.* Group practice is becoming more common among behavioral health care providers and will become the norm. The reasons for this restructuring are not the result simply of managed care, but of the increasing complexity of behavioral health practice and, with it, the importance of subspecialization. Collaborative practice, as compared with the loose affiliation (or competition) among solo practitioners who may be part of the same network, maximizes the treatment armamentarium while minimizing the risk of losing the patient to the subspecialist. Group practice optimizes the opportunity for communication and increases the likelihood that treatment will be scrutinized and reviewed. Insofar as the group is accountable for monitoring and improving quality, the possibility for risk management as a cultural value is enhanced, and the possibility of "continuous risk improvement" becomes a corollary.

3. *The clinician should address the matter of learning how to function within a managed care setting.* As Michael Balint (1972, p. 299) informed us, when asked what it took for physicians to learn to perform psychotherapy, it takes a "limited, though consider-

able, change in the doctor's personality." The same may be said about managed behavioral health practice. Behavioral health practitioners have thus far largely resisted the retraining required in order to accommodate to the care of populations. As curricula in training programs are revised in order to prepare trainees for life in a managed clinical environment, current practitioners will need to update their skills in order not only to remain relevant, but to survive. Continuing education that is focused on the requirements of practice within a managed care system will encourage the adoption of many of the principles of practice described in this chapter–none of which are new.

The Place of Risk Management in Managed Care

As we look ahead, we should assume that virtually all behavioral health care will be managed; that is, that most care will be financed prospectively and provided in organized systems featuring both horizontal and vertical integration of services. Although the agents managing care may change, and we will learn more about how to provide services efficiently, the principles will be the same. How should we think about risk management comprehensively in such contexts?

To start, risk management should be considered a key function standing alongside quality improvement (to which it can contribute), legal services (for which it serves as the intermediary to clinical services), and clinical services. A single clinical manager with risk-management experience should be charged with responsibility in this area and be in a position to advocate for it. Risk management should be part of the organization's ongoing programs for educating case managers, clinicians, and those whose roles place them in contact with patients. Inspection should remain an aspect of the risk-management program; audits of adverse incidents remain a powerful tool to raise consciousness, identify gaps, and track improvements through effective links with the QI function. Because of the variety of risks assumed by a managed care entity–many of which have implications for practice–risk-management directors can support other functions assigned to the legal department (for example, the writing of provider contracts) or to marketing or other departments. These directors' main functions should nevertheless remain that of clinical-risk management. A committee comprising clinicians and legal, information-processing, and administrative staff can help coordinate risk-management activities and develop the necessary policies and procedures.

What is clinical-risk management in such a setting? A major criticism of managed care has been its emphasis on cost containment. At the core of this concern is the cost-benefit analysis that takes place systemically and, in fact, during each clinical encounter. Utilization management, for example, implies such analysis. I suggest that we replace *cost-benefit* analysis with *risk-benefit* analysis and make this concept explicit rather than implicit. At the clinical heart of the system, the balancing of risk versus benefit becomes a guiding and explicit part of the organizational mission. How does this work?

First, the clinical encounter must be associated with informed consent. Our patients come to us with expectations, some based on fact, some not. To understand that the obligation of the health care system is to prioritize allocations based on need—a principle much discussed but little implemented (outside, perhaps, of Oregon)—is to understand the type of weighing that a clinician will be expected to make. What are the risks of treating versus not treating—to the patient, his or her family, society? What are the risks versus benefits of one type of treatment versus another—one site or intensity versus another, one drug versus another? What is the threshold for including a new technology? It will be expected that clinicians consider risks to the organization, *including but not limited to* financial costs, as well as risks to themselves.

The last concern mentioned—risk to the clinician—is the one that is most promoted through the risk-management training clinicians currently receive (if they receive any at all); that is, clinicians are taught to protect themselves, a consideration that is important but not exclusive, and that should be balanced against all the others. Achieving this type of balance requires a broader advocacy than is usually understood, accepted, and practiced by clinicians. It can be inculcated through training designed to teach the basics of comprehensive risk management, including the ethical considerations associated with it. Such training will encourage the internalization of the balance—and tension—between allocation to the individual patient and planning for the needs of the population. It is this balance that is at the heart of properly managed care.

The purpose of inspection, education, and supervision is to shape the culture and bring it into alignment with the mission of the larger organization, which is to deliver effective care to a population, allocated based on need and in a manner that is affordable and safe. Safety, in turn, is defined comprehensively—to the individual, the population, the organization, and society. The professional community cries out for a restoration of its autonomy. The price is assumption of accountability for managing society's resources.

SUMMARY

Managed care is relatively new phenomenon, though its antecedents date back many years. Pressures to contain costs have led us to manage care, initially through managing benefits and controlling access to the most costly resources, especially hospitals. More recent phases of managed care have begun to address serious matters of access, allocation, effectiveness, and the value and quality of services.

The past decade has seen the rise and then the dominance of the MBHO, primarily the for-profit carve-out, in managed behavioral health care. There are reasons to believe that this era is transitional and may be drawing to a close. These reasons include widespread dissatisfaction in the provider community, leading to unionization and other forms of resistance to policies that are essential to MBHO profitability; a further squeeze on profits that is created by increasing performance requirements in the face of declining reimbursement and capitation rates; trends toward increased benefits and choices for members, which also increase costs; challenges to the legal barriers to lawsuits by disaffected patients; and the renewed thrust toward reintegrating behavioral health care with general medical care, a trend that reflects both the rise of biological psychiatry and the evolution of the concept of parity (which may reflect, in turn, the "democratization" of behavioral health). Perhaps the most ominous indicator is the dramatic decline in shareholder values common to the largest players in the carve-out field.

Assuming that the era of the carve-out is drawing to a close, other configurations will very likely emerge as part of the necessary process of updating our models of behavioral health care to integrate psychosocial theories of health and illness with advances in genetics, neurochemistry, learning theory, rehabilitation, and alternative medicine. Reintegration of behavioral and physical health care is likely in such a scenario. Whether the current enthusiasm for behavioral health treatment by primary care providers proves to be any more successful than it has in the past remains to be seen. What is clear, however, is that the increasing sophistication of consumers and payers about behavioral health issues, the explosion of mass means of education and communication, and the reduced stigma associated with behavioral health interventions have increased demand and made many of the old methods for containing costs anachronistic. These changes may presage a growing public investment in behavioral health care and an increased interest both in its successful management and in retrieving control of it from the business community. Government's increasing interest in behavioral health care suggests, too, a progressively growing role.

New ways must be found to deal with the vast, unmet need in the population at large for behavioral health services. This need is especially great with regard to the elderly, who are not only at risk for mental disorder, but highly at risk for suicide (Bharucha & Satlin, 1997). At the other end of the spectrum, recent concerns about escalating acts of violence among the young point to the needs of this segment of the population. MBHOs, which have evolved very little beyond being utilization managers and have focused on providing acute care and eliminating excess, have failed to develop a vision of what good care ought to look like. Further, because of the methods of financing involved, MBHOs have had little incentive to identify needy individuals or to expand the access to care to those who remain silently at need. We are about to enter a new era, in which the management both of risk and of outcome will become preeminent considerations in the management of care, whoever the agents are who oversee it.

Defining risk management as the avoidance of adverse consequences while optimizing care for a population, I have presented a model based on a three-year experience in one MBHO. Developed from a program for auditing serious adverse incidents–mainly, patient suicides–the program involved the creation of a risk-management committee and the development of policies and procedures designed to increase the safety of clinical operations from both a clinical and liability perspective. Essential features of the program were drawn from the audits, which identified nine parameters found to be persistently or repeatedly deficient. Proceeding from such findings, quality ratings were prepared and distributed to the various administrative units, offering a portrait of how well the unit functioned relative to other units in the same organization. The aim was to inspire a closer look at the identified gaps through extant QI mechanisms–an attempt that proved only partially successful until reinforced by the presence of regulatory mechanisms from other sources. In an effort to improve the MBHO's case oversight and help shape behavior among participating (network) clinicians, risk management was introduced as a set of expectations for case management and psychiatric supervision. Most policies and procedures pertained to the assessment and management of the suicidal patient (the most common audited adverse event), but training sessions also addressed a full range of other risk-management issues.

Because of the nature of the relationship with the provider community, it was not possible to train clinicians at large to manage risk effectively, and we had to settle for a case-by-case correction of patterns manifested in an audit. Thus, correction was always directed to the next case, and there is no way of determining its effectiveness. From the outset, based on the literature about suicide prevention–which repeatedly cautions us that we have not yet learned to predict suicide in the individual case–the purpose was not to prevent suicides per se, but to use the event as a marker that might enlighten us as to gaps that required correction and, if correction occurred, opportunities to improve the overall function of our system. Though the suicides per 100,000 members were found progressively to diminish over the period studied, there is no way to relate that finding to the program. What appears to have happened, however, is that certain valued strategies became part of the clinical culture of the organization: protocols for limiting gun access for patients in treatment for depression; routine provision of services to survivors; thoroughness of substance use and lethality assessments; increased communication among concurrent clinicians; increased collaboration of the family in treatment; and development of a longitudinal dimension to discharge planning for patients with severe disorders.

As managed care continues to evolve, the next generation will provide a context more favorable to inculcating values such as those described. There is general agreement that we will increasingly focus our attention on achieving a desired outcome, but we have a lot to learn about how to measure and document this dimension of care. Clinical-risk management, which may be understood as the quest for maximal outcome at minimal risk, will be our most important tool in achieving this goal. Continuous risk improvement should become a corollary of continuous quality improvement as we move into this new century.

REFERENCES

Appelbaum, P. (1993). Legal liability and managed care. *American Psychologist, 48* (3), 251–257.

Balint, M. (1972). *The doctor, his patient and the illness.* New York: International Universities Press.

Bennett, M. (1992). Managed mental health care in health maintenance organizations. In S. Feldman (Ed.), *Managed Mental Health Services* (pp. 61–82). Springfield, IL: Charles C Thomas.

Bennett, M. (1994). Are competing psychotherapists manageable? *Managed Care Quarterly, 2* (2), 36–42.

Bennett, M. (1996). *Best practices: Assessing and managing the suicidal patient.* Maryland Heights, MO: Merit Behavioral Care Corporation.

Bennett, M. J. (1996). Is psychotherapy ever medically necessary? *Psychiatric Services, 47,* 966–970.

Bharucha, A. J., & Satlin, A. (1997). Late-life suicide: A review. *Harvard Review of Psychiatry, 5* (2), 55–65.

Budman, S. H., & Armstrong, E. (1993). Training for managed care settings: How to make it happen. *Psychotherapy, 29* (3), 416–421.

Cox, B. J., Direnfeld, D. M., Swinson R. P., & Norton, G. R. (1994). Suicidal ideation and suicide attempts in panic disorder and social phobia. *American Journal of Psychiatry, 151* (6), 882–887.

Fawcett, J., Clark, D. C., & Busch, K. (1993). Assessing and treating the patient at risk for suicide. *Psychiatric Annals, 23* (5), 244–255.

Keller, M. B., Lavori, P. W., Klerman G. L., Andreason, N. C., Endicott, J., Coryell, W., Fawcett, J., Rice J. P., & Hirschfeld, R. M. (1986). Low levels and lack of predictors of somatotherapy and psychotherapy received by depressed patients. *Archives of General Psychiatry 43,* 458–466.

Kinzie, J. D., Maricle, R. A., Bloom, J. D., Leung, P. K., Goetz, R. R., & Singer, C. M. (1992). Improving quality assurance through psychiatric mortality and morbidity conferences in a university hospital. *Hospital and Community Psychiatry, 43* (5), 470–474.

Marzuk, P. M., & Mann, J. J. (1988). Suicide and substance abuse. *Psychiatric Annals, 18,* 639–645.

Murphy, G. E. (1988). Suicide and substance abuse. *Archives of General Psychiatry, 45,* 593–594.

Oquendo, M. A., Malone, K. M., Ellis, S. P., Sackeim, H. A., & Mann, J. J. (1999). Inadequacy of antidepressant treatment for patients with major depression who are at risk for suicidal behavior. *American Journal of Psychiatry, 156* (2), 190–194.

Sabin, J., & Daniels, N. (1994). Determining "medical necessity" in mental health practice. *Hastings Center Report, 24* (6), 5–13.

Sederer, L., & Bennett, M. (1996). Managed mental health care in the United States: A status report. *Administration and Policy in Mental Health, 23* (4), 289–306.

Simon, R. I. (1991). The suicide prevention pact: Clinical and legal considerations. In R. I. Simon (Ed.), *Review of Clinical Psychiatry and the Law* (Vol. 2, pp. 441–451). Washington, DC: American Psychiatric Press.

Simon, R. I. (1992). *Psychiatry and law for clinicians.* Washington, DC: American Psychiatric Press.

Weiss, R. D., & Stephens, P. S. (1992). Substance abuse and suicide. In D. Jacobs (Ed.), *Suicide and clinical practice: Multiple perspectives* (pp. 101–114). Washington, DC: American Psychiatric Press.

Chapter 4

TRAINING

Michael A. Hoge

It can be argued that in an ideal world, treatment approaches for mental illness and addictions would be research driven and evidence based. Services would evolve as a product of scientific investigation. The academicians who conduct the research would simultaneously educate students about state-of-the-art practices. Practicing clinicians would stay current with changes in the field of behavioral health through a process of lifelong learning.

In actuality, however, the evolution of clinical services has not been principally research driven. Economics, health care financing, professional theories, and guild interests have had a heavy influence in shaping the field. Research has tended to follow, rather than drive, innovation—providing the justification, as it were, for changes that have already occurred in clinical practice (Hoge, Davidson, & Hill, 1993).

This time differential has significant implications for the process of educating professionals. As academic research and training centers strive to complete the complex process of funding and conducting studies of selected clinical interventions or approaches, they may lag behind changes in the field. Simultaneously, the clinical training

Note: The author would like to thank the following individuals for their time in providing information about current professional training and workforce retraining activities: Kay Davidson, Michael Freeman, William Goldman, Judith Krauss, Anita Lightburn, Jo Linder-Crow, Ronald Manderscheid, Monica Oss, Kimberly Strom-Gottfried, Sarah Raphel, Gail Sicilia, Jeanne Spruill, Deborah Teplow, Warwick Troy, Douglas Walter, Richard Weiner, and Susan Zlotlow. The opinions expressed in this chapter are the sole responsibility of the author.

offered in these sites is likely to lag behind the current health care environment (Feldman, 1978). This lag may subsequently continue into trainees' lives as working professionals. Practice patterns, which are established early in a career, are not easily changed; after training is completed, professionals tend to maintain minimal contact with academic centers and spend only a small percentage of their time on continuing education.

If our era were one in which approaches to treatment are evolving slowly, these dynamics would probably be tolerable. But it is not. Managed care has radically reshaped the field of behavioral health care over the past decade. When change is so dramatic, the gulf between practice realities and professionals' training and skills can become enormous.

The purpose of this chapter is to examine the implications of managed behavioral health care for professional education and workforce retraining. The efforts to revamp graduate training programs and to reeducate professionals are considered in light of a set of training objectives that are driven by changes in the health care marketplace. The status of these issues in each of the four major behavioral health disciplines–psychiatry, (clinical) psychology, and subfields within social work and nursing–is considered, as are some innovative educational approaches.

TRAINING OBJECTIVES

To function effectively as a professional, an individual needs appropriate values, knowledge, and skills. Managed care has challenged the traditional values of behavioral health care professionals. It has also rewarded, through reimbursement, those who have a knowledge base and skill set that are compatible with managed care principles and practices.

No matter what the fate of managed care, it is reasonable to conclude that the values, knowledge, and skills necessary to survive–and thrive–in practice are changing substantially and that educational programs must therefore also change. In the absence of definitive data on the clinical effectiveness of managed and nonmanaged approaches to service delivery, the educational objective should be to teach both traditional and managed approaches to care. The justification for teaching about managed care is a pragmatic one, however, that is rejected by many faculty, who maintain that educating students and working professionals about managed care is akin to surrendering to it.

Values

The objective of instilling relevant values illustrates the balance that must be achieved in the educational process. Given the controversy about traditional versus managed care approaches, Ross (1997) has argued that the most fundamental value to instill is that of "academic integrity," which he defines as a questioning attitude coupled with a frank acknowledgment of what we know and do not know about the treatment of mental illness and substance abuse.

Educators will undoubtedly continue to teach and model the traditional values that emphasize delivering quality care and meeting the needs of individual patients. From a managed care perspective, the professional values that are taught and modeled should also emphasize the need to use scare resources in an efficient manner to meet the treatment needs of individuals and of populations. Students and working professionals need to understand how the traditional value placed on professional autonomy or the independence of clinical judgment is being challenged by a more contemporary emphasis on adherence to standards. These standards take the form of level-of-care guidelines crafted by managed care organizations and of practice guidelines published by professional organizations and government agencies.

Knowledge and Skills

There is a growing body of literature that identifies the knowledge and skill base that practitioners must possess in order to function effectively and to be successful in this health care climate (American Nurses Association, 1997; Coursey, 1998; Feldman & Goldman, 1997; Gabbard, 1992; Ross, 1997; Sabin, 1991; Schreter, 1997; Schuster, Lovell, & Trachta, 1997; Strom & Gingerich, 1993; Tasman & Minkoff, 1997; Yager, Docherty, & Tischler, 1996). Much of that which is taught in graduate schools (including professional schools and training programs) or has been learned by active practitioners remains relevant. There are new topics and skills, however, that need to be addressed in educational programs, and there are some traditional topics whose content needs to be revised and updated to reflect changes in the field.

The recommendations that have been made regarding the knowledge base for psychiatrists have been integrated by Hoge, Jacobs, and Belitsky (2000). The new topic areas that optimally would be covered in curricula include: health care regulation and reform; the economics of behavioral health care; an overview of managed care covering its history, developmental phases, procedures, and impact; a review of various health care structures such as carve-outs, HMOs, PPOs, PHOs, IPAs, and group practices; the utilization-management process, including a review of level-of-care criteria and of the concept of medical necessity; practical strategies for working with managed care organizations; practice guidelines; quality-management strategies; and the interface between behavioral health and primary medical care.

Revised approaches to topics traditionally covered in professional education are needed in a range of areas. These include: an historical overview of the forces that have shaped clinical service delivery; the expanded continuum of care; practice models and settings; legal and ethical issues; and the changing nature of professional roles and inter-disciplinary relationships.

In considering the new skills and new approaches to traditional skills that practitioners should ideally possess, it is useful to employ a categorization scheme adapted from Schreter (1997). The first category, *clinical skills*, includes a variety of basic clinical competencies that are important in a managed care environment. These skills include: efficient, multiaxial assessment and differential diagnosis; goal-focused and problem-oriented treatment planning; and facility with a broad range of clinical interventions such as psychopharmacology, brief treatments, behavioral and cognitive interventions, and various "alternatives" to inpatient care (Hoge et al., 2000).

The second category, *clinical-management skills*, involves competencies specifically related to managing care. These skills include: determining medical necessity and appropriate levels of care; utilizing research evidence and guidelines when selecting treatments; coordinating care and managing the cases of "high utilizers"; and responding to ethical dilemmas faced by practitioners as a consequence of managed care.

The final category, *administrative skills*, focuses on the need for competence in collaborating with utilization reviewers, in documenting care in compliance with applicable regulations and requirements, in accurately completing credentialing materials and billing forms, and in advocating for patients' rights within treatment systems and managed care organizations.

PROFESSIONAL TRAINING

Across all disciplines, the status of professional education about managed care and related aspects of contemporary clinical practice is very similar. The curriculum contains, at best, a small number of lectures about managed care. There is generally no attention to the business side of health care delivery and only modest attention to the changing nature of professional roles. Students receive little training or experience in modalities that managed care has promoted, including brief treatment, intensive outpatient treatment, and ambulatory detoxification. Because of reimbursement issues, trainees are often excluded from working with patients whose care is managed. Whatever involvement there is with such patients typically occurs in inpatient settings where managed care tends to be the most intrusive, thus fostering negative attitudes towards managed care among the trainees.

Enhancing the relevance of professional education to managed care involves addressing a range of issues, including the following: faculty attitudes, interests, and skills; access to curricular time; access to an expanded range of training sites; constraints imposed by accreditation bodies; reimbursement and funding issues; and the diversity of supervisory pools. Each of these issues is considered in turn.

Faculty Interests, Attitudes, and Skills

At best, most faculty members in professional schools merely tolerate managed care. At worst, they disdain it. By and large, the faculty have been insulated from, and consequently have not embraced the changes in practice patterns prompted by, managed care. As a consequence, the professional training provided by faculty lacks a certain relevance to practice realities. The faculty foster negative attitudes among students about managed care and about related changes in health care delivery. In a recent survey published in the *New England Journal of Medicine* (Simon et al., 1999), half of the medical school faculty members acknowledged giving negative messages to students about managed care, and 60% of the medical students and residents stated that their negative assessment of managed care was influenced by the faculty. Few efforts have been made to educate faculty about managed care.

Clinical care has long been the least valued mission of academic departments, which give primary importance to research and education. Nevertheless, clinical activities have remained prominent (particularly in psychiatry departments) because of their ability to cross-subsidize academic departments' other, primary missions. Now that such cross-subsidies are dwindling, many departments are implicitly or explicitly questioning their commitment to clinical care. By the same token, attitudes toward managed approaches to clinical services have worsened, and departments are increasingly hostile toward educating students about these approaches.

For those departments that remain committed to clinical care and choose to address the need for faculty who interested in, and capable of teaching about, contemporary practice, the strategies are fairly straightforward. Adjunct faculty members who are immersed in managed care can be employed to teach. Recruiting or retraining one or two full-time faculty members is an alternative way to build a department's expertise in managed approaches to care delivery. The most direct mechanism for altering faculty behavior is to eliminate faculty's isolation from marketplace realities and to modify compensation systems in order to tie at least a portion of faculty income to the financial performance of their clinically related activities. The latter has been most easily accomplished in departments where clinical care has a long and strong tradition (Meyer, 1998).

Access to Curricular Time

Although it is relatively straightforward to identify the new didactic material that needs to be taught, gaining access to student time in the curriculum has been extraordinarily difficult. Competition for this time is intense as programs strive to meet the mandates of accreditation bodies and as faculty vie to have their specialties and interests represented in the formal educational program. The debate about curricular content evokes strong feelings among faculty: it symbolizes the values, orientation, and philosophy of the program or department.

In view of faculty attitudes and interests, topics related to managed care have been largely blocked from inclusion in formal curricula. Faculty interested in broadening the curriculum have succeeded in adding lectures, but seldom courses, to the educational program. Some have offered elective seminars, although students—facing the multiple demands of a program—have infrequently opted for such electives. Top-down strategies of change—in which the department's leadership requires a modification of the curriculum to keep it relevant and current—have seldom been employed; such strategies run contrary to the culture of academia, in which faculty independence and consensual decision making are strongly held values. As a consequence, the updating of curricula will continue to be slow, driven by the few faculty and department chairs pressing for such change.

Accreditation

External review and accreditation are necessities for all professional schools that wish to be competitive and to produce highly marketable graduates. Accreditation standards are developed through consensus and evolve slowly; in order to be changed, they must undergo a complicated, highly political process of review and approval. This process, too, lags behind changes in the field.

Although accreditation standards do not prohibit efforts to educate students about managed approaches to behavioral health care, they may impede such efforts. At worst, they overemphasize training in areas of practice that are becoming less central, such as inpatient care. At best, the need to meet mandated accreditation requirements limits the amount of faculty energy and curricular time available to teach about the changing health care environment.

Training Sites

Student attitudes, knowledge, and skills are largely developed through their clinical placements. Most rotations involve a single site and emphasize a single modality such as outpatient or inpatient care. Unfortunately, students are less frequently exposed to the sites and modalities that managed care has favored—for example, ones involving partial hospitalization, intensive outpatient treatment, brief treatment, substance abuse, dual diagnosis, and hospital diversion. Students who become familiar with these issues through their rotations will have skills that enhance their marketability upon completing the training program.

A more fundamental concern is that students are almost always placed in treatment systems where there is considerable discontinuity of care; although patients are often transferred from one program to another, staff members work within the confines of a single program. A fundamental alternative to this structure involves placing students on continuous-treatment teams, in which staff members and students follow patients through a range of services, providing continuity to the treatment plan. This type of structure has the potential to bring to life for students the principles of continuity and coordination of care that have been espoused by both the managed care industry and the community mental health movement. Although still uncommon, such structures have been successfully employed in public sector clinics, such as one run by the University of Louisville (Tasman & Minkoff, 1997), and in the VA system, which adopted the "firm model" of continuous treatment that was imported from Great Britain (Meyer & McLaughlin, 1998). Continuous-treatment teams have also been implemented in the academic medical center at Dartmouth (Meyer, 1998).

A handful of opportunities have been created around the country for trainees to rotate through managed care organizations. These opportunities are generally reserved for advanced students, and most often in the discipline of psychiatry. Most of these rotations are within the managed behavioral health divisions of academic medical centers. A few, such as the University of Maryland program described below in the section on innovation, involve rotations through a for-profit managed behavioral health organization.

Funding and Reimbursement

As the pressure grows to contain health care costs, the funding base for graduate education is increasingly threatened. Cross-subsidies of education from clinical care are dwindling, and the federal government, through the Balanced Budget Act of 1997, is reducing the teaching hospital revenue that supports medical education (Krakower,

Williams, & Jones, 1999).

With respect to the objective of preparing graduates to practice in a managed care environment, a major funding obstacle is the exclusion of students from the panels of managed care organizations. In ambulatory care sites, it is generally not possible to deploy students to treat patients whose care is managed, because students are ineligible for reimbursement. Managed care organizations typically require licensure and two to five years of postgraduate experience for panel membership. Psychiatrists are typically required to have board certification. When pressed about allowing students to treat individuals covered under managed care plans, the executives of managed care organizations maintain that this restriction is one demanded by payers.

The American Managed Behavioral Healthcare Association (AMBHA) and the American Association of Chairmen of Departments of Psychiatry (AACDP) attempted to draft a position paper on advanced residents' participation in panels. The negotiation process regarding the draft language was contentious and at times drifted into debates about the ethics of managed care and the relevance of academic psychiatry. The resulting white paper (AACDP/AMBHA, n.d.) appears never to have received formal approval by either AMBHA or AACDP. There has been a recent effort, however, to resurrect the draft and to secure approvals. The strategy is to negotiate an agreement between managed behavioral health organizations and academia, and then to present a model to payers regarding both student participation in ambulatory care delivery and their eligibility for reimbursement. Achieving a workable overall agreement will undoubtedly prove difficult.

Supervisor Skills and Attitudes

Much of the clinical supervision received by graduate students is delivered by adjunct clinical faculty and field-placement supervisors. Serving as adjunct faculty members and providing supervision to students have been considered sources of prestige and also of intellectual stimulation. Many members of the supervisory pools have been engaged in this form of service since long before the advent of managed care.

Because managed care has decreased their professional autonomy and often also their incomes, the attitudes of many supervisors toward changes in the organization and financing of behavioral health services is very negative. Thus, they often convey to students strong negative views about managed care organizations and about treatment approaches that are driven by managed care principles. Since supervisors serve as role models, the impact of their messages on trainees' values, attitudes, and practice patterns cannot be underestimated.

Just as diversity among the full-time faculty should be an objective for academic training programs, so, too, should programs strive to achieve diversity among clinical supervisors. Students should be exposed to a range of supervisors who represent both traditional and more contemporary approaches to practice. Programs consequently need to recruit new adjunct faculty members and field supervisors who can model approaches to treatment that are driven by managed care's focus on cost-effectiveness, accountability, practice standards, and outcomes.

WORKFORCE RETRAINING

The changes wrought by managed care have challenged some of the most basic values, professional theories, and core practice patterns of those who completed their graduate training before the advent of managed care. Their professional autonomy and independence were also threatened as utilization reviewers began to question their clinical judgments and treatment recommendations. Further, many practitioners saw reimbursement, and perhaps total income, decline as a direct result of managed care.

The reactions of working professionals to managed care have been diverse. Many maintain that it is nothing more than an unconscionable and unethical attempt to cut costs by depriving patients of needed services. This subgroup has attempted to continue practicing in a traditional manner and has fought managed care or avoided it altogether by refusing to accept patients with managed benefits. Other working professionals have attempted to learn about managed care and its impact, and to adapt in various ways to the changes in the health care marketplace.

Managed care was such a major departure from traditional practice that it created an enormous gulf between the demands of payers and the knowledge and skills of professionals. Foreign to most practitioners were the assumptions underlying managed care, the concept of medical necessity, and the new methods of financing and administering behavioral health care.

As many practitioners grappled with trying to understand the new marketplace, there was a rapid growth of organized efforts to provide continuing education about managed care. Because academic centers took a back seat in the continuing education process, however, for-profit organizations moved in to fill the void, offering a range of conferences, seminars, and workshops designed to help clinicians understand and adapt to managed care. What began as relatively low-cost educational sessions soon blossomed into high-priced events that often cost over a thousand dollars for registration alone. To varying degrees, the professional associations representing the major disciplines also began to address the needs of their members by incorporating seminars and workshops on managed care into their national and regional meetings, and by offering separate conferences focused exclusively on managed care.

These continuing education offerings on managed care appear to have run their course. For the last few years, there has been a shift away from the formal topic of managed care, and toward an emphasis on specific skills or treatment approaches that may be particularly useful or marketable in a managed care environment. Brief treatments, cognitive therapies, and cognitive-behavioral interventions have been popular topics. Detailed workshops on the business aspects of practice, such as the marketing and pricing of services, are also being offered.

A critical question is whether all of this continuing education has had an impact on the existing workforce. The vast majority of continuing education activities has been limited to didactic presentations. Although such presentations may influence attitudes and knowledge, research on continuing education in medicine indicates that didactic conferences and workshops have no demonstrated impact on the behavior of the professionals participating or on the health outcomes of the patients that these professionals treat. In a comprehensive review and meta-analysis of studies on continuing medical education, Davis and colleagues (1999) concluded that the absence of positive findings for the effect of didactic, noninteractive education are so consistent that professionals should receive little, if any, credit for participating in such activities. The authors argued that this approach to continuing education persists only because it is easy to organize, profitable, and heavily underwritten by the pharmaceutical industry.

Both theory and research in adult learning and continuing education have long recognized the limitations of didactic approaches. The evidence suggests that interactive methods, sequenced over time, are required in order to change behavior (Schon, 1990). Davis and colleagues (1999) concluded from their review that change in medical practice is achieved through interactive sessions involving techniques such as case discussions, role playing, problem solving, practice, and sequenced "learn-work-learn" activities. To a lesser extent, these techniques also produce changes in health care outcomes. Although assessment of continuing education in managed behavioral health care, in particular, has generally been limited to studies of knowledge acquisition and participant satisfaction, there is no reason to believe that future findings on the impact of continuing education in behavioral health care would differ from those in the field of general medicine.

The impact of continuing education on professionals' skills and behavior may be heavily influenced by their attitudes and motivations, as well as by the environment to which they return after completing a course (Davis et al., 1999). Although the impact of continuing education about managed care is unclear, it appears that a portion of the existing workforce in behavioral health care has learned about, adapted to, and perhaps even embraced—in practice—a managed care philosophy. Managed care organizations have become increasingly sophisticated at identifying these practitioners and in directing referrals to them.

With respect to the future, there is near consensus among experts in the field of medicine and managed behavioral health care that education, including continuing education, will be technology driven and rely heavily on the Internet, other distance-learning approaches, and perhaps simulation devices (Issenberg et al., 1999). There is a sense of optimism and promise, which has been accompanied by some preliminary efforts to realize that promise. *Behavior.net* is a Web site designed to foster interactive discussions by professionals—facilitated by topic experts—on a range of behavioral health topics. *Audio-Psych.com* offers online continuing education courses that comprise expert lectures (audio portions only), synchronized slide shows, course outlines, quizzes, satisfaction surveys, and links to related materials. Although the site is sophisticated in concept, offers continuing education credits, and charges modestly for accessing its materials, it has generated little interest. Perhaps the most daunting challenge to these distance-learning and technology-driven approaches to education will be to incorporate the teaching strategies identified as essential for behavioral change, including modeling, role playing, practice, and feedback.

DISCIPLINARY PERSPECTIVES

Psychiatry

Managed care has had a range of effects on the discipline of psychiatry. Roles have shifted as prior-authorization procedures and restructured fee schedules have increased psychiatrists' focus on psychopharmacology and decreased their involvement in providing psychotherapy and other psychosocial interventions. As physicians, psychiatrists have been incensed by what they view as managed care's constraints on the independence of their medical judgments and on their determinations regarding medical necessity.

With respect to educational issues, the most notable response from the discipline has been the effort by the American Psychiatric Association (APA) to develop and disseminate practice guidelines. Through an elaborate process of literature review, expert panels, and comment by a broad range of stakeholders, the APA has produced practice guidelines for a range of illnesses—including, for example, major depressive, bipolar, and substance use disorders (APA, 1996). The primary limitation of these guidelines is that many see them as "broadly permissive" and as therefore providing practitioners too much latitude. The impact of the guidelines on practice patterns and clinical outcomes has not been demonstrated (Yager, Zarin, Pincus, & McIntyre, 1997). Nevertheless, the guidelines mark a serious step forward by the discipline of psychiatry to embrace the notion of evidence-based medicine—a notion largely promulgated by managed care. The APA has, moreover, widely disseminated the guidelines to its membership and is promoting their use in undergraduate, graduate, and continuing medical education (Yager et al., 1997).

With respect to residency training, it appears that relatively few academic departments of psychiatry have made substantial modifications to their educational programs in response to managed care. The most common changes include the addition of didactic course work on managed care and the diversification of clinical rotations to include modalities, such as brief treatment and intensive outpatient programs, that are marketable in a managed care environment. The most progressive changes, described below in the section on innovative training initiatives, have included case-oriented managed care seminars, administrative fellowships in managed care organizations, and the pedagogical use of videoconferencing to access national experts on managed care.

A group of academic departments of psychiatry—intent on responding to managed care—have formed a loosely organized consortium to share information and ideas about strategies for surviving and thriving in the current health care environment. Improving residency education about managed care and contemporary clinical practice was identified as a common and important need by these departments, which also formed a training committee to draft a model curriculum and to pursue funding for its development. The drafting is under way, and additional meetings are scheduled to review curricular content and explore options for funding the development of training materials.

With respect to continuing education, the APA has offered its members workshops and seminars on managed care topics, including overviews of managed care, strategies for competing in the managed care marketplace, and ethical and legal issues. As with other disciplines, there appears to have been declining interest in educational events focused specifically on managed care.

At present, continuing education for psychiatrists is largely funded and influenced by pharmaceutical companies, which underwrite educational events as a marketing strategy designed to increase the visibility of the companies and their products. A focus on psychopharmacology may fit well with the role definition for psychiatrists that has been promulgated by managed care. There continues to be concern, however, that these industry-sponsored events may convey biased information and exert undue influence on practice patterns.

Psychology

Psychologists believe that their discipline has been affected quite negatively by managed care. With respect to the delivery of psychotherapy and other psychosocial interventions, there is a perception that provider organizations and some managed care organizations have increasingly turned to other disciplines, such as social work, that can deliver similar services at lower cost. Psychological testing, which is the unique purview of the discipline, is seldom considered medically necessary by managed care organizations.

Organized psychology, working through its professional organizations, has been vociferous in its opposition to managed care. It has lobbied actively for legislation to control managed care and has initiated and supported suits against managed care organizations. There have also been two failed efforts to create within the American Psychological Association a division for psychologists working in managed care.

With respect to the graduate education of psychology students, little has changed. In 1995, the American Psychological Association convened a Presidential Task Force on Education and Training for Work in Organized Delivery Systems to examine training needs in light of managed care (Troy, 1997). The final report of recommendations lingered in committee review. Ultimately, the recommendations were never formally endorsed, and it appears that the process, as a whole, had no impact.

A subsequent task force issued a detailed report on training needs that was disseminated to all graduate programs (Spruill, Kohout, & Gehlman, 1997). The report highlighted the importance of educating students about the following: organized delivery systems; ethical issues pertinent to managed care; strategies for working in multidisciplinary and interdisciplinary environments; applied research and evaluation techniques; management and business skills; and a range of treatment and case-management interventions considered especially relevant in a managed care environment. The authors acknowledged, however, that the report was not an official policy statement of the American Psychological Association and that there remained considerable diversity of opinion among the organization's members about how to respond to managed care. The impact of the report to date appears to have been minimal. Graduate programs in psychology have generally added a few lectures about managed care but have made no extensive or systematic changes to their training programs in response to the changing health care environment. Accreditation standards for graduate programs and internships in psychology do not address managed care.

In terms of the existing workforce in psychology, the American Psychological Association expends considerable effort to keep it informed about issues related to managed care. Much of the information, however, is focused on the profession's activities opposing managed care. With respect to continuing education, the organization has offered members workshops and seminars on managed care. Such offerings have followed the recent trend of focusing less on managed care as such and more on treatment approaches, such as brief therapies, that are relevant in a managed health care marketplace.

At its 1999 annual convention, the American Psychological Association, through its Education Directorate, completed a lengthy process of developing and approving a revised definition of continuing education. The previous definition limited the content of activities eligible for continuing education credit to those that were clinically focused. The new definition broadens the acceptable range of topics and recognizes that it is important for psychologists to be educated in the business aspects of health care delivery.

Somewhat unique to the American Psychological Association's response to the needs of the current workforce has been the organization's initiative to educate practicing psychologists about career alternatives that bypass managed care. The educational model that the association is using involves conducting large conferences, each of which highlights an opportunity for psychologists. Featured as presenters are various psychologists who have been successful in the particular career path in question. For example, a conference cohosted with the American Bar Association was attended by over a thousand psychologists and attorneys, and showcased professional opportunities for psychologists in the field of law. A similar conference is planned that will focus on opportunities for psychologists in medical centers.

Social Work

Over the past decade the profession of social work has been successful in extending licensure or certification status to every state, and in expanding social workers' eligibility for third-party reimbursement (Strom & Gingerich, 1993). Given that social workers are among the lowest salaried of all professionals, the provider organizations that have adapted to managed care by trimming costs have increasingly given preference to social workers when hiring clinical staff. There is also evidence that in a managed (versus fee-for-service) environment, social workers have been providing a significantly increased proportion of outpatient behavioral health services (Vandivort-Warren, 1998). On the downside, there is considerable anecdotal evidence that an increasing percentage of social workers are being offered nonsalaried, per diem, or contract work, all without benefits. Private practitioners in many areas have seen incomes decline by up to 50% due to shorter lengths of stay and declining reimbursement rates.

As in the other major behavioral health disciplines, academic programs in social work have made few changes in their formal curricula in order to educate students about managed care (Strom-Gottfried, 1997). Most social work faculty members have been insulated from the impact of managed care and have negative attitudes toward it. The major texts used in clinical training do not address managed care and its implications for practice. The Council of Social Work Education, which accredits programs, does not specifically address managed care in its accreditation standards. The council, along with the National Association of Social Work (NASW), did convene a task force to examine the impact of managed care on social work training. The final report identified needs and barriers to educating students (CSWE/NASW, 1996), but the report is not considered to have had substantial impact.

Because field placements are a core element of social work training, supervisors in the field placements have been clamoring for academic social work to respond to the impact that managed care is having on fieldwork. At present, course work does not adequately prepare students for the realities of their placements; students are increasingly excluded from seeing patients alone because students are ineligible to participate in panels; and field supervisors have less time to devote to mentoring because of the economic strain faced by their agencies (Brooks & Riley, 1996; Raskin & Blome, 1998). Despite these complexities, the heavy emphasis placed on fieldwork does mean that social work students gain some significant exposure to practice realities during their graduate education.

Like other professional organizations, the NASW has conducted a range of continuing education programs (both at the national level and through local chapters) on managed care. This educational activity has decreased significantly in the last few years as members' interest in managed care training has declined. The focus of continuing education has shifted to contemporary clinical and administrative issues such as youth violence, the use of technology in social work practice, risk management, addiction treatment, and grant writing.

There are two unique challenges faced by social work in educating its students about managed care and contemporary practice. First, the profession has historically rejected the medical model in favor of an ecological model. Thus, there is an ideological conflict between social work tradition and the current emphasis on the concept of medical necessity that permeates managed care. Second, social workers specializing in behavioral health receive a common or generic "foundation" year as the first of two years of master's-level education. This year must meet the needs of social workers specializing in nonbehavioral areas such as medical social work and social welfare. In the context of this generic introductory year designed for a diverse student body, it is a complicated challenge to provide an adequate education to social workers specializing in behavioral health.

Nursing

The impact of managed care on psychiatric nurses has been very mixed. On the one hand, the managed care industry has offered a range of opportunities to bachelor's- and master's-level nurses in the area of utilization management. On the other hand, consultative-liaison nursing in many medical centers has been radically downsized or eliminated. The medical centers can no longer afford to subsidize the activity, and direct reimbursement for such services has been difficult to obtain. Declining rates of reimbursement and difficulty getting onto panels have also had a negative impact on nurse psychotherapists; it appears that an increasing percentage is choosing to deliver services to patients on a self-pay, sliding-scale basis rather than accepting payment from managed care organizations.

Nursing has recognized the need to make graduate education more relevant to the current managed health care environment. The

American Nurses Association (ANA) created a task force that produced the *Managed Behavioral Health Care: Curriculum Guidelines for Psychiatric–Mental Health and Addictions Nurses* (ANA, 1997). The guidelines contain learning objectives, teaching strategies, and content to be covered for six modules: managed care delivery models; administrative issues such as contracting, utilization management, and information systems; financing and reimbursement; clinical practice issues such as brief-treatment strategies and approaches to measuring outcomes; ethical issues related to managed care; and legal issues such as confidentiality, liability, and patients' rights. These guidelines were released in 1996 and distributed to all graduate programs. Follow-up one year later revealed that 5 of the 98 master's-level psychiatric nursing programs had attempted to implement the recommended curriculum.

One of nursing's principal strategies has been to increase the scope of practice available to master's-level nurses. Through intense lobbying, nurses with specialized training have obtained the right in many states to prescribe medications cither independently or under supervisory or collaborative relationships with physicians. A second strategy for broadening the scope of practice has been for graduate programs to train selected students as both psychiatric nurses and nurse practitioners. With such training, graduates are qualified to care for both the psychiatric and general medical needs of patients.

These two trends in training seem to fit with a managed care ideology that emphasizes cost-effectiveness and the coordination of psychiatric and medical services. In practice, however, managed care organizations have been reluctant to authorize and reimburse such nurses for psychopharmacology and primary medical care. The reasons are unclear, although many nurses attribute the resistance to physician opposition. A second impediment may be the lack of uniformity in nursing degrees, in advanced training, and in certification— all of which complicate efforts by managed care organizations to set credentialing standards for nurses with advanced training. Despite the obstacles, there is an increasing trend to employ such nurses in public sector settings, where there is less dependence on reimbursement from the managed care industry.

Retraining of the existing workforce of nurses does not appear to have been given a great deal of attention. As in other disciplines, there have been workshops and conferences focused on managed care.

More recently, these educational activities have focused on clinical skills that are relevant in a managed care environment.

INNOVATIVE TRAINING INITIATIVES

There have been some creative attempts to address the challenges of training students and of retraining professionals in managed approaches to care. Examples of these innovative initiatives are described below.

Mobilizing Faculty

In 1997, 13 schools of social work convened a meeting to educate faculty about managed care. The objective was to influence faculty's attitudes, knowledge, course offerings, and research related to managed care and contemporary practice. The meeting—the First Managed Behavioral Health Care Invitational Conference for New England Graduate Social Work Faculty—lasted a day and a half, and was funded by the Robert Wood Johnson Foundation and the National Institute of Mental Health. The program was heavily didactic. It included a review of changes in the organization and financing of health care, of the impact of these changes on social work, and of the opportunities for social workers in this new environment. The program covered ethical issues relating to managed care, as well as strategies for educating social work students for contemporary clinical practice. Selected papers from the conference were published as a book, *Humane Managed Care?* (Schamess & Lightburn, 1998). A second conference is planned as part of the deans' efforts to improve the relevance of social work education and research.

Videoconferencing in Residency Training

Douglas Walter and colleagues (2000) conducted a videoconferencing project in 1998 that was focused on educating psychiatric residents about managed care. Experts from around the country delivered presentations on managed care and on related topics such as quality management, ethics, and legal issues. A number of these presentations were delivered live, through video links, to residents in participating departments. Other lectures were videotaped and distributed to the departments for later viewing. An effort was made to assess residents' knowledge acquisition through, and satisfaction with, the program. A plan to expand this initiative is under development.

Teaching Clinical-Management Skills

Sabin and Borus (1992) have introduced two valuable concepts in teaching psychiatric residents to practice in a staff-model HMO. They have fostered a population-based approach to care by teaching students about *individual practice management and collaborative program development.* The first concept involves learning to manage a caseload, accommodate new patients, and deal with the "crunch" that occurs when commitments to current patients preclude new patients from gaining access. The second concept involves learning to collaborate with colleagues in a practice setting in order to develop and offer a sufficiently broad range of services to meet the needs of the group of patients requesting services. Strategies that can be employed to accomplish this objective include designing groups or tracks for patients with similar problems and the specialization of clinicians within the practice to complement the skills of their colleagues. These teaching concepts are designed to help residents achieve an efficient, goal-oriented approach to treatment that is demanded by, and rewarded in, a managed care environment.

Administrative Fellowship in Managed Care

The Department of Psychiatry at the University of Maryland has collaborated with Magellan Behavioral Health to offer a postresidency fellowship in managed care. The objectives of this one-year program are to build fellows' practice skills for managed care settings and to give them experience, within a managed care organization, in arranging services for a population. The fellowship includes didactic instruction through managed care seminars and case conferences. Clinical rotations occur in mental health and addiction-treatment settings, where practice patterns are heavily influenced by managed care principles. Administrative and leadership experience is gained by implementing, under supervision, a continuous quality improvement project within the private managed care organization. Fellows also work as apprentices to senior physician advisors in the managed care organization, which enables fellows to observe and learn about the application of criteria for medical necessity and level of care.

Case-Oriented Managed Care Seminar

A group of faculty at Thomas Jefferson University Hospital and Einstein Hospital in Philadelphia developed a seminar designed to teach to medical students and psychiatric residents the application of criteria for medical necessity (Chester, Sanguineti, & Best, 1998). The seminar also helps students to identify the common deficiencies in documenting care and presenting cases that hinder providers' efforts to obtain authorization for the requested level or duration of service. Participants first receive didactic material on managed care and the utilization-review process. During the case-based portion of the seminar, one student is assigned to review the chart of a patient being treated by another student. In the next seminar session, the student "reviewer" interviews the student caregiver, probing the issue of medical necessity and appropriate level of care. Faculty members also discuss selected cases that highlight complicated clinical, ethical, or legal issues.

Educating a Provider Network

In 1995 and 1996, United Behavioral Health attempted to improve the skills of its providers in diagnosing and treating depression. This managed behavioral health company organized a daylong workshop on this topic and offered it at four locations around the country. Approximately one thousand providers participated. An informal evaluation was conducted and revealed that satisfaction with the training was fairly high, with master's-level professionals finding it somewhat more helpful than doctoral-level professionals and physicians. The company was not able to assess the impact of the training on practice patterns or clinical outcomes.

DISCUSSION

A number of key themes emerge from this review of the current status of professional education and workforce training as they relate to managed care.

1. Academic departments across all disciplines have lost their leadership positions as educators for contemporary clinical practice. Their training programs have not kept pace with the dramatic changes in the field, leaving the relevance of their educational programs in serious question and their graduates unprepared for the realities of clinical practice. There is some evidence that academic departments are beginning to respond to changes in the field, but modifications to curricula have been minor. There is no evidence that these departments will regain their leadership edge in the near future.

2. Without strong leadership from academia, educating professionals about managed care and contemporary practice has become largely a for-profit industry. Education is being provided on a "hit and run" basis involving brief workshops and seminars offered at exorbitant prices. Unfortunately, available research evidence suggests that these brief encounters are unlikely to change professionals' behavior or to affect the health outcomes of those whom they treat. Like other professions, the behavioral health disciplines have ignored the literature on the necessary components of effective adult education and have favored approaches that are profitable and easy to implement.

3. Leaders in the managed behavioral health industry do believe that a subset of professionals has become knowledgeable about managed care and has adopted practice patterns that are congruent with the assumptions and philosophy of managed care. The role that continuing education played in shaping these practice patterns remains unclear.

4. There is concern that a significant portion of the workforce that is contracted with managed care organizations has learned the language of managed care but has not adapted effectively to the new health care environment. For example, many providers seem to be practicing a truncated version of traditional practice in which they approach treatment as they always have, but ter-

minate treatment earlier when additional authorizations cannot be secured. This pattern is not optimal either from a managed care or traditional treatment perspective.

5. The training needs related to managed care and contemporary clinical practice are, by and large, not discipline-specific. With few exceptions, such as a national interdisciplinary colloquium on training issues related to managed care (Feldman & Goldman, 1997) and a government-sponsored initiative to identify core competencies (Coursey, 1998), the disciplines are not working together on the development of graduate-level curricula or continuing education programs. The politics of trying to induce change within a single discipline are so daunting that simultaneously tackling the politics of interdisciplinary differences has seemed, to many, insurmountable.

6. A principal lesson of managed care has been the need for providers to attend to the economics of service delivery. An equally critical lesson is that managed care organizations and the disciplines must attend to the economics of professional training. Trainees will not be prepared to work in a managed care environment if, during training, they do not have the opportunity both to treat patients whose care is managed and to be reimbursed for those services.

CONCLUSION

The recent backlash against managed care in public and political circles leaves its future somewhat uncertain. Nonetheless, the field of behavioral health care has been permanently altered by the past decade of experimentation with managed care and health care reform. The assumptions, values, knowledge base, and skills emphasized by managed care will continue to have relevance to the delivery of mental health and substance abuse services for the foreseeable future, no matter what the fate of managed care. Thus, students and working professionals should be increasingly exposed to these contemporary ideas about behavioral health care through redesigned curricula in graduate schools and training programs, and through innovative continuing education initiatives.

REFERENCES

American Association of Chairmen of Departments of Psychiatry & American Managed Behavioral Healthcare Association. (n.d.). *Joint AACDP/AMBHA white paper on using licensed psychiatric resident physicians who are post-internship for managed care services* [3rd draft]. Washington, DC: Author.

American Nurses Association. (1997). *Managed behavioral health care: Curriculum guidelines for psychiatric–mental health and addictions nurses.* Washington, DC: Author.

American Psychiatric Association. (1996). *Practice Guidelines.* Washington, DC: Author.

Brooks, D., & Riley, P. (1996). The impact of managed health care policy on student field training. *Smith College Studies in Social Work, 66,* 307–316.

Chester, J. G., Sanguineti, V. R., & Best, K. (1998). Teaching managed care: Philosophy and technique. *Academic Psychiatry, 22,* 36–40.

Coursey, R. D. (1998). *Competencies for direct service staff who work with adults with serious mental illness in public mental health services.* Rockville, MD: Center for Mental Health Services.

Council on Social Work Education & National Association of Social Workers. (1996). *Managed care and workforce training: Social work strategic action plan.* Washington, DC: National Association of Social Workers.

Davis, D., O'Brien, M. A. T., Freemantle, N., Wolf, F. M., Mazmanian, P., & Taylor-Vaisey, A. (1999). Impact of formal continuing medical education: Do conferences, workshops, rounds, and other traditional continuing education activities change physician behavior or health care outcomes? *Journal of the American Medical Association, 282,* 867–874.

Feldman, S. (1978). Promises, promises or community mental health services and training: Ships that pass in the night. *Community Mental Health Journal, 14,* 83–91.

Feldman, S., & Goldman, W. (Eds.). (1997). Managed behavioral health and academia: Is there a "fit" between services and training? [Special issue]. *Administration and Policy in Mental Health, 25,* 3–98.

Gabbard, G. O. (1992). The big chill: The transition from residency to managed care nightmare. *Academic Psychiatry, 16,* 119–126.

Hoge, M. A., Davidson, L., & Hill, W. L. (1993). The evolution of mental health services: Partial hospitalization as a case example. *The Journal of Mental Health Administration, 20,* 161–168.

Hoge, M. A., Jacobs, S. C., & Belitsky, R. (2000). Psychiatric residency training, managed care, and contemporary clinical practice. *Psychiatric Services, 51,* 1001–1005.

Issenberg, S. B., McGaghie, W. C., Hart, I. R., Mayer, J. W., Felner, J. M., Petrusa, E. R., Waugh, R. A., Brown, D. D., Safford, R. R., Gessner, I. H., Gordon, D. L., & Ewy, G. A. (1999). Simulation technology for health care professional skills training and assessment. *Journal of the American Medical Association, 282,* 861–866.

Krakower, J. Y., Williams, D. J., & Jones, R. F. (1999). Review of US medical school finances, 1997–1998. *Journal of the American Medical Association, 282,* 847–854.

Meyer, R .E. (Ed.). (1998). Appendices: Case studies. In R. E. Meyer, & C. J. McLaughlin (Eds.), *Between mind, brain, and managed care: The now and future world of academic psychiatry* (pp. 177–253). Washington, DC: American Psychiatric Press.

Meyer, R. E., & McLaughlin, C. J. (1998). The educational missions of academic psychiatry. In R. E. Meyer & C. J. McLaughlin (Eds.), *Between mind, brain, and managed care: The now and future world of academic psychiatry* (pp. 49–76). Washington, DC: American Psychiatric Press.

Raskin, M. S., & Blome, W. W. (1998). The impact of managed care on field instruction. *Journal of Social Work Education, 34,* 365–374.

Ross, D. R. (1997). Training residents in the era of managed care. In R. K. Schreter, S. S. Sharfstein, & C. A. Schreter (Eds.), *Managing care, not dollars* (pp. 299–315). Washington, DC: American Psychiatric Press.

Sabin, J. E. (1991). Clinical skills for the 1990s: Six lessons from HMO practice. *Hospital and Community Psychiatry, 42,* 605–608.

Sabin, J. E., & Borus, J. F. (1992). Mental health teaching and research in managed care. In J. Feldman & R. J. Fitzpatrick (Eds.), *Managed mental health care: Administrative and clinical issues* (1st ed.) (pp. 185–199). Washington, DC: American Psychiatric Press.

Schamess, G., & Lightburn, A. (Eds.). (1998). *Humane managed care?* Washington, DC: National Association of Social Workers.

Schon, D. A. (1990). *Educating the reflective practitioner: Toward a new design for teaching and learning in the professions.* San Francisco: Jossey-Bass.

Schreter, R. K. (1997). Essential skills for managed behavioral health care. *Psychiatric Services, 48,* 653–658.

Schuster, J. M., Lovell, M. R., & Trachta, A. M. (Eds.). (1997). *Training behavioral healthcare professionals: Higher learning in the era of managed care.* San Francisco: Jossey-Bass.

Simon S. R., Pan, R. J. D., Sullivan, A. M., Clark-Chiarelli, N., Connelley, M. T., Peters, A. S., Singer, J. D., Inui, T. S., & Block, S. D. (1999). Views of managed care: A survey of students, residents, faculty, and deans at medical schools in the United States. *New England Journal of Medicine, 340,* 928–936.

Spruill, J., Kohout, J., & Gehlman, M. S. (1997). *Changes in the health care delivery system: Recommendations for the education, training, and continuing professional education of psychologists.* Washington, DC: American Psychological Association.

Strom, K., & Gingerich, W. J. (1993). Educating students for the new market realities. *Journal of Social Work Education, 29,* 78–87.

Strom-Gottfried, K. (1997). The implications of managed care for social work education. *Journal of Social Work Education, 33,* 7–18.

Tasman, A., & Minkoff, K. (1997). Educational and training issues in public sector managed mental health care. In K. Minkoff, & D. Pollack (Eds.), *Managed mental health care in the public sector* (pp. 321–330). Amsterdam: Harwood Academic Publishers.

Troy, W. G. (1997). Training the trainees: The new imperatives. *Administration and Policy in Mental Health, 25,* 27–35.

Vandivort-Warren, R. (1998). How social workers can manage managed care. In G. Schamess & A. Lightburn (Eds.), *Humane managed care?* (pp. 255–267). Washington, DC: National Association of Social Workers.

Walter, D. A., deGroot, C. M., Ulven, T. P., Rosenquist, P., Daniels, A., Dewan, N. A., & Weathers, V. (2000). A new teaching program: Telemedicine, psychiatric residents, and issues germane to managed care. *Academic Psychiatry, 24,* 209–213.

Yager, J., Docherty, J., & Tischler, G. L. (1996, Fall). Training psychiatric residents for managed care: Fundamental values and proficiencies, and an outline for a model curriculum. *American Association of Directors of Psychiatric Residency Training Newsletter,* 3–6.

Yager, J., Zarin, D. A., Pincus, H. A., & McIntyre, J. S. (1997). Practice guidelines and psychiatric education. *Academic Psychiatry, 21,* 226–233.

Chapter 5

EFFECT ON PHYSICAL HEALTH CARE

Sherry A. Glied

Most Americans who have insurance—nearly 80%—obtain coverage for physical health service costs through one vendor and coverage for behavioral health service costs through a different, specialized behavioral health care vendor (Findlay, 1999). These "carve-out" arrangements explicitly separate the financing of physical health care from that of behavioral health care. In so doing, they have re-ignited long-standing concerns about the lack of coordination between physical and behavioral health services.

Fragmentation of behavioral and physical health services can generate two types of problems. First, because behavioral health problems often co-occur with physical health problems, fragmentation of services may reduce the overall quality of care. People who initially seek care from a general practitioner for physical health problems may fail to have their behavioral health problems recognized and treated. Conversely, people who are under the regular care of a behavioral health professional may fail to receive needed physical health services (McFarland, Johnson, & Hornbrook, 1996). Second, because the physical health care and behavioral health care sectors sometimes provide similar services, fragmentation can lead to boundary problems. These boundary problems can make it difficult to assess the effectiveness of policy changes, such as the implementation of managed care. They can also lead to an inappropriate allocation of health care resources between the physical and behavioral health sectors. Some observers believe that such inappropriate allocations are most likely to occur when carve-outs are negotiated by employers rather than by managed care firms (Olfson, Sing, & Schlesinger, 1999).

Specialization in medicine has always generated concerns about service fragmentation–among specialists and also between specialty and general medical care (and with respect to both physical and behavioral health). Although carve-out plans are new, the potential lack of harmonization of physical and behavioral health services is not. The systems of care that provide services to people with behavioral health problems have generally been distinct from those that provide care to people with physical health problems. This distinction has existed at all levels of severity. People with serious physical health problems are treated in general hospitals. Those with serious behavioral health problems are treated in psychiatric hospitals and residential treatment facilities, as well as in specialized psychiatric units of general hospitals. People with less serious physical health problems see generalist and specialist physicians in their offices. Those with less serious behavioral health problems may also see generalist and specialist physicians, but they are often treated by psychologists and psychiatric social workers–practitioners who play no part in providing physical health services.

The structures of financing and regulation for the two systems have also been quite different. Physical health treatment (for the population under 65) is most often financed by private health insurance and provided in private institutions. Behavioral health care is often provided in institutions that are publicly funded, and outpatient treatment of the seriously ill is often financed through public insurance. For those with less serious behavioral health problems, much of the cost of treatment is paid by patients themselves. Most states separate their departments of health and mental health, and federal expenditures for the two areas are also quite separate.

This evident demarcation between the treatment of physical and behavioral health problems has always been a cause for concern. In an 1894 speech to the American Medico-Psychological Association, S. Weir Mitchell, a prominent neurologist, assailed his mental health colleagues: "Your hospitals are not our hospitals; your ways are not our ways" (Grob, 1994, p. 136). In the 1920s, critics of psychiatry complained of the discipline's lack of integration with, and of its isolation from, general medicine (Grob, p. 162). Similarly, the increased attention today within primary care medicine to the recognition and treatment of depression and other mental illnesses suggests that behavioral health care and physical health care would both benefit if service provision were less separated.

The rise of managed care in both the private and public sectors appeared to offer an opportunity to unite the provision of physical and behavioral health care. In the private sector, novel approaches to the organization and financing of services could foster a new, more coordinated model. Traditional HMOs (group- and staff-model plans) typically provided physical and behavioral health services within a single, capitated environment, with primary care physicians usually acting as gatekeepers. In principle, primary care gatekeepers both provide care themselves and coordinate the care provided by an array of specialists, including behavioral health specialists.

In the public sector, the rise of Medicaid managed care explicitly requires pooling of historically distinct state funding streams for physical and behavioral health. Behavioral and physical health agencies therefore must work together to develop contracting requirements for health plans that will, in principle, offer coordinated care to the Medicaid population. For example, faced with the goal of implementing managed care in the Massachusetts Medicaid program, the state's Department of Mental Health and its Division of Medical Assistance created a joint planning and purchasing initiative that coordinated care across systems that already existed (Elias & Navon, 1995). Managed care, which breaks down the organizational and financing barriers between state departments of health and mental health, requires genuine collaboration among institutions and practitioners in both fields.

Actual practice, however, belies the apparent promise of the service integration prompted by managed care. Rather than offering integrated physical and behavioral health services, most managed care firms, employers, and public systems have carved out the provision of behavioral health services to firms specializing in that type of care. Increasingly, even HMOs carve out their behavioral health benefits to such firms (Durham, 1995).

ADVANTAGES OF CARVE-OUTS

Carve-outs offer three types of advantages in behavioral health care markets. First, specialized behavioral health firms benefit from their managerial specialization. By focusing on just one aspect of health care for many enrollees, these carve-outs may be able to develop better specialty networks. Managed care plans that have expertise in contracting with and managing physicians and general hospitals may have no comparable expertise in contracting with and managing psychologists, psychiatric social workers, psychiatric hospitals, and residential treatment facilities. Behavioral health carve-out plans have proven to be more effective than unified contracts at reducing moral hazard—the additional use of services that occurs because people have health insurance—and at controlling behavioral health care costs.

This need for specialization—and the strong distinctions between providers of physical health and behavioral health services—explains, in part, why the financing and management of behavioral health services have historically been separated from the financing and management of physical health services. In this respect, behavioral health carve-out plans reproduce the specialized knowledge that state departments of mental health developed in working with the same groups of specialists.

A second advantage of carve-outs is that they increase accountability for behavioral health outcomes. Relatively few members of any single managed care plan will ever use behavioral health services. Quality measures computed from the experience of the few patients who use specialty behavioral health services may not be very precise, and they may not, in any case, play a part in the decisions of most plan members. Members who do have behavioral health problems may pay attention to these statistics, but the nature of behavioral health problems—more than with other chronic diseases—makes it especially difficult for those who use these services to advocate improvements in their quality. Because of the improved accountability of the carve-out model, advocates for people with other chronic conditions (such as children with serious illnesses) have been led to propose similar models in other contexts (Glied, 1998). The spread of the carve-out model to other sectors of health care provides further evidence of the value of specialization.

As in the case of managerial specialization, the importance of accountability contributes to the historical separation of mental health agencies from departments of health (Grob, 1994; Frank & McGuire, 2000). Because of the difficulty that behavioral health patients have in seeking better care for themselves—especially in public systems—it was necessary to design institutional structures with clear lines of accountability.

The third advantage, which is peculiar to today's environment of competition between health plans, is that carving out behavioral health to a single company limits problems of adverse selection. In general, people prefer to be offered a choice of health plans. Individuals may vary in their preferences concerning the style of health care delivery and the use of financial and managerial mechanisms for limiting the amount of care. Nevertheless, although allowing people a choice between health plans is often a good idea, it may also encourage those who anticipate using the services to choose more generous plans. Conversely, those who do not anticipate ever using the services may choose narrower plans (Hogan, 1997). This problem of self-sorting can be very serious in the case of behavioral health. Since many mental illnesses are chronic conditions, there is considerable potential for those who know they are ill to self-sort into more—or less—generous plans; since there is considerable variation in people's propensity to seek help from behavioral health professionals, some people choose plans that offer no behavioral health benefits at all. This process of self-selection can drive generous plans out of the market altogether. Consequently, by requiring all members of an insured group to join a single behavioral health plan, carve-outs can help sustain a market for behavioral health insurance (Frank, Huskamp, McGuire, & Newhouse, 1996).

Although these three arguments are powerful ones in support of carve-out plans, the problems that motivate concern about fragmentation of services are also serious and legitimate. Physical and behavioral health problems are intertwined in ways that suggest that better harmonization could both enhance quality and reduce costs. In economic terms, there are important complementarities between the provision of physical and behavioral health care. These complementarities may take the form of enhanced recognition and treatment of physical (or behavioral) health problems by behavioral health (physical health) service providers. There are also possibilities that services provided in one sector can substitute for those provided in the other. Primary care practitioners can (and do) offer behavioral health services, and medical pharmacy coverage can (and does) cover psychiatric prescriptions. Sometimes these possibilities for substitution can lead to overall cost savings. The cost of additional behavioral health services may be more than offset by reductions in the cost of medical services for the same patients, the "cost-offset" effect.

POSSIBLE DISADVANTAGES OF CARVE-OUTS

As has been suggested, the success and predominance of carve-outs have reawakened historic concerns about the separation of physical and behavioral health care. Analysts assert that the separation of behavioral and physical health through carve-outs may reduce the incentive to respond, or the feasibility of responding, to these quality and financing concerns.

Recognition and Treatment of Psychiatric Disorders in the Medical Sector

Most people who meet diagnostic criteria for mental illness receive no formal treatment for their problems. Estimates suggest that fewer than one in five of those with diagnosable illness obtain treatment (Kessler et al., 1994). This gap between need and service use makes it critical to exploit all opportunities to identify and treat persons with mental illness. One obvious locus for recognition and treatment is general health care.

Most people–including most people with mental illness–see a generalist health care provider regularly. People with mental health problems are much more likely to make such visits than are those without such problems. An estimated 5 to 20% of patients seen by generalist providers are estimated to have major depressive disorder, and the prevalences of other psychiatric disorders are also elevated (Katon & Schulberg, 1992; Lyness, Caine, King, Cox, & Yoedino, 1999). Integration of physical and behavioral health services would provide an opportunity to address the problems of these patients. Offering opportunities for behavioral health treatment in primary care may be especially important for those patients who do not see themselves as mentally ill and who might therefore not seek out carve-out services (Bennett, 1992).

If behavioral health care is separate from the capitation payment, generalist physicians may have little incentive, however, to treat patients diagnosed with behavioral health problems. Moreover, if generalists have no incentive to treat patients with behavioral health problems, they may also have little incentive to learn more about the recognition and treatment such problems in primary care. Because carve-out plans separate diagnosis from treatment and define the scope of service responsibility by condition, the existence of such plans can encourage physical health providers to diagnose people with behavioral health problems, thereby moving them out of the basic capitation pool. Referral to the carve-out plan costs the generalist no money and saves her practice effort, while also improving the quality of patient care. (It should also be noted, however, that if she cannot make a direct referral but must, instead, refer a patient to an 800 number, she may feel a loss of control over the treatment process.)

Physical Health Problems Among the Severely Mentally Ill

People with mental illness, especially those with severe illness, have high rates of untreated, and often preventable, physical health problems. For example, in one study of severely mentally ill HMO patients, the level of other chronic diseases was significantly higher than among non-mentally ill controls (McFarland et al., 1996). The often poor living conditions of people with severe mental illness may place them at higher risk for the development of infectious disease, such as tuberculosis and HIV.

The treatments provided to people with severe mental illness may affect their physical health. Several psychotropic medications have potentially serious consequences for physical health. For example, clozapine, a valuable new drug for the treatment of schizophrenia, can lead to a fatal blood disorder; patients using this drug need to be regularly monitored (Lehman, 1999). Furthermore, psychotropic medications may interact with medications prescribed for physical health ailments.

Providers of behavioral health services, by virtue of their regular contact with patients, may have unique opportunities to recognize physical health problems. Such regular contact also presents them with opportunities to provide, or refer patients for, preventive health interventions. In some cases, as with drug side effects, these physical health services are a necessary part of providing psychiatric treatment. More problematic are situations where physical health services are not directly related to behavioral health conditions. Morbidity and mortality associated with physical health problems is relatively high among people with serious mental illness, but behavioral health providers may not focus on these aspects of their patients' health (there is very little evidence on this point). These populations are at high risk of infectious disease (including tuberculosis and HIV, as previously noted) and may need not only treatment, but counseling. Reductions in general-health risk behaviors, such as smoking, may improve both behavioral and physical health (Yassa, Lal, Korpassy, & Ally, 1987). Again, harmonization of behavioral and physical health services could be very useful in addressing this array of problems (McFarland et al., 1996).

Under carve-out plans, behavioral health care providers may have little reason to attend to the physical health problems of their patients. If they are paid capitated rates, they do not benefit financially from providing such treatment themselves. Although they might wish to refer patients back to their general health providers, such referrals may be administratively difficult. Under behavioral health carve-outs, referrals to specialty behavioral health providers generally operate through a central coordinating arrangement, rather than through individual physicians. Thus, behavioral health care providers may not have established relationships with particular general health providers, and may not even know where to refer a particular patient for physical health care services.

Substitution between the Behavioral Health and Physical Health Sectors

General health providers may sometimes provide care that substitutes for that provided by behavioral health professionals (and vice versa). When the two types of care are covered by separate contracts, there is a risk that care will be inappropriately shifted between sectors (Frank & McGuire, 2000; Norton, Lindrooth, & Dickey, 1999). Under a carve-out arrangement, the plan financing physical health services has incentives to shift care to the behavioral health plan, while the behavioral health plan has incentives to shift costs back to the general health plan (Chang et al., 1998). For example, observers have argued that managed care plans may overuse psychopharmaceuticals (relative to other therapies) because the cost of drugs is included in the general health contract, whereas the cost of other therapies is covered by the behavioral health contract (Jellinek, 1998).

In some cases, substituting behavioral health services for physical health services may reduce overall costs. In several well-documented contexts (and perhaps also in other contexts) increased behavioral health spending may actually reduce physical health spending. For example, psychiatric consultation for patients with somatization disorder can lead to substantially reduced medical care costs (Olfson et al., 1999). In general, these savings are likely to occur in contexts where patients have less severe behavioral health disorders. Such cost offsets suggest that health plans can profit from maintaining behavioral health spending at adequate levels. For this reason, the integration of financing decisions can reduce the total health care bill.

The possibility of substituting services across the behavioral health/physical health boundary can make it difficult to determine the appropriate payment level for carve-out plans versus the plans from which behavioral health has been carved out. If financing decisions lead to an inappropriate choice of sector for providing treatment, or if such decisions limit the use of services that generate cost offsets, they may even lead to increased total costs. Some analysts argue that the existence of carve-out plans is to blame for an inefficiently low allocation of funds to behavioral health care and behavioral health providers under managed care arrangements (Jellinek, 1998); behavioral health care costs have fallen substantially as a share of medical plan costs since 1989 (Buck, Teich, Umland, & Stein, 1999).

The Difficulties of Empirical Assessment

There is almost no evidence to date estimating the prevalence of problems generated by carve-out plans with respect to the potential complementarities between physical and behavioral health. There is very little evidence that addresses the potential substitution possibilities. That is not to say that the dangers of fragmentation through carve-out arrangements are illusory. For example, the Tennessee Partners Managed Medicaid experience suggests that poorly designed carve-out arrangements can lead to just the types of substitution problems described above.

In 1996, in the wake of poor experience with respect to behavioral health care in its original Medicaid managed care program, Tennessee began a carve-out called TennCare Partners. The carve-out was implemented in a hurry—over a period of just eight months. Each enrollee chose a general managed care plan and was assigned to a separately capitated behavioral health carve-out plan. Since the demarcation lines between the responsibilities of each plan were not well defined, the plans tried to shift costs to one another. The result was chaotic: patients were confused, spending declined precipitously, and money flowed away from the seriously mentally ill (Chang et al., 1998).

The Tennessee example points to serious perils, but the poor implementation of the program makes it difficult to draw any general conclusions. In addition to carving out behavioral health care, the state reduced funding and capped enrollment in TennCare—which had the effect of further limiting funding to the behavioral health organizations. Failure to risk-adjust payments to the carve-out plans for caring for those with the most serious illnesses may also have contributed to the disaster. As is apparent from what happened in Tennessee, the incentive structures of carve-out plans present the risk of generating poor outcomes. Nevertheless, this risk has not, by and large, been realized. Other carve-out experiences (such as that in Massachussetts) have been successes—at least in the sense that they have reduced spending without clearly reducing either access or quality (Goldman, McCulloch, & Sturm, 1998).

Only a few studies have examined the extent of cost shifting from carve-out plans to other sectors, and the results are ambiguous. A study of the Aid to Families with Dependent Children population found that the introduction of a behavioral health carve-out had no implications for care in the medical sector or for pharmacy costs (Norton, Lindrooth, & Dickey, 1997). A study of people with histories of substance abuse found increases in the use of general hospitals under carve-outs (Brisson, 1998, as cited in Frank & McGuire, 2000). Finally, a study of the Massachusetts Medicaid carve-out for those with psychiatric disabilities found increases in the use of both pharmaceutical and nonpsychiatric medical services, particularly among the most seriously ill (see Norton et al., 1999, though that study did not find cost shifting from the carve-out plan to the state-funded mental hospital system).

Other evidence suggests that carve-out plans may improve the use of behavioral health services among the populations that might generate cost offsets. By using effective management instead of high financial barriers to initial care, behavioral health carve-outs have typically drawn more patients into behavioral health services. For example, the proportion of beneficiaries seen by behavioral health professionals increased among Medicaid enrollees under the Massachusetts behavioral health carve-out and also among state employees under Ohio's carve-out program (Feldman, 1998). Marginal patients who were not receiving any behavioral health treatment prior to the carve-out are most likely to be the ones who generate cost offsets.

Although carve-out plans may well set up incentives that do not encourage collaboration, it is far from obvious that they actually have this effect or, conversely, that formal integration of behavioral and physical health delivery does better at generating effective collaboration (Frank & McGuire, 2000). Although integration is a laudable goal, the actual experience of fully integrated delivery of physical and behavioral health services—whether organized through a single entry point or through an integrated delivery system—has not been encouraging.

There has been relatively little research on the effectiveness of traditional, fully integrated HMO arrangements in achieving appropriate use of behavioral health services. Moreover, the existing evidence is contradictory. Researchers at the Yale site of the adult Epidemiological Catchment Area study found that people with behavioral health problems who were HMO members, when compared with those with fee-for-service insurance coverage, had more physician visits and were more likely to see specialists (Leaf et al., 1988). The RAND Medical Outcomes Study, however—which examined an adult population with current depressive disorder in three different sites in 1986—found that HMO members were less likely to see a behavioral health specialist than were those covered by fee-for-service insurance (Wells et al., 1989). The latter group typically self-referred to specialists for behavioral health care. Some recent data suggests that integrated HMOs also use much lower levels of behavioral health staffing than do other plans (Scheffler & Ivey, 1998)—which suggests, again, that these plans rely on generalist practitioners to deliver much of that care.

Part of the reason for the unimpressive experience of HMOs in delivering behavioral health care may be their reliance on detection and treatment through primary care. A considerable body of research indicates that primary care practitioners often fail to recognize and treat mental illness in their patients (Leaf, 1994). Whereas behavioral

health specialists usually recognize depression and other mental illnesses, primary care providers fail to diagnose between 45 and 90% of
cases of mental illness (Eisenberg, 1992). For example, the RAND
Medical Outcomes Study found that only about half of all cases of
depression were recognized by primary care practitioners (Wells et al.,
1989).

Efforts to improve recognition–for example, through feedback
interventions and guidelines dissemination–have not led to substantial
improvements (Rubenstein et al., 1999). Even when primary care
physicians recognize mental illness, they often fail to treat patients
with appropriate therapies (Mechanic, 1990; Rogers, Wells, Meredith,
Sturm, & Burnam, 1993). Primary care physicians rely heavily on psychotropic medications, often prescribe these medications in less than
therapeutically acceptable dosages (Eisenberg, 1992; Morlock, 1989),
and rarely refer patients with mental illness for specialty treatment
(Morlock; see also Mechanic; Rogers et al.). One recent study found
that primary care doctors referred as few as 10% of their depressed
patients to specialists (Rogers et al.).

Although improving the detection and treatment of disorders in
primary care is a desirable goal, the available data suggest caution in
encouraging integration of services through a primary care model
(Glied & Kofman, 1997). The studies described above that compare
treatment under HMOs (which formally integrate treatment) and
unmanaged fee-for-service arrangements (which do not) are consistent
with this caution.

There has been relatively little research concerning the effects of
formally integrated models on the physical health of people with serious mental illness, mainly because such arrangements are so rare. One
example–a short-lived experiment in Hennepin County, Minnesota–
enrolled seriously mentally ill people into an integrated, prepaid
health plan. Overall differences between the groups were small, but
prepaid patients were less likely to receive outpatient and inpatient
physical health care (Mechanic, Schlesinger, & McAlpine, 1995).

It is difficult to measure the effect of integration on the incentive to
capture cost-offset effects. Populations enrolled in different health care
arrangements differ in their underlying risks, making comparisons of
per capita spending difficult. The available evidence suggests, however, that behavioral health care spending in integrated health care sys-

tems tends to be a smaller percentage of total health care spending than in less integrated arrangements (Mechanic et al., 1995).

It is also not clear that even the strongest financial incentives will greatly encourage the use of behavioral health interventions that could lead to cost offsets. One of the best documented cost offsets that has been identified in the literature involves behavioral health interventions for elderly medical inpatients (Olfson et al., 1999). Hospitals, which are paid prospective rates under Medicare's DRG system, already bear full financial risk for the cost of inpatient care. This incentive has not been enough, however, to encourage widespread use of behavioral health interventions among inpatients.

Finally, it is important to recognize that the problem of balancing spending on physical and behavioral health care would arise under almost any conceivable organizational arrangement because of the nature of the professionals who provide behavioral health services. Whereas other medical specialists are often packaged with generalists through existing physician groups or hospital affiliations, behavioral health professionals often stand entirely outside the professional loop involved in providing physical health care. In one study of 75 carve-out plans, 72% of claims were paid to nonphysician providers, chiefly psychologists and social workers (Sturm & Klap, 1999). The effective use of such nonphysician professionals appears to be more difficult in a fully integrated system. In particular, integrated HMOs appear to use lower levels of highly skilled nonphysician professionals (doctoral-level psychologists) than do carve-out plans (Scheffler & Ivey, 1998).

This distinction implies that contracting with and managing behavioral health providers would likely be a separate line responsibility even in a plan that combined financing for the two types of plans. In a taxonomy of the practices of carved-in managed behavioral health plans, for example, Mihalik and Scherer (1998) describe two forms of organization. In one, the managed care plan contracts with a carve-out plan to manage behavioral health services on its behalf. In the other, apparently more integrated form of organization, the managed care plan establishes a separate division or department to manage behavioral health benefits. As Mihalik and Scherer note, interdepartmental negotiations are generally, but not always or necessarily, easier than interfirm negotiations. Proponents of managed behavioral health carve-outs assert that these plans can enhance behavioral health spending because they sequester funds for this specific purpose

(Bennett, 1992). In interdepartmental negotiations, behavioral health care might suffer.

Other Efforts to Integrate
Physical and Behavioral Health Care

The evidence suggests that full integration of behavioral and physical health services through a managed care gatekeeper or staff plan is not an ideal solution to the concerns discussed above. Several other approaches to integration have also been considered, including team approaches (in which a behavioral health care provider works jointly with a physical health care provider) and resource arrangements (in which a behavioral health resource person is made available to a physical health care provider).

Team approaches have been used both to enhance the delivery of behavioral health services to patients seen in primary care, and to improve the delivery of services to people with serious mental illness. In an HMO context, behavioral health professionals form part of a team of practitioners (and specialists) to provide care to a defined population at one site. Although in a staff-model HMO, all services may be provided at the same location, full integration cannot be achieved; primary care providers do not supervise psychiatric treatment (Budman, 1981). In practice, the declining share of the HMO market held by staff-model plans suggests that they will not (coupled with the team approach) serve as a model for the future delivery of behavioral health services.

Another team approach–the "partner in care" model–uses quality improvement techniques in ongoing primary care practices. The "partner" is a nurse specialist in depression (or other behavioral health care provider) who helps physicians provide therapy to patients with depression. In the past, these models appeared successful in research settings, but efforts to use them in standard practice settings were disappointing. A recent effectiveness trial, however, shows significant improvements in outcomes under this model (Rubenstein et al., 1999; Wells et al., 2000). Although the results of this study are encouraging (for example, the study found improved employment outcomes), only half of the patients with depression received counseling or had antidepressant medications prescribed at an appropriate dosage (Wells et al., 2000).

A more intensive team approach geared toward the seriously mentally ill who would otherwise require hospitalization–the Program of Assertive Community Treatment–uses a range of physical health, behavioral health, and social service providers. Although psychiatrists generally provide frontline primary care under this program, they may also coordinate the provision of services from other health professionals. The program has proved successful in keeping those with serious mental illnesses in the community (Lehman, 1999). Its effect on physical health outcomes has not been directly evaluated.

Resource enhancement approaches add a behavioral health professional to the primary care staff. Managed care plans in the private sector have experimented with this type of arrangement. One such approach, which placed behavioral health professionals (usually social workers) into primary medical care clinics as consultants to other staff, proved to be unsuccessful, however: primary care providers often did not have the time or inclination to treat patients with behavioral health problems, and behavioral health professionals resented the implication that behavioral health services could readily be provided by primary care practitioners who had received minimal consultation assistance and training (Budman, 1981).

Innovative efforts to coordinate physical and behavioral health care in the public sector were introduced in the context of Community Mental Health Centers (CMHCs). Beginning in 1978, CMHCs were offered funding to hire behavioral-health-linkage workers. In 1980, CMHCs were also eligible to receive grants if they established affiliation agreements with health centers (Marks & Broskowski, 1981). Several centers proceeded to develop linkage programs, but implementation of the programs ran into several barriers. For example, while many CMHCs felt that the linkage workers increased referrals to the CMHCs, there were no resources made available to handle the additional referrals. It was also difficult to identify the appropriate level of expertise and experience for linkage staff (Burns, Burke, & Kessler, 1981).

The preponderance of evidence suggests that neither full integration nor any of the partial-integration models is successful in addressing the concerns raised by fragmentation of physical and behavioral health services. The growth of carve-outs may simply illuminate problems that were largely in the shadows in earlier systems of care.

The vigor of carve-out arrangements suggests, however, that integration of physical and behavioral health care may not be a critical feature of effective behavioral health service delivery. In separating physical and behavioral health care, carve-out plans are just the latest manifestation of a long tradition. Integrated services do not have a better track record with respect to any of the concerns voiced by advocates. In fact, many carve-out arrangements go further than prior institutional arrangements in integrating service delivery–though not across the physical/behavioral health divide. Instead, carve-out plans are distinct from other type of health plans, and from the arrangements that preceded them, in that they play a substantial role in providing care (and referrals) within employer groups. Nearly 70% of all Americans with depression in each year are in the labor force (England, 1999). About 40% of those with schizophrenia are in the labor force (McFarland et al., 1996). A substantial proportion of American workers suffers from a diagnosable mental illness. Although diagnosis and treatment of mental illness in the workplace raises troubling issues of privacy, job safety, and coercion, the workplace nevertheless offers opportunities to diagnose mental illness that are at least as good as those provided by a visit to a primary care physician.

In addition to their main business of managing behavioral health services, many carve-out plans also staff and manage Employee Assistance Programs (EAPs) within companies. These programs, which are usually distinct from health insurance benefits, offer counseling services to employees with mental health and substance abuse problems. Today, about half of the employees in medium and large companies have EAPS available to them (Institute of Medicine, 1993). Over 14 million Americans are enrolled in EAPs that are integrated with behavioral health carve-outs (Findlay, 1999). EAP counselors are likely to see individuals early in the course of their problems and have more opportunity to observe them on a regular basis (Kongstvedt, 1997).

Integration of workplace services and health plan benefits may also be very important with respect to cost offsets. Although mental illness may increase patients' likelihood to seek physical health care, a growing literature documents that such illness also has negative effects on workplace productivity. Indeed, mental illness leads to significant reductions not only in productivity, but in employment and earnings (Frank & McGuire, 2000). If managed behavioral health firms can document the workplace savings from behavioral health treatment, they have an extremely powerful tool to encourage greater spending on behavioral health services. For example, a recent study found that the costs of psychiatric disability claims are lower among employers with good outpatient behavioral health service benefits (England, 1999). Such findings have prompted a number of employers to work with health plans to increase the rate of diagnosing and treating mental illness (England). Although cost offsets between physical and behavioral health may be harder to calculate when employers negotiate carve-outs directly, the indirect cost-offset effects are likely to be most salient in precisely such situations.

The example of integrating EAPs and behavioral health services suggests that alternative forms of integration may be generally more important than a physical health/behavioral health link. For example, most children who are treated for a mental illness receive treatment through their schools. Pediatricians treat only a minute fraction of children with such disorders. By contrast, although schools also provide some physical health services, health care providers outside the schools provide the bulk of these services. Given this situation, it may be more useful to focus efforts on coordinating behavioral health services with schools, rather than with pediatricians. Carve-out plans may be well positioned to forge such linkages with nonmedical providers (Bennett, 1992).

FUTURE STEPS

Carve-out plans did not invent poor coordination of behavioral and physical health care, and they do not seem to have appreciably worsened the existing fragmentation. Nonetheless, the poor quality of service coordination today, coupled with the growth of carve-outs and the renewed interest in service integration, presents opportunities for improvement.

Behavioral health plans should be active participants in efforts to encourage primary care practitioners to diagnose and treat—or to refer for treatment—behavioral health problems. These efforts may take two forms. First, managed care plans can be encouraged to develop ties to their behavioral health partners. These ties can be encouraged whether the partnership is initiated by the managed care plan or by the employer. For example, quality assessment measures can require that primary care providers know where to refer patients with psychiatric disorders. Second, behavioral health plans should be encouraged to experiment with referral systems that permit primary care providers to make initial referrals directly to behavioral health care providers within behavioral health networks—just as primary care providers do with other specialty referrals.

Coordination of physical health care for seriously mentally ill patients between behavioral health professionals and primary care (or other physical health) physicians is a thornier problem. The high prevalence of physical illness among the seriously mentally ill suggests that team or resource approaches may be applicable here, although methods for coordinating and financing these services could be complex. Some writers support the adoption of formal agreements to coordinate care (Lehman, 1999). Unfortunately, the history of such formal agreements in other sectors suggests that they may work better on paper than they do in practice.

One alternative would be to hold the carve-out behavioral health care provider accountable for ensuring that patients with severe mental illness receive routine physical health care. For example, the carve-out plan could be required to record a primary care physician contact for all patients. The plan could be also required to provide an annual referral to primary care for all patients with specific severe mental health diagnoses.

Boundary problems can lead to wasted efforts as different plans vie to shift costs rather than provide cost-effective care. The best way around boundary problems is to write clear contracts having well-defined lines of demarcation. Recognizing and quantifying the extent of such problems is a necessary first step.

Finally, with respect to payment levels, the most effective way to ensure adequate payment for behavioral health services is to show that they are a cost-effective means of improving the health and well-being of the population. Behavioral health firms should use their data and resources to make this case.

Coordination of behavioral and physical health services is a sound goal for health policy, but it is not one that is easily attained. The problems of organizing and managing physical and behavioral health services are in many respects quite distinct from one another. Few institutions seem capable of doing both well. The existence of carve-out plans is a symptom of this underlying intractability.

The problems that arise because of service fragmentation are unlikely to be solved by a wholesale abandonment of the carve-out model. Evidence suggests that the problems are, if anything, worse under fully integrated approaches. Instead, improvements in policy will come only through a focus on the most serious problems of care coordination. These problems include the need to address the significant physical health problems of the seriously mentally ill; to assist those primary care practitioners who are trying to improve diagnosis and treatment of mental illness; and to produce evidence that would justify higher levels of spending on behavioral health care.

REFERENCES

Bennett, M. J. (1992). Managed mental health in health maintenance organizations. In S. Feldman (Ed.), *Managed mental health services* (pp. 61–82). Springfield, IL: Charles C Thomas.

Buck, J. A., Teich, J. L., Umland, B., & Stein, M. (1999). Behavioral health benefits in employer-sponsored health plans, 1997. *Health Affairs, 18* (2), 67–78.

Budman, S. H. (1981). Mental health services in the health maintenance organization. In A. Broskowski, E. Marks, & S. H. Budman (Eds.), *Linking health and mental health* (pp. 103–114). Beverly Hills, CA: Sage Publications.

Burns, B. J., Burke, J. D., Jr., & Kessler, L. G. (1981). Promoting health–mental health coordination: Federal efforts. In A. Broskowski, E. Marks, & S. H. Budman (Eds.), *Linking health and mental health* (pp. 27–44). Beverly Hills, CA: Sage Publications.

Chang, C. F., Kiser, L. J., Bailey, J. E., Martins, M., Gibson, W. C., Schaberg, K. A., Mirvis, D. M., & Applegate, W. B. (1998). Tennessee's failed managed care program for mental health and substance abuse services. *Journal of the American Medical Association, 279,* 864–869.

Durham, M. L. (1995). Can HMOs manage the mental health benefit? *Health Affairs, 14* (3), 116–123.

Eisenberg, L. (1992). Treating depression and anxiety in primary care: Closing the gap between knowledge and practice. *New England Journal of Medicine, 327* (10), 1080–1084.

Elias, E., & Navon, M. (1995). The Massachusetts experience with managed mental health care and Medicaid. *Health Affairs, 14* (3), 46–49.

England, M. J. (1999). Capturing mental health cost offsets. *Health Affairs, 18* (2), 91–93.

Feldman, S. (1998). Behavioral health services: Carved out and managed. *American Journal of Managed Care, 4,* SP59–SP67.

Findlay, S. (1999). Managed behavioral health care in 1999: An industry at a cross-roads. *Health Affairs, 18* (5), 116–124.

Frank, R. G., & McGuire, T. G. (2000). Economics and mental health. In A. J. Culyer & J. P. Newhouse (Eds.), *Handbook of health economics*. New York: Elsevier.

Frank, R. G., Huskamp, H. A., McGuire, T. G., & Newhouse, J. P. (1996). Some economics of mental health "carve-outs." *Archives of General Psychiatry, 53,* 933–937.

Glied, S. (1998). Getting the incentives right for children. *Health Services Research, 33* (4), 1143–1159.

Glied, S., & Kofman, S. (1997). Women's mental health: An introduction. *Compensation and Benefits Management, 13* (4), 43–51.

Goldman, W., McCulloch, J., & Sturm, R. (1998). Costs and use of mental health services before and after managed care. *Health Affairs, 17* (2), 40–52.

Grob, G. N. (1994). *The mad among us*. Cambridge, MA: Harvard University Press.

Hogan, M. (1997). Organization and financing of mental health care. In A. Tasman, J. Kay, & J. Lieberman (Eds.), *Psychiatry* (pp. 1781–1802). Philadelphia: W. B. Saunders.

Institute of Medicine. (1993). *Employment and health benefits: A connection at risk*. Washington, DC: National Academy Press.

Jellinek, M. S. (1998). Mental health care costs–not the whole story [letter]. *Health Affairs, 17* (4), 241–242.

Katon, W., & Schulberg, H. C. (1992). Epidemiology of depression in primary care. *General Hospital Psychiatry, 14* (4), 237–247.

Kessler, R. C., McGonagle, K. A., Zhao, S., Nelson, C. B., Hughes, M., Eshleman, S., Wittchen, H., & Kendler, K. S. (1994). Lifetime and 12-month prevalence of DSM-III-R psychiatric disorders in the United States. *Archives of General Psychiatry, 51,* 8–19.

Kongstvedt, P. (1997). *Essentials of managed health care* (2nd ed.). Gaithersburg, MD: Aspen.

Leaf, P. J. (1994). Psychiatric disorders and the use of health services. In J. Miranda, C. Hohmann, C. C. Attkisson, & D. B. Larson, (Eds.), *Mental disorders in primary care* (pp. 377–401). San Francisco: Jossey-Bass.

Leaf, P. J., Bruce, M. L., Tischler, G. L., Freeman, D. H., Jr., Weissman, M. M., & Myers, J. K. (1988). Factors affecting the utilization of specialty and general medical mental health services. *Medical Care, 26* (1), 9–26.

Lehman, A. F. (1999). Quality of care in mental health: The case of schizophrenia. *Health Affairs, 18* (5), 52–65.

Lyness, J. M., Caine, E. D., King, D. A., Cox, C., & Yoediono, Z. (1999). Psychiatric disorders in older primary care patients. *Journal of General Internal Medicine, 14* (4), 249–254.

Marks, E., & Broskowski, A. (1981). Community mental health and organized health care linkages. In A. Broskowski, E. Marks, & S. H. Budman (Eds.), *Linking health and mental health* (pp. 159–182). Beverly Hills, CA: Sage Publications.

McFarland, B. H., Johnson, R. E., & Hornbrook, M. C. (1996). Enrollment duration, service use, and costs of care for severely mentally ill members of a health maintenance organization. *Archives of General Psychiatry, 53* (10), 938–944.

Mechanic, D., Schlesinger, M., & McAlpine, D. D. (1995). Management of mental health and substance abuse services: State of the art and early results. *Milbank Quarterly, 73* (1), 19–55.

Mechanic, D. (1990). Treating mental illness: Generalist versus specialist. *Health Affairs, 9* (4), 61–75.

Mihalik, G., & Scherer, M. (1998). Fundamental mechanisms of managed behavioral health care. *Journal of Health Care Finance, 24* (3), 1–15.

Morlock, L. L. (1989). Recognition and treatment of mental health problems in the general health sector. In C. A. Taube, D. Mechanic, & A. Hohmann (Eds.), *The future of mental health services research* (pp. 39–62). Washington, DC: U.S. Government Printing Office.

Norton, E. C., Lindrooth, R. C., & Dickey, B. (1997). Cost shifting in a mental health carve-out for the AFDC population. *Health Care Financing Review, 18* (3), 95–108.

Norton, E. C., Lindrooth, R. C., & Dickey, B. (1999). Cost-shifting in managed care. *Mental Health Services Research, 1* (3), 185–196.

Olfson, M., Sing, M., & Schlesinger, H. J. (1999). Mental health/medical care cost offsets: Opportunities for managed care. *Health Affairs, 18* (2), 79–90.

Rogers, W. H., Wells, K. B., Meredith, L. S., Sturm, R., & Burnam, M. A. (1993). Outcomes for adult outpatients with depression under prepaid or fee-for-service financing. *Archives of General Psychiatry, 50,* 517–525.

Rubenstein, L. V., Jackson-Triche, M., Unutzer, J., Miranda, J., Minnim, K., Pearson, M. L., & Wells, K. B. (1999). Evidence-based care for depression in managed primary care practices. *Health Affairs, 18* (5), 89–105.

Scheffler, R., & Ivey, S. L. (1998). Mental health staffing in managed care organizations: A case study. *Psychiatric Services, 49* (10), 1303–1308.

Sturm, R., & Klap, R. (1999). Use of psychiatrists, psychologists, and master's-level therapists in managed behavioral health care carve-out plans. *Psychiatric Services, 50* (4), 504–508.

Wells, K. B., Hays, R. D., Burnam, M. A., Rogers, W., Greenfield, S., & Ware, J. E. (1989). Detection of depressive disorder for patients receiving prepaid or fee-for-service care: Results from the medical outcomes study. *Journal of the American Medical Association, 262,* 3298–3302.

Wells, K. B., Sherbourne, C., Schoenbaum, M., Duan, N., Meredith, L., Unützer, J., Miranda, J., Carney, M. F., & Rubenstein, L. V. (2000). Impact of disseminating quality improvement programs for depression in managed primary care: A randomized controlled trial. *Journal of the American Medical Association, 283,* 212–220.

Yassa, R., Lal, S., Korpassy, A., & Ally, J. (1987). Nicotine exposure and tardive dyskinesia. *Biological Psychiatry, 22,* 67–72.

Chapter 6

ECONOMICS

Richard G. Frank and Judith R. Lave

Managed care organizations have become the dominant institutions in the U.S. health care delivery system. As managed care has evolved, separate institutions have emerged to manage the delivery of general medical care and of mental health and substance abuse services (together known as behavioral health care). Today, the majority of American behavioral health care is "managed" by specialized managed behavioral health care organizations (MBHOs) under managed behavioral health carve-out contracts. Thus, MBHOs contract with employers, public payers, or health plans to take responsibility for a segment of services covered by insurance, namely, those related to specialty mental health and substance abuse (MH/SA) care. In order to understand and evaluate the delivery of MH/SA services, it is necessary to understand how MBHOs perform with respect to cost, access, and quality of care.

Research on the effects of specialty managed behavioral health care has been under way for less than a decade. The research community has responded energetically to the emergence of these new institutions that serve to "ration" and to "rationalize" mental health and substance abuse care. By and large, the research strategy adopted by the field has been to conduct a series of empirical case studies that examine aspects of the use of MH/SA services before and after an

Note: The authors gratefully acknowledge financial support from the Alfred P. Sloan Foundation, the National Institute of Mental Health (MH43703 and MH56925), and the National Institute on Drug Abuse (DA10233).

146

MBHO has taken on the responsibility for managing the care for the insured population under study. These case studies have been conducted in a variety of contexts. The types of organizations contracting with MBHOs have differed: in some cases, the contracting organizations have been payers (for example, a state Medicaid program or an employer), and in other cases the contracting organizations have been health plans. Studies have focused on different components of behavioral health care: whereas some analysts have focused on all behavioral health services, others have looked at substance abuse or mental health only. Different studies have targeted different segments of the life cycle (children, adults, or the elderly). The performance of MBHOs has been measured in terms of their impact on specialty behavioral health care costs, on access to specialty care, and (occasionally) on indicators of treatment quality.

In this essay we focus on the results reported in the literature and take stock of what has been learned. Because of the rapid pace of research in this area, our review is unlikely to be comprehensive. Thus, we give special attention to assessing the current findings, with special attention to the needs of public and private policymakers. Our review will examine the findings from the literature in three categories. (1) What is the net impact of managed behavioral health carve-out contracts on spending, quality, and access to MH/SA care? (2) To the extent that savings were realized, how were they achieved (lower prices, reduced intensity of care, reduced volume of care, and so on)? (3) What features of MBHOs (network structure, utilization management, payment methods) led to the savings and to the changes in access and quality?

In the first section, we discuss some of the preliminary empirical issues that provide the context for discussing the three questions set out above. In second section, we review the empirical evidence relating to those questions themselves. In the final section, we consider what has been learned and what open questions remain.

WHAT EVIDENCE IS REQUIRED
TO ANSWER OUR QUESTIONS?

As noted above, researchers have examined the performance of MBHOs by conducting interrupted-time-series or before-and-after evaluations. Such studies are fraught with well-known methodological difficulties, however, and one must be careful in interpreting their findings. The inferences to be drawn from the experiences with managed behavioral health care to date depend critically on the dimensions of performance that are measured, on the ability of researchers to control for factors such as secular trends and technical change, and on the strategic behavior of MBHOs. In this section we will discuss these issues with regard to the cost, access, and quality dimensions of MBHO performance.

The Cost Question

What impact has managed behavioral health care had on spending for health care services? Conceptually, there are three different levels at which this spending can be measured: spending on overall health care services, spending for MH/SA services, and spending on MH/SA services provided by specialty-care providers. Since carve-out contracts generally involve management of the use of, and spending associated with, specialty inpatient, outpatient, residential, and intensive outpatient services for the treatment of MH/SA problems, first-generation researchers tended to focus on the impact of managed behavioral health care on the services provided and on the categories of spending that an MBHO was responsible for managing. Determining this impact was an important policy question; in the late 1980s and early 1990s, spending on specialty MH/SA care had grown rapidly and was a concern of both private and public payers (Frank, Salkever, & Sharfstein, 1991). The answer to the cost question has been largely settled. Private payers and health plans achieve significant savings by entering into managed behavioral health contracts for specialty MH/SA care. Studies of the Medicaid experience include those by Callahan, Shepard, Beinecke, Larson, and Cavanaugh (1995) and Stoner, Manning, and Christianson (1997). Studies in private insurance include those by Goldman, McCulloch, and Sturm (1998), Grazier, Eselius, Hu, Shore, and G'sell (1999), and Ma and McGuire (1998).

A more relevant measure of performance for most payers is the effect of carve-out plans on the total health care costs of payers' enrolled populations. Measuring this effect is complicated by a number of factors. Of particular importance in this context are expenditures for prescription drugs and for primary care. Most managed behavioral health carve-out contracts do not, for example, cover prescription drugs. Nonetheless, pharmocotherapies are key components of the modern treatment of depression, schizophrenia, alcoholism, and some anxiety disorders. Spending on antidepressant medication has been identified as one of the three fastest growing areas of prescription drug spending (Novartis, 1999a). By 1998, HMOs' spending per member per month on antidepressants and antipsychotic drugs averaged $1.95. Spending per member per month on psychotropropic medications increases to $2.50 if antianxiety drugs and mood stabilizers are included in the calculation (Novartis, 1999b; IMS Health Inc., 1998). The spending on MH/SA services (excluding prescription drugs) in HMOs and other private carve-out programs (those involving contracts with PPOs or direct contracts with employers) typically ranges from about $2.00 to $4.50 per member per month (Sturm, Goldman, & McCulloch, 1998). Thus, HMOs currently spend about the same amount for psychotropic medications as they do for all specialty MH/SA inpatient and outpatient services. Moreover, much treatment for MH/SA problems remains the responsibility of primary care physicians and, as such, is not counted as part of specialty care. Recent estimates suggest that 40 to 50% of all MH/SA care delivered by the health care system takes place in general medical settings (Satcher, 1999, chap. 6).

A systematic problem underlying MB/SA expenditures for prescription drug services and primary care services is that under a carve-out plan, the MBHO—which is held accountable only for specialty MH/SA services—can effectively view these two types of services as "free goods"; since spending for these services does not count against the carve-out budget, there is an incentive for MBHOs to encourage their use and possibly to overuse them. Some of the decrease in costs observed in the specialty-care sector may therefore be a result of shifting costs to other sectors. Some researchers have noted this issue in general discussions of "cost shifting," but it has received only limited attention in empirical estimates of the impact of managed behavioral health care on spending (see, for example, Norton, Lindrooth, & Dickey, 1999; Sturm, 1999b).

An additional factor making it difficult to assess the effect of carve-out plans on total MH/SA costs is the continuing development of innovative pharmacotherapeutic treatments for mental disorders.

These innovations would have led (and will continue to lead) to changes in the patterns and costs of MH/SA care even in the absence of institutional changes in health care delivery. That is, since advances in pharmacotherapy have taken place simultaneous with the growth of behavioral health carve-out plans, it is difficult to determine the differential impact of therapeutic advances (and the patterns of care associated with them) and of the changes grounded in the rationing methods of managed care.

Further complicating the problem of determining the effect of MHBOs on overall health care costs for payers is the possibility that there may be some interactions between the use and effects of behavioral health services and physical health services: one result of better (worse) treatment of MH/SA problems may be a decrease (increase) in expenditures on physical health problems. A final complication in calculating MH/SA costs is the uncertain degree to which those costs are being shifted from the private sector to the public behavioral health sector. There has long been a shifting of financial responsibility for behavioral health care from the private financing system (insurance) to the public behavioral health system (Frank & McGuire, 2000). This shift has been caused, in part, by the setting of limits on coverage for inpatient days and for visits under traditional health insurance. The management of MH/SA care can well be expected to have a similar, though presently indeterminate, effect.

In attempting to evaluate the empirical literature on managed MB/SA care, one further note of caution is in order. It is possible that there is some selection bias in the matching of contracts and MBHOs. Firms do not bid on all contracts, and MBHOs may learn that there are specific types of contracts under which they can perform well. In order to generalize research findings, it is therefore imperative to observe a number of companies operating under a variety of contractual arrangements. As we shall see, however, the experience to date is based on a limited set of observations.

Interpretation of Changes in Patterns of Care: Cost and Access

Under fee-for-service indemnity arrangements, the delivery of behavioral health services was criticized for inefficiency. The inefficiencies took a variety of forms, three of which are important here: an overemphasis on inpatient care for the treatment of many mental and addictive disorders (Mechanic, 1989); wide variation in the number of days for which patients with a given condition were hospitalized, though with no observable differences in outcomes; the inappropriate treatment of many illnesses, such as major depression (Well et al., 1996; Lehman & Steinwachs, 1998), coupled with relatively frequent failure to observe accepted standards of care (Busch, 2000). In view of these considerations, it is difficult to interpret the observed shifts in patterns of care under a managed behavioral health carve-out. For instance, does the observed shift from psychotherapy alone to drug treatment result from more appropriate management of care or from cost shifting? Similarly, does a reduction in inpatient care result from more appropriate management of care or from an inappropriate reduction in access to inpatient care?

As noted above, most analyses of the impact of managed behavioral health care have focused on its effect on the use of specialty services. In large part, researchers were required to focus on specialty services because they had access only to information about services covered under the carve-out. As a consequence, it is difficult to interpret the findings of the impact of managed behavioral health care on nonfinancial outcomes such as access to care. For example, several studies found increases in rates of utilization for MH/SA services following implementation of a carve-out program (see Callahan et al., 1995; Goldman et al., 1998). If, however, under fee-for-service indemnity arrangements, many patients received behavioral health care from the primary care physicians in the form of counseling and pharmacotherapy during routine office visits, then studies focusing on the difference in the use of specialty behavioral health services between fee-for-service and carve-out arrangements may be quite misleading. In particular, such studies will tend to undercount the rate of behavioral health treatment prior to the carve-out, thereby mistaking a shift in setting of care for a change in access to care.

Both in studying and designing carve-outs, it needs to be kept in mind that the incentives are different for primary care physicians and for MBHOs. MBHOs have obvious incentives to shift MH/SA care to primary care physicians. Primary care physicians, however, have even stronger incentives to shift care to MBHOs. Many primary care physicians receive capitated payments. Moreover, because the very purpose of MBHOs is to shift MH/SA care to the specialized sector, some plans will not reimburse primary care physicians for claims that have an ICD MH/SA diagnosis.

What Features of Managed Behavioral Health Contracts Affect Costs and Quality?

Researchers and policymakers would like to be able to identify the specific features of managed behavioral health contracts that affect costs and quality. There are many features of such contracts, however, that might affect performance–which makes it difficult to isolate particular features and to measure, in turn, the associated impact.

An essential aspect of managed care is that it introduces new techniques for rationing care. These techniques, most of which are designed to influence the treatments that patients receive, include: specialized forms of utilization management; disease management; level-of-care guidelines; and provider profiling. MBHOs also develop specialized networks of providers whose treatment philosophies tend to be consistent with those of the MBHOs. These organizations have also introduced a number of new methods of paying providers, such as case-based payments, that contain incentives to limit the volume of care.

Purchasers of managed behavioral health care, in turn, use a number of methods to obtain favorable performance from vendors of such care. Both health plans and private payers use competitive procurements to select an MBHO. In addition, purchasers use mechanisms–such as capitation payment, risk-sharing contracts, and so-called administrative-services-only (ASO) contracts–to pay MBHOs. Purchasers also require that MBHOs produce a variety of performance reports, including: measures of administrative performance, such as efficiency of claims processing; indicators of access to care, such as penetration rates (specialty MH/SA users/enrollees); and quality measures, such as the process of medication management for depression (a HEDIS measure). Contracts also contain information–which varies across contracts–on the level of covered services and on the associated cost-sharing for the enrolled population.

Contracts for managed behavioral health care are consequently quite complex, which makes it difficult to determine the effect of specific contract features on performance. Suppose that one wanted to determine whether performance was influenced by payment method (capitation, risk sharing, or ASO). The estimated effect of a capitation contract will depend on how that contract is structured. For example, many capitation contracts are accompanied by reinsurance requirements. A common type of reinsurance protects plans or MBHOs from the costs of individual cases that exceed $30,000. In such cases, the MBHO actually bears far less financial risk than is implied by simple conceptions of capitation. Other contract features also serve to reduce risk. In some contracts, future rates are based on current performance. Thus, if a plan saves substantial money this year, its rates will be lower next year. Consequently, the actual incentives to reduce spending may be far weaker than would be suggested by the MBHO's being paid a strict capitation payment (sometimes called "100% supply-side cost sharing") (Frank & McGuire, 1997). Since the introduction of managed behavioral health contracts typically involves the simultaneous change of many parameters governing the organization, management, and financing of care, it can be difficult to identify the impact of specific contract features.

Several researchers have made efforts to circumvent this problem by examining different contracts within a single MBHO. By studying a single company, one implicitly controls for variation in administrative rationing methods such as levels-of-care protocols and network structure. Nevertheless, identification of a single element can still remain elusive because of the complexity of individual contracts and because of the impact of competitive dynamics. Since the market for managed behavioral health care is so competitive, the awarding of contracts appears to have been, and to a lesser degree still is, sensitive to the reputation of vendors for performance. Therefore, contracts with different payment and data-monitoring provisions may yield similar performance with respect to costs and quality if vendors believe that future business depends on their performance in these areas.

WHAT IS THE EVIDENCE TO DATE?

We examine results from the literature on managed behavioral health carve-out programs to assess what is known about the impact of these institutions on MH/SA spending, access, and quality.

Evidence on Overall Spending: Private Payers

Table 1 reports results from the evaluations of introducing managed behavioral health carve-out plans to privately insured populations. The table includes only those studies that reported the *aggregate* impact of the carve-outs. Many of the efforts to evaluate the impact of introducing carve-out plans have been published as separate papers on different facets of that impact. For instance, some studies focused on the effect of the carve-out on the use of different types of behavioral health services, whereas others have addressed the effect of spending for different subpopulations. Table 1 does not present the results of such studies, but only of those that report estimates of broader impacts on spending of the managed behavioral health carve-out.

Table 1

PRIVATE INSURANCE: CARVE-OUT ANALYSIS

Study	Sample	MBHO	Spending Type	Cost Impact
Goldman et al., 1998	Non-elderly enrollees from HMO and FFS plans	UBH	Specialty inpatient, outpatient, IOP, residential MH/SA claims	-40%
Ma & McGuire, 1998	Non-elderly FFS and PPO enrollees from Massachusetts state employees	OPTIONS	Inpatient, outpatient, IOP, residential MH/SA claims	-30% to -40%
Grazier et al., 1999	Employees enrolled in PPO/POS	PNA	Outpatient claims for visits with an ICD-9 MH/SA diagnosis	-30% to -42%
Sturm et al., 1998	Enrollees covered by state of Ohio health plans	UBH	Specialty inpatient, outpatient, IOP, residential MH/SA claims	Non-HMO carve-out: -38% HMO: 0%
Brisson et al., 2000	Non-elderly in an HMO carve-out	PNA	All MH/SA claims defined by ICD-9 and procedures	-48%

The studies in Table 1 are notably consistent in the estimated impacts of the carve-out on behavioral health spending–despite several significant differences in the studies' institutional contexts and in their definitions of MH/SA spending. Four of the five studies include estimates of changes in spending for non-HMO carve-out enrollees.

All four estimates suggest spending reductions for MH/SA services of 30 to 40%, using indemnity or PPO-type arrangements as a baseline. Two studies report results for the implementation of carve-out arrangements for HMO enrollees. One reports no change in spending, whereas the other reports a 48% reduction in MH/SA spending. The studies differ somewhat in how MH/SA services are defined. All exclude spending on prescription drugs. Goldman and colleagues (1998), Ma and McGuire (1998), and Sturm and colleagues (1998) define MH/SA services as those services that are covered by the carve-out–that is, as services provided by specialty providers. Grazier and colleagues (1999) and Brisson, Frank, Berenbaum, and Gazmararian (2000) define MH/SA services by the ICD-9 diagnosis and procedure codes. In particular, they track services that are associated with care of MH/SA problems as defined by ICD-9 codes, not by the organization that manages the claims. Grazier and colleagues examined only outpatient MH/SA services. All other studies examined both inpatient and outpatient services.

The components of spending that change as a result of introducing a managed behavioral health carve-out are quite similar across studies. All studies in Table 1 that included inpatient services found that there was a significant decrease in the use of inpatient care. All studies found that there was a decrease in the number of visits per episode of outpatient care. All studies reported that the prices paid to providers were lower after the carve-out than they were before. The effect of the carve-out on the overall access to care, however–that is, the probability of using any MH/SA services–differed across the studies. This result is not surprising; one would expect that the impact of the carve-out on access would depend, in part, on utilization rates prior to the implementation of the carve-out. Thus, for example, the carve-out plan may have reduced the rate of use of all MH/SA services for Massachusetts state employees because their baseline utilization rates were already very high.

As discussed earlier, in order to interpret these results, we also need to know how much MH/SA care continues to be delivered in the general medical sector subsequent to the carve-out.

Three of the five studies in Table 1 examined the effect of the carve-out on MH/SA specialty care, whereas two looked at the effect on MH/SA care as identified by the ICD codes across all settings. The similarity of results across the studies using total payments for claims based on ICD-9 MH/SA diagnoses and for carve-out claims offers some reassurance that there have been no major shifts in spending away from carve-out budgets towards the general medical care sector. Thus, we have not found evidence suggesting that primary care providers are substantially increasing their supply of MH/SA care in response to carve-out structures.

The evidence on shifts in spending patterns in the areas of prescription drugs, however, offers a somewhat different story. Two studies of private insurance carve-out arrangements examined the impact of the managed behavioral health carve-outs on the use of drug treatments for depression. Both studies found that there was an increased use of antidepressant medication stemming from the implementation of a managed behavioral health carve-out (Berndt, Frank, & McGuire, 1997; Busch, 2000). In the more complete study, Busch estimated that carve-out arrangements led to an increase of between 30 and 50% in the share of episodes of depression treated with antidepressant medication. The growth in use of antidepressant medication took the form of a doubling in the share of episodes treated with selective serotonin reuptake inhibitors (SSRIs) alone and a 60% reduction in the use of psychotherapy alone. These results suggest that there is likely to be some substantial growth in prescription drug spending on psychoactive drugs as a consequence of choosing to use a managed behavioral health carve-out. Although these data point in the direction of increased spending, there are no reported results that directly estimate the impact of carve-outs on spending for psychoactive drugs.

A study by Rosenthal (1999), which examined the use of case rates to pay providers for services within the context of a managed behavioral health carve-out, also found some indication of cost-shifting behavior. She found that the shift from fee-for-service to a case-rate payment (with an MBHO) was accompanied by a significant decrease in payments. She also found, however, that the reduction in use of services associated with the case-rate payment method was accompanied by the increased likelihood both of receiving a prescription and of being referred to a publicly funded community mental health program.

Given the overall evidence, we conclude that current estimates of savings from managed behavioral health carve-outs should be viewed as defining upper limits.

Evidence on Savings: Public Payers

Studies of the implementation of managed behavioral health care in the Medicaid context have been more concerned with measurement of net impacts of carve-out arrangements on overall MH/SA costs than have private-insurance studies. Table 2 summarizes the findings from a number of studies that have evaluated the impact of carve-out programs under Medicaid.

Table 2

PUBLIC INSURANCE: CARVE-OUT ANALYSIS

Study	Sample	MBHO	Spending	Cost Impact
Callahan et al., 1995 Frank & McGuire, 1997 Norton et al., 1999	Massachusetts Medicaid	MHMA	Specialty inpatient, outpatient, residential MH/SA claims	-22%
Christianson et al., 1995 Stoner et al., 1997	Utah Medicaid	Community Mental Health Centers	Specialty inpatient and outpatient claims	-17%
Burns et al., 1999	North Carolina Medicaid (children)	Community programs	Specialty inpatient, outpatient, partial-wrap-around case management, residential	-33%*
Bloom et al., 1998	Colorado Medicaid	CMHC/MBHO partnerships	Specialty inpatient, outpatient care, including state hospitals	27%

* Authors' calculation of difference in differences estimates.

There are several important points highlighted by Table 2. First, the carve-out programs all led to large reductions in spending on specialty MH/SA services. The estimated savings for services that were carved out range from about 17% in Utah to 33% for children's services in North Carolina. Second, the savings were realized under a variety of organizational arrangements. Massachusetts organized its managed behavioral health carve-out along the lines used in the private sector. The state conducted a competitive procurement process and selected a private for-profit vendor to manage behavioral health services under Medicaid. Utah delegated all financial, administrative, and clinical responsibility for MH/SA care to community mental health centers. Colorado contracted with partnerships between community mental health centers and private, for-profit MBHOs. North Carolina contracted with community-based systems of care. Third, the evaluations of the Massachusetts and Colorado carve-out plans took account of some services (residential facilities, state hospitals, medical services, and pharmacy) that were delivered outside of the carve-out program.

The components of spending that changed as a result of introducing the managed behavioral health carve-outs were similar across sites and similar to those found for the private sector. As in the private sector, most of the savings to public payers resulted from the reduced use of inpatient care and reduced intensity of outpatient treatment. In some cases, payments to providers were reduced (Massachusetts). It was less common to find expanded rates of overall utilization of MH/SA care in the public sector than it was in private sector. This difference is difficult to interpret.

The evidence on cost shifting is mixed. The researchers detected little shifting of care to public mental hospitals in either Colorado or Massachusetts. Although the researchers who studied Massachusetts did not find any shifting of MH/SA treatment from specialty services to general medical care or prescription drugs for the Aid to Families with Dependent Children population, they did observe such shifts for the disabled (Supplemental Security Income) populations (Norton, Lindrooth, & Dickey, 1997). One finding was that spending on both general medical services and prescription drugs for the disabled population increased. The increase in prescription drug expenditures resulted from an increase in prescription drug expenditures per user rather than from an increase in the number of users (Norton et al., 1999). It is not surprising that the number of users did not increase; nearly all people with severe mental illnesses were using psychotropic medications prior to the introduction of the carve-out. It is difficult to determine, however, whether the increase in prescription drug expenditures resulted from the carve-out itself. As noted earlier, new (and expensive) antipsychotic medications were being introduced into the market during the study period. It is therefore not possible to distinguish between secular trends in drug spending and the impact of the carve-out on expenditures on prescription drugs.

We conclude that the estimates in Table 2 provide upper limits on net MH/SA savings resulting from the implementation of managed behavioral health carve-outs.

We should note that the savings resulting from the implementation of a carve-out plan are likely to vary depending upon the period during which the studies were conducted. The studies of the early 1990s compared the outcomes (cost, quality, access) resulting from a carve-out with those of a completely unmanaged, fee-for-service indemnity plan. Later studies (beginning in the mid-1990s) have compared outcomes to general HMO or to PPO care. During this later period, however, HMOs, PPOs, and even fee-for-service indemnity arrangements involved much more management than they did early in the decade. Thus, it is unlikely that current estimates of the savings resulting from a shift to a carve-out would be as large as those reported in Table 1.

A related point is that most analyses have treated the impact of managed behavioral health carve-outs as being largely one-time effects. A recent paper by Sturm (1999a) highlights the significance of considering the ability of MBHOs to learn and to adapt their techniques to produce additional savings over a number of years.

For the above reasons, introducing managed behavioral health care into an HMO or aggressively managed PPO in 1999 may have produced very different results than introducing managed behavioral health care into a fee-for-service indemnity plan or a PPO early in the decade. Furthermore, one needs to assess the savings over a number of years to obtain a complete assessment of the impact on spending.

Evidence on Quality

Very little research has examined changes in the quality of care stemming from implementation of a managed behavioral health carve-out program in either the public or private sector. In the few studies that have been conducted, the quality measures examined have varied. Merrick (1998), in her study of the carve-out for Massachusetts state employees, focused on a measure of coordination of care following the discharge from a hospital for major depression. She found that there was a significant increase in linkages to community-based care following a hospital discharge for treatment of depression. Sturm (1999a), in his study of the carve-out by the state of Ohio for its public employees, focused on rehospitalization rates as a quality indicator. He found that the large decrease in spending was associated with a nonsignificant increase in rehospitalization rates. Busch (2000), in her study of the introduction of a carve-out to a regional HMO, determined the likelihood that an episode of care for treatment of depression adhered to the guidelines of the American Psychiatric Association and Agency for Health Care Policy and Research. She estimated that, holding other factors constant, episodes treated under the carve-out arrangements were about twice as likely to meet guideline-level care as episodes treated through an integrated HMO.

Dickey and colleagues (1998) examined continuity of care for people with severe mental illness that were enrolled in the Medicaid program in Massachusetts before and after a carve-out was introduced. Dickey found that follow-up care after a hospital discharge remained constant throughout the study period. The rate of rehospitalization, however, increased somewhat after the carve-out was introduced. The researchers attributed this change to possible increases in the severity of the illness for which patients were initially admitted for hospital care under the carve-out. The changing severity of illness confounds the interpretation of readmission as a quality indicator.

In one of the few studies that analyzed treatment outcomes, Manning and colleagues (1999) compared the outcomes for patients with schizophrenia served under the Utah Medicaid carve-out with outcomes for similar patients served under fee-for-service arrangements in the state. On the basis of several clinical outcome measures, the mental health status of both populations improved, but patients covered under the carve-out improved less than those who remained in the fee-for-service sector.

The evidence on quality of care is mixed for both publicly and privately insured people. It is notable, however—given the negative treatment of managed behavioral health care in the popular press—that no study has found dramatic shifts in quality following the introduction of a carve-out plan. One wonders, though, whether the carve-outs studied to date are representative of the universe of such arrangements.

Mechanisms Affecting Patterns of Care

Researchers have hypothesized that a variety of mechanisms have caused the observed changes in costs, utilization, and quality of MH/SA care under managed behavioral health carve-out arrangements. They have posited that the evolving treatment patterns for MH/SA problems have been influenced by factors such as network effects, utilization management, clinical guidelines, reputation effects, competition, and the explicit financial incentives built into the carve-out contracts. As we discussed earlier, however, because carve-outs involve complex organizational and contractual elements, it is difficult to identify the impact of individual factors on patterns of utilization and spending.

There has been a great deal of interest in identifying the impact of financial incentives on cost and quality of MH/SA care. Powerful financial incentives such as capitation payments have been shown in other contexts to exert strong influences on patterns of treatment. Critics of managed-care practices have pointed out that capitation incentives may lead to undertreatment and reduced quality of care. In the managed behavioral health context, however, it has been surprisingly difficult to estimate the impact of financial incentives on the behavior of MBHOs; as discussed above, a managed behavioral health intervention involves a bundle of rationing methods.

Two studies provide some empirical clues about the impact of financial incentives. Huskamp's (1998) analysis of the Massachusetts state employees' experience assessed the effect of a change in risk bearing within an existing managed behavioral health program. She found that a small change in the level of risk borne by an MBHO had a significant effect on outpatient MH/SA spending. Brisson and colleagues (2000) studied the change within an MBHO of a shift from discounted per diem payment of hospital MH/SA care to a capitation contract. They found that even though hospital-utilization rates were low to begin with, the implementation of capitation led to a significant reduction in spending on inpatient care.

As for the impact of other mechanisms, Ma and McGuire (1999) identified the combined effect of network structure and benefit-design copayments, deductibles, and limits. They found that strong network effects accompanied the benefit-design expansions that occurred in the Massachusetts state employees' health plan. Wickizer and Lessler

(1998) studied hospital utilization for 50,000 patients and estimated the separate effects of prior authorization and concurrent review on hospital care. They reported that the MBHO denied very few requests for admission to hospital. They also found, however, that concurrent review of psychiatric cases had strong effects on the length of hospital stays, which fell by about 47% (compared to about 24% for all hospital cases). Finally, Rosenthal (1999) assessed the impact of a change in provider-payment arrangements from a discounted fee-for-service system to a case rate within a carve-out plan. She estimated that a 25% reduction in patient visits could be attributed to the new incentive. This study indicates the powerful impact that a single financial incentive may have on the use of services.

In sum, because the information on particular mechanisms is quite limited, the vast majority of what is known about the quantitative effect of managed behavioral health carve-outs on utilization and costs is nonspecific.

CONCLUDING OBSERVATIONS

The landscape of the delivery of mental health and substance abuse services is dramatically different in the year 2000 than it was in 1990. The delivery system has come to be populated by managed care organizations, and the carve-out model has come to dominate the delivery of behavioral health care in the private sector. The carve-out is also of central importance in the public sector. Nevertheless, fear of change, threats to entrenched economic interests, and concern for vulnerable patient populations have all led to calls for oversight and regulation of the MBHOs that are exerting control over the resources for MH/SA care. The task of research on managed behavioral health care is to provide information for policymakers interested in using or regulating the use of managed behavioral health carve-outs.

Research on managed behavioral health carve-outs has expanded quickly in the 1990s, and our understanding of carve-outs has advanced dramatically. The basic facts about these MBHOs have been established. The basic structural features of carve-outs have been described. The economic functions of MBHOs are understood. The first-order effects of managed behavioral health carve-outs have been estimated in a number of case studies. There is substantial agreement about their impact on specialty MH/SA services and spending.

There remains a variety of fundamental questions that need to be addressed. What is the net impact of managed behavioral health carve-outs on total MH/SA spending across all settings in which MH/SA care is delivered? How are the delivery of primary care and the use of prescription drugs affected by introducing a managed behavioral health carve-out to an insured population? Are MBHOs sensitive to the different needs and preferences of patients concerning the treatment they receive and where they receive it? What is the effect of carve-out plans on the quality of care?

A critical issue that needs more work is the implication of the redrawn boundaries of specialty versus primary care in the delivery of MH/SA services. As noted earlier, a significant proportion of patients with MH/SA problems is seen in the general medical sector. In response to such reports and to evidence that MH/SA problems are not recognized (and if recognized, inadequately treated) by primary care physicians, there has been a large-scale effort to train these physicians to assist more effectively in the management of MH/SA patients. There has been little discussion, however, about the appropriate interaction of primary care physicians and managed care carve-out plans, or about how to structure payments to primary care physicians for their role in the care of MH/SA patients.

Finally, for public and private purchasers to make good choices on behalf of the populations they serve, we need a much fuller understanding of the impact of specific features of managed behavioral health carve-out programs. Purchasers must make choices about how to organize the procurement of managed behavioral health services, how to pay MBHOs, and what constraints should be placed on network design. Purchasers also need to know which utilization-management and clinical protocols are worthwhile, and how data should flow between the primary care sector, the carve-out plans, and the pharmacy plans. In order to advance, research will have to move beyond the case study of a global change in managed MH/SA care. Studies will need to focus on more specific variations in the design of managed behavioral health carve-outs by using data that integrates information on health care, MH/SA care, and prescription drug treatment.

REFERENCES

Berndt, E. R., Frank, R. G., & McGuire, T. G. (1997). Alternative insurance arrangements and the treatment of depression: What are the facts? *American Journal of Managed Care, 3* (2), 243–250.

Bloom, J. R., Hu, T. W., Wallace, N., Cuffel, B., Hausmann, J., & Scheffer, R. (1998). Mental health costs and outcomes under alternative capitation system in Colorado: Early results. *Journal of Mental Health Policy and Economic, 1* (1), 3–14.

Brisson, A. S., Frank, R. G., Berenbaum, P. A., & Gazmararian, J. A. (2000). Changes in a MBHC carve-out: Impact on MH/SA spending and utilization. Unpublished working paper.

Burns, B. J., Teagle, S. E., Schwartz, M., Angold, A., & Holtzman, A. (1999). Managed behavioral health care: A Medicaid carve-out for youth. *Health Affairs, 18* (5), 214–225.

Busch, S. H. (2000). *The impact of a carve-out on quality of care in treatment of depression.* Working paper, Harvard University.

Callahan, J. J., Jr., Shepard, D. S., Beinecke, R. H., Larson, M. J., & Cavanaugh, D. (1995). Mental health and substance abuse treatment in managed care: The Massachusetts Medicaid experience. *Health Affairs, 14* (3):173–184.

Christianson J. B., Manning, W., Lurie, N., Stoner, T. J., Gray, D. Z., Popkin, M., & Marriott, S. (1995). Utah's prepaid mental health plan: The first year. *Health Affairs, 14* (3), 150–172.

Dickey, B., Norton, E., Normand, S. L., Azeni, H., & Fisher, W. (1998). Managed mental health experience in Massachusetts. In D. Mechanic (Ed.), *Managed behavioral health care: Current realities and future potential* (pp. 115–122). San Francisco: Jossey-Bass.

Frank, R. G., & McGuire, T. G. (1997). Savings from a Medicaid carve-out for mental health and substance abuse care. *Psychiatric Services, 48* (9), 1147–1152.

Frank, R. G., & McGuire, T. G. (2000). Economics and mental health. In J. P. Newhouse & A. T. Culyer (Eds.), *The Handbook of Health Economics.* Amsterdam: North Holland Press.

Frank, R. G., Salkever, D. S., & Sharfstein, S. S. (1991). A look at rising mental health insurance costs. *Health Affairs, 10* (2), 116–124.

Goldman, W., McCulloch, J., & Sturm, R. (1998). Costs and use of mental health services before and after managed care. *Health Affairs, 17* (2), 40–52.

Grazier, K. L., Eselius, L. L., Hu, T., Shore, K. K., & G'sell, W. A. (1999). Effects of a mental health carve-out on use, costs and payers: A four-year study. *Journal of Behavioral Health Services and Research, 26* (4), 381–389.

Huskamp, H. A. (1998). How managed care carve-out plans affect spending for episodes of treatment. *Psychiatric Services, 49* (12), 1559–1562.

IMS Health Inc. (1998). Unpublished data (on file with author).

Lehman, A. F., & Steinwachs, D. M. (1998). Patterns of usual care for schizophrenia: Initial results from the schizophrenia PORT. *Schizophrenia Bulletin, 24,* 1–10.

Ma, C., & McGuire, T. G. (1998). Costs and incentives in a mental health carve-out. *Health Affairs, 17* (2), 53–69.

Ma, C., & McGuire, T. G. (1999). *Network effects in managed behavioral health care.* Working paper, Boston University.

Manning, W. G., Liu, C., Stoner, T. J., Gray, D. Z., Lurie, N., Popkin, M., & Christianson, J. B. (1999). Outcomes for Medicaid beneficiaries with schizophrenia under a pre-paid mental health carve-out. *Journal of Behavioral Health Services and Research, 26* (4), 442–450.

Mechanic, D. (1989). The evolution of mental health services and mental health services research. In C. Taube, D. Mechanic, & A. Hohmann (Eds.), *The future of mental health services research.* Washington, DC: U.S. Government Printing Office.

Merrick, E. (1998). Treatment of major depression before and after implementation of a behavioral health carve-out plan. *Psychiatric Services, 49* (11), 1563–1567.

Norton, E. C., Lindrooth, R. C., & Dickey, B. (1997). Cost shifting in a mental health carve-out for the AFDC population. *Health Care Financing Review, 18* (3), 95–108.

Norton, E. C., Lindrooth, R. C., & Dickey, B. (1999). Cost-shifting in managed care. *Mental Health Services Research, 1* (3), 185–196.

Novartis. (1999a). *Fact and Figures 1999.*

Novartis. (1999b). *Pharmacy Benefit Report: 1999 Facts and Figures.*

Rosenthal, M. B. (1999). Risk sharing in managed behavioral health care. *Health Affairs, 16* (5), 204–213.

Satcher, D. (1999). *Mental health: A report of the surgeon general.* Rockville, MD: National Institute of Mental Health.

Stoner, T., Manning, W. G., & Christianson, J. (1997). Expenditures for mental health services in Utah's prepaid mental health plan. *Health Care Financing Review, 18* (3), 73–93.

Sturm, R. (1999a). Cost and quality trends under managed care: Is there a learning curve in behavioral health carve-out plans? *Journal of Health Economics, 18* (5), 593–604.

Sturm, R. (1999b). Tracking changes in behavioral health services: How have carve-outs changed care? *Journal of Behavioral Services and Research, 26* (4), 360–371.

Sturm, R., Goldman, W., & McCulloch, J. (1998). Mental health and substance abuse parity: A case study of Ohio's state employee's program. *Journal of Mental Health Policy and Economics 1,* 129–134.

Well, K., et al. (1996). *Caring for depression.* Cambridge, MA: Harvard University Press.

Wickizer, T. M., & Lessler, D. (1998). Effects of utilization management on patterns of hospital care among privately insured adults. *Medical Care, 36* (11), 1545–1554.

Chapter 7

QUALITY MANAGEMENT

Sharon A. Shueman and Warwick G. Troy

This chapter provides an overview of quality management issues and activities in managed behavioral health care. Beginning with an historical overview, the chapter describes some significant precursors of current managed behavioral health programs. It includes a discussion of how quality management programs have expanded, especially within the last decade, from a primarily audit-focused orientation to one that embraces a much broader range of activities that provide the tools required to effect improvements in the quality of care. The chapter presents a discussion of the kinds of activities typical of managed behavioral health, and of the contributions made by these activities to improving the care and services provided to consumers. A concluding section details the challenges confronting, and the potential promise of, quality management in managed behavioral health.

WHAT IS QUALITY MANAGEMENT?

The phrase *quality management* denotes, first, that the mechanisms and structures used in advancing the cause of quality within an organization are the product of a clear design or plan. A second characteristic of the quality management approach is that the application of an organization's plan is *constant*; the process involves a continuous cycle of applying measures for quality assessment, which are followed, in turn, by strategies for taking corrective actions based on the assessment findings. A third characteristic of the quality management approach is that it is *systemic:* it is integrated into all aspects of an organization's operations, and the responsibility for ensuring quality is "owned" by virtually everyone within the organization. It is this last aspect of the ongoing management of quality improvement that most clearly distinguishes current approaches from the earlier, mechanistic tradition of quality "assurance."

MANAGED BEHAVIORAL HEALTH CARE: "IN THE BEGINNING . . ."

The bulk of behavioral health services in the United States is provided through systems that are managed in some way. Typically, these systems take the form of managed behavioral health organizations (MBHOs), proprietary specialty companies that contract with employers and other purchasers of behavioral health care to ensure that consumers receive access to services that are considered, on the basis of operational criteria, to be necessary, appropriate, and of adequate quality. MBHOs play both intermediary and facilitator roles as part of a nexus between consumers and the providers of care. In this context, the term "managed" is used to signify both a planned and an integrated approach to services, one that involves varying degrees of direct and indirect control over providers. Such control is manifest through the establishment of guidelines that address various types of contingencies and that thereby affect how providers practice and how they document service encounters. The phrase "managed behavioral health" thus denotes the diverse mix of potential arrangements for the organization, financing, and provision of behavioral health services (Marquis & Long, 1999). Driving this array of different approaches is a commitment to service coordination, which is intended to bring operational coherence to behavioral health care.

Historically, formal efforts to assess and improve the quality of behavioral health services was predominantly limited to inpatient facilities and publicly funded, organized care settings such as community mental health centers. Within these service settings, demands for assessing and improving quality came from state and federal regulatory agencies, as well as from accrediting bodies, most notably the Joint

Commission for the Accreditation of Hospitals (JCAH, now JCAHO), which acted in a quasi-regulatory capacity. Because of the emphasis on compliance, the kinds of activities carried on in the name of quality within these settings tended to be mechanistic, retrospective, and isolated from service delivery. As a consequence, these compliance-related activities rarely had a consistently positive effect on the quality of services delivered. Moreover, such top-down compliance systems tended to have little effect on the practice patterns of providers.

In sites where most specialty outpatient behavioral health services were delivered–the offices of independent practitioners and small group practices–quality-focused activities were virtually unknown. Practitioners operating out of such sites were accountable to no external entity for the quality of services they provided. Furthermore, practitioners were, by and large, uninformed about even the most basic aspects of quality assessment and improvement. Few programs training behavioral health professionals attached much importance to such issues. And there was typically little in professional education and training that imbued practitioners with an appreciation for the role of objective self-evaluation in the cause of quality improvement.

In the 1970s, however, the regulatory environment began to change in the wake of important new initiatives by the Civilian Health and Medical Program of the Uniformed Services (CHAMPUS)–a federal entitlement program, under the Department of Defense, to provide health benefits to dependents of military personnel on active duty and also to military retirees. CHAMPUS beneficiaries received behavioral health services primarily through a network of independent practitioners, hospitals, and residential treatment centers (RTCs) for children, but the program was seen to have two sets of serious problems, both of which caught the attention of the U.S. Congress. The first involved widespread overutilization, poor quality of care, and, in some cases, flagrant abuse of children in CHAMPUS-sponsored RTCs. The second, not unrelated, set of problems was an alarming rate of cost increase in the program due to provider-driven overutilization (not only in RTCs, but also in other inpatient and outpatient behavioral health service settings). In certain geographic areas, more than 25% of CHAMPUS's entire services budget was consumed by behavioral health care.

Responding to these quality and cost problems, CHAMPUS instituted formal monitoring programs, using principles of peer review and aiming to ensure that services paid for by the program were necessary and appropriate. As quality management programs, these peer review activities were primitive, but they marked the first serious effort by a third-party entity to elicit accountability from independent practitioners. The prevailing reaction from the national community of providers to these CHAMPUS initiatives was extremely negative: providers' professional autonomy had been violated. Nevertheless, a precedent had been set: the federal government established a model under which a payer could make reimbursement contingent upon independent practitioners' supplying documentary evidence that the services they provided were necessary and appropriate.

Despite the early encounter with regulation under CHAMPUS, the implementation of quality management in behavioral health care has been much more recent and less common than in general health care. Of all providers, behavioral health practitioners have been the most resistant to external scrutiny of their services—let alone to the use of evidence-based guidelines. These same practitioners continue to be particularly hostile to organized efforts to impose management structures and processes on the delivery of services. The major professional associations in behavioral health have devoted significant resources to finding ways to return to the days when provider incomes were predictable, and the level of professional control, high. Perhaps what they are seeking is a return to the halcyon days when fee-for-service reimbursement prevailed.

The federal government's CHAMPUS experience of uncontrolled cost escalation in behavioral health was not unlike what would later be experienced by many employers and other third-party payers with respect to general health care. As a consequence, throughout the 1980s a number of entities sprang up to help purchasers stem the rate of cost increase. The mission of these organizations—some corporate, some not—was not quality improvement, but cost control through utilization review: a determination that services being paid for were necessary and appropriate.

As is now well-known, the interventions aimed at reducing inappropriate utilization were highly successful. This revolt of the payers against the wild escalation of health benefit costs yielded dramatically reduced health care premiums for many purchasers of care. With the focus on cost containment, managed care companies "delivered" for their clients, who, it must be stressed, were generally not seeking improvements in the quality of care as a concomitant or even secondary goal.

Over a period of years, practitioners and, eventually, consumers and purchasers became increasingly dissatisfied with what many perceived as an exclusive and draconian focus on cost control by MBHOs. In particular, these various constituencies perceived cost control as posing a significant threat to quality, and began to seek assurances that pressures to contain costs were not compromising quality (Iglehart, 1997). Over time, criteria for the business success of MBHOs increasingly included demonstrations not only of effectively controlling costs, but of delivering quality services. Very slowly, purchasers themselves came to regard successful quality management as value enhancing. Fortunately, the capital then available to the for-profit health care industry permitted acquisition of the resources necessary for the development both of formal programs focused on quality and of the adjunctive technologies of quality assessment and improvement.

Whether managed care companies were guilty of compromising quality by overzealous attempts to reduce utilization—and therefore costs—has not been definitively settled. Overutilization was generally recognized as a serious problem, as was the inappropriate use of intensive and highly restrictive levels of care. These utilization patterns not only were unnecessarily costly but, to the extent that they were clinically inappropriate, were themselves a threat to quality. In other words, reductions in the use of certain kinds of treatment, coupled with the use of more appropriate alternatives, led to an improvement in quality.

Regardless of the truth about cost versus quality, the perception that reducing costs compromised quality became entrenched, and by the early 1990s, payers were beginning to demand that MBHOs broaden their mission to include quality of care. By that time, however, the industry was already maturing; companies were expanding their focus to include, and increasing their expertise in, quality assessment and management. And at present there is a strong consensus among purchasers, payers, and consumers that efforts should be made to enhance the quality of care. As a consequence, the companies responsible for managing behavioral health care have come to be centrally concerned with issues of quality.

The Contributions of Accreditation

Corresponding to, and facilitated by, the growing demand by payers for accountability in behavioral health care, independent accrediting organizations have exerted an increasing influence on MBHOs. Their influence has been especially strong during in the last decade. Most notable among these organizations are the National Committee for Quality Assurance (NCQA) and the Joint Commission for the Accreditation of Healthcare Organizations (JCAHO). Both organizations have had a significant impact on the structure and process of health care delivery systems, as well as on the development of strategies for monitoring and improving quality.

The standards promulgated by these organizations (JCAHO, 1997; NCQA, 1999b) have extended the quality landscape by emphasizing that quality management should be understood within a broader organizational context—that is, that it be extended to include all aspects of the organization and its operations that have a direct impact on the consumers of health care. The development of such a systematic and inclusive approach had been supported by many practitioners and by most policy specialists (see, e.g., Berwick, 1989), but it was the growing influence of external accreditation organizations that led to the widespread adoption of this more inclusive approach.

A consequence of these developments has been the increasing standardization of ways that health care organizations operate and of how they report their performance. This standardization, in turn, has resulted in increased opportunities for purchasers of behavioral health services to select among suppliers on the basis of quality measures. Therein lies much of the promise of accreditation: not only to improve the quality of services provided, but also to allow purchasers and consumers to "comparison shop" for health services.

Accrediting bodies have been subject to criticism for being unduly focused on structure and process, and insufficiently focused on outcome. These organizations have become increasingly concerned, however, about quality improvement, in general, and about outcomes, in particular. This change reflects what is, perhaps, the biggest practice advance in quality management over the last several decades: stakeholders—including public and private payers, consumer groups and advocates, and state and federal regulatory agencies—have embraced external review with enthusiasm and have given special emphasis to assessing outcomes.

The View from the Quality Committee

From the perspective of professionals working day to day on ensuring quality within an MBHO, the changes in philosophy and in the approach to quality have required profound changes in both attitude and technical competence. A step back in time would show, for example, that matters of quality, once relegated to the quality committee (an entity of little status and less power), have now become central to the operation of all health care organizations, including MBHOs. Any organizational activity or structure that affects patients has become subject to quality monitoring and improvement. Quality indicators focus both on clinical variables and on service issues such as access to care and service systems' responsiveness to cultural differences. Indicators deal with factors as varied as timeliness of phone responses, accuracy of benefit information, and adequacy of other consumer communications; quality of the provider network; adherence to clinical practice guidelines; and adequacy and effectiveness of the complaints-and-appeal process.

Assuring quality once the primary responsibility of line staff (mostly nurses), with the oversight of an (often reluctant) physician—has increasingly come to be perceived as the responsibility of everyone within the organization, at all levels. Indeed, the driving force of the quality management program in many organizations is the board of directors or another high-level entity (for example, a quality council) directly accountable to the board. Moreover, instead of being marginalized within the organization and regarded as little more than a nuisance by practitioners, quality management is emerging as a fundamentally important activity, the success of which can have a significant impact on an organization's position in a fiercely competitive marketplace.

Finally, once conceptualized primarily as a series of relatively simple, episodic audit activities, the process of ensuring quality management (often referred to as "QM") has evolved to embrace a set of technically complex and ongoing activities. Successful implementation requires the expertise of professionals sophisticated in the use of management information systems, statistical analysis, services research, clinical epidemiology, and program development and evaluation. Table 1 contrasts characteristics of traditional quality-assurance programs with newer programs that reflect a quality management approach.

Table 1

**TRADITIONAL AND EMERGING CHARACTERISTICS OF QUALITY
MANAGEMENT IN MENTAL HEALTH SERVICES**

Traditional	*Emerging*
1. External	1. Internal, participatory
2. Regulatory	2. Proactive, "owned" from within
3. Ancillary, isolated from service delivery	3. Integrated within service delivery
4. Sole "expert"	4. Integrated team performance
5. Single stakeholder	5. Multiple stakeholders
6. Focus on finding and "fixing" problems	6. Focus on improvement
7. "Top-down," compliance-oriented	7. "Bottom-up" process "owned" by service system
8. Episodic	8. Continuous, ongoing
9. Retrospective	9. Concurrent
10. Ad hoc, non-theoretical	10. Systematic, possessing a technology
11. Focus on "assuring" quality	11. Focus on management of quality

Not surprisingly, the emphasis on quality management and its attendant sophistication has spawned the development of an industry specializing in the creation of quality-enhancing systems and technologies. Taking advantage to these systems and technologies has increased costs for health care organizations despite the lack of compelling evidence that these additional expenditures are generating substantial benefits either to the organizations themselves or to the consumers of health care.

CONTRIBUTIONS OF MBHOS TO QUALITY

Managed behavioral health programs, as developed by MBHOs, have initiated many changes in behavioral health services–changes that are said to have resulted in improved quality at the level of service operations. There have been changes, for example, in the types and level of care delivered; in the way it is delivered, documented, monitored, and evaluated; and in the role of the consumer as conceptualized in services planning and evaluation. Many of the most important MBHO-sponsored program initiatives are direct outgrowths or byproducts of what is, in effect, an enhanced technology of clinical management: a "science of practice." This enhanced technology of management is itself the byproduct of the *virtual delivery system* that was developed by large MBHOs as they sought to bring coherence and consistency to the service-delivery process.

The virtual delivery system comprises the structures and processes that have been superimposed on the heterogeneous networks of independent clinicians, group practices, and institutional providers that deliver most specialty behavioral health services. For example, MBHOs promulgate clinical standards, implement strategies for measuring and monitoring care, encourage interdisciplinary communication, and set reporting requirements. All such initiatives are aimed at reducing variation in service delivery and at facilitating the reporting of critical process and outcome indicators. It is these virtual systems that have enabled MBHOs to respond to the accountability imperatives of stakeholders, and that have consequently been the driving force behind MBHO-related innovations in clinical-management technology and in service planning and delivery.

A Developing Technology of Clinical Management

It is in through the development of a technology of clinical management that MBHOs have most visibly exerted their influence over clinical practice. Because behavioral health treatment has been characterized by a lack of precision and consequently by a lack of replicability, it has typically been difficult not only evaluate outcomes, but to define the process of care itself. The situation is changing, however, as a result of the development of the clinical technologies that are usually known as "practice guidelines." These empirically derived guidelines define the desired treatment process, enable the establishment of indicators that can be used to determine whether practitioners are implementing the appropriate process, and allow the measurement of outcomes based on standardized criteria. Four critical components of an enhanced technology of clinical management are considered below.

1. *Empirically supported treatment protocols.* "Evidence-based" clinical procedures, or practice guidelines (Eddy, 1990a, 1990b; Shueman & Lane, 2000), are at the heart of the new technology of clinical management. They represent a critical example of the potential gains to be made from the development and systematic use of appropriate mechanisms for the translation of clinical outcomes and research findings into replicable therapeutic procedures accessible to individual providers and large care systems alike.

   MBHOs have adopted guidelines—some developed by the MBHOs themselves, some by others—and distributed them to practitioners, usually as part of an educational strategy. The companies subsequently monitor clinicians' adherence to selected aspects of the guidelines in an attempt to increase the level of compliance. Such efforts have played a significant role in raising practitioners' awareness of the importance of evidence-based approaches to clinical practice. To date, the guidelines have also contributed in a limited way to reducing variation in the relevant aspects of clinical practice.

2. *Treatment monitoring.* The use of simple measurements and of treatment-planning methods (such as goal-attainment scaling, which was once considered an arcane, behaviorist approach used only in community mental health centers) are becoming routine as more organizations respond to calls for accountability. These and other data-based strategies may be tailored to the needs of the service system. In addition, health services researchers, often with the support of the managed care industry, have emphasized the development and use of standardized measures for monitoring the process and outcome of treatment (Lambert, Heufner, & Reisinger, 2000). Although these measurement tools have been difficult to implement in the real world of managed behavioral health service delivery, they have the potential to facilitate comparisons of quality across service settings.

   The process of implementation presents a variety of vexing and complex challenges. Behavioral health practitioners, for example, are generally reluctant to embrace the tools of science-based practice. The source of this reluctance, we believe, is to be found in the inadequacies of professional training programs: in the presentation and interpretation of treatment modalities, in student selection, and in negative attitudes that develop toward performance monitoring (Broskowski, 1995; Troy, 1994).

3. *The use of automated information systems.* As integrated systems of care evolve, the use both of electronic media for case tracking and of management information systems is becoming increasingly common (Meredith, Bair, & Ford, 2000). Such systems, if they are to be useful and effective, must continuously provide the mix of information required for clinical management. Such data, appropriately used, provide the substantive basis for monitoring various aspects of the treatment process, as well as progress toward the achievement of designated outcomes. The availability of such flexible systems will facilitate the development of metrics for better monitoring the process and outcomes of care, and of benchmarks for judging relative quality.

4. *Clinical benchmarking.* "Best practices" approaches are increasingly common in health care. They provide a comparative framework for providers—and especially for health care systems—to assess how well they are performing. Currently, benchmarks tend to address the process of care. A common example of this type of benchmark is the percentage of patients discharged from acute psychiatric care who subsequently receive behavioral health outpatient services within a specified period after discharge (NCQA, 1999a). As the use of standardized outcome measures becomes more widespread, it will be possible to establish benchmarks defining the desired outcome—and not just the process—of treating specific disorders.

Applications of the Technology

The application of these new technologies has enabled MBHOs to define innovative strategies that have had a marked impact on service delivery. What follows are some of the ways in which the quality of services has been affected.

Changing the Service Profile

Possibly the most visible impact of MBHOs has been on the service profile of the U.S. behavioral health system (a service profile is defined by the types, levels, and amounts of service delivered and by the settings in which service delivery occurs). In particular, MBHOs have been responsible for the decreased use of traditional, institutional, intensive, and high-cost services. These services have been replaced by less intensive, less costly, community-based, and–most importantly–empirically supported alternatives. Examples include:

- reduction in the incidence of acute inpatient hospitalization and a corresponding increase in use of alternatives such as intensive outpatient care and day treatment
- reduction in the average length of stay for acute care hospitalization, coupled with the increased use of alternatives such as day and intensive outpatient treatment
- routine use of outpatient treatment programs for substance abuse, in lieu of standard 28-day inpatient or residential programs
- use of community based "wrap-around" services in lieu of residential treatment for emotionally disturbed children and adolescents
- use of goal-focused, time-sensitive outpatient therapy in lieu of open-ended, uncovering treatment

Elimination of Clinical Outliers

The application of the principles of treatment monitoring and reporting, as discussed above, has resulted in elimination of the most egregious cases of poor quality care, commonly known as "outliers." In particular, an outlier is a clinical practice substantially at variance with a mean or norm (in statistical terms, greater than 1.5 standard deviations from the mean). Simple examples of outliers are an acute hospital stay of 60 days, daily outpatient psychotherapy, and failure to evaluate for antidepressant medication a patient with a long history of recurrent major depression. In any single case, a clinical outlier may be justified based on the specific circumstances of the patient and on his or her particular life situation. Nevertheless, a pattern of such variations–especially in relation to a particular practitioner or treatment program–is more likely to be an indication of inappropriate, poor quality care. MBHOs' case-management function, coupled with the information systems typically used by these organizations, makes it relatively simple to identify such cases and to intervene when necessary.

Interprofessional Communication to Achieve Continuity and Coordination of Care.

In an effort to improve continuity and coordination of care, MBHOs implement structures intended to facilitate communication between practitioners. These practitioners may be two behavioral health professionals who are serving the same patient (for example, a psychiatrist monitoring medications and a nonmedical professional providing psychotherapy). They may be two behavioral health practitioners serving the same patient at different points in time (for example, an inpatient practitioner handing over a case to an outpatient therapist). Or they may be a behavioral health practitioner and a nonpsychiatric medical professional (for example, a treating psychologist and a primary care physician). The focus of communication may be to ensure a smooth transition from one type or level of care to another or, more generally, to ensure the all relevant practitioners are working together in the context of a unified and rational treatment plan designed to achieve desired outcomes. MBHOs have mandated such communications within the limitations imposed by patient confidentiality and consent.

Functional Treatment Planning

One of the earliest contributions of MBHOs was to require the use of "plain language" in the reporting of clinical encounters. Attempts to provide effective oversight in behavioral health care had long been stymied by practitioners' use of jargon that was based on their own theoretical orientations. MBHOs began to require providers to express plans in terms of patient functioning. Although not asking that practitioners adopt a strictly behavior-theoretic orientation, MBHOs did require them to express goals and progress in terms of patient behaviors. This modest development has increased the use of simple rating scales in assessing progress toward goals, while enhancing patients' understanding of, and involvement in, their own treatment.

Facilitating Interdisciplinary Collaboration

One effect of managed behavioral health care has been to accentuate the differences in skill sets across practitioner types–particularly between medical and nonmedical professionals. MBHOs tend to perceive behavioral health professionals somewhat more as specialists than these professionals often see themselves. For example, most psychiatrists regard themselves as skilled in the provision of verbal psychotherapy. MBHOs, however, often view psychiatrists as specialists in medication evaluation and monitoring—and not in the provision of psychotherapy, which is considered the domain of nonmedical practitioners, namely, psychologists, social workers, and counselors.

Under such a specialist approach, it is incumbent upon practitioners to understand their own role in relation to those of their colleagues. Nonmedical professionals therefore need to have a basic understanding of psychoactive medications and of the kinds of clinical situations that warrant a consultation with a psychiatrist. By the same token, psychiatrists need to be able to recognize cases in which a dual approach to treatment (medication and psychotherapy) may be appropriate. And all professionals need to acquire the skills necessary to develop and maintain ongoing consultative relationships in the interest of patient outcomes. Ultimately, the success of such a collaborative approach requires putting the welfare of patients ahead of the welfare of practitioners, even—and especially—those who resist seeking consultation out of a fear of "losing" their patients to another professional.

MBHOs often provide educational opportunities to help practitioners understand issues related to interprofessional collaboration. For example, one MBHO hosted a series of workshops for their nonmedical-network practitioners that was focused on the use of psychoactive medications. Another company hosted a similar series of sessions focused on the recognition and specialty treatment of substance abuse. The goal of such educational programs is to improve practitioners' capacity to recognize the need for specialty care, as well as to facilitate effective collaboration with specialists.

Profiling Providers

The information systems available to MBHOs allow them to develop a "picture," constructed from aggregated data, of a practitioner's or treatment program's practice patterns. These pictures are usually referred to as "provider profiles" (Shueman & Lane, 2000). Depending on the nature of the database, a picture might include: the distribution of diagnoses that practitioners assign to their patients, duration and frequency of outpatient treatment episodes; cost of treatment episodes; patient outcomes as reflected by standardized measures; patients' self-ratings of outcomes; and patients' satisfaction ratings. These profiles are usually used for educational purposes or in a professional-development context to inform practitioners about their own performance on indicators deemed important by the MBHO, payers, or consumers. In addition, practitioners may be given comparative data reflecting the profiles of other practitioners, which allows them to evaluate their performance against that of their peers. It has been shown that providing feedback through peer data is an effective strategy for changing practitioner behaviors.

A Focus on Customer Service

With the advent of managed care organizations and the systems they create has come an increased emphasis on quality of customer service. Variables such as ease of making clinical appointments, timeliness of phone response, and handling of complaints and appeals have come to be given equal status with clinical quality. Although clinicians have traditionally regarded such variables as inconsequential, consumers and payers regard them as critically important. These variables also tend to be relatively simple for MBHOs to monitor and report, and easy for consumers and payers to understand. Hence, MBHOs have come to favor these variables as important indicators of their own performance. Moreover, accreditation bodies commonly include such variables among their standards and criteria.

Protecting Consumers from Unqualified Professionals

All MBHOs maintain processes for credentialing individual and institutional providers who contract with them as part of their service networks. Initially, a determination is made whether providers satisfy the minimum requirements for network membership. Requirements typically relate to education, training, professional license, malpractice history, and professional liability coverage. MBHOs also conduct ongoing monitoring of the National Practitioner Data Bank, state licensing boards, and other regulatory agencies to ensure that providers maintain their licenses in good standing. As a quality improvement tool, this kind of activity is a very blunt instrument, but it does offer consumers some level of protection against manifestly unscrupulous, incompetent, or impaired professionals.

Expanded Role for Consumers

MBHOs attempt to expand the role of consumers in the treatment relationship. Of the two most common methods, the first is through mandating patients' direct involvement in the development of treatment plans. A patient's involvement would typically be signified by his or her signature on the treatment plan. The plan would either be submitted to the MBHO or maintained in the patient's record. In the latter case, the record would be subject to audit by the MBHO, and patient involvement would be one of the indicators audited. The second common type of involvement is in the evaluation of services. Sometimes the patient rates his or her own progress or outcome on measures mandated by the MBHO, but, more commonly, patients complete patient-satisfaction surveys. These survey instruments are often unique to the MBHOs that develop them, but the Agency for Health Care Policy and Research has recently coordinated a national effort to develop a standardized instrument for general health care (AHCPR, 1997). A similar survey instrument for behavioral health is in development.

What Hath Quality Management Wrought?

We are currently faced with a health system in transition. This transition is characterized by movement away from a fee-for-service, independent practice model and toward a more systemic approach to service delivery and monitoring. Modern quality management, an integral component of the modern health care system, is a result of the evolution of organized approaches to quality assessment and improvement that are gradually bringing to behavioral health care common standards, a common language, and common ways of measuring what is done. With these changes are coming new attitudes toward the importance of accountability, the need for coordination of services within the behavioral health system (as well as between the behavioral health and general health systems), the importance of consumers' role in the treatment relationship, and the value of an evidence-based approach to practice. Although it may be disingenuous to claim that these innovations have resulted in meaningful improvement in the quality of behavioral health care, it must be acknowledged that they have provided us with the tools to work toward this goal.

FUTURE CHALLENGES

Even the most committed advocates of managed behavioral health care would concede that in the last decade, the pace of change has created a chaotic behavioral health services environment, and that this chaos has affected providers, consumers, and payers. It is uncertain what the overall impact of MBHO systems has been on quality improvement in behavioral health services. Nevertheless, these systems have induced critical changes within a clinical technology of practice. The next step–modifying practice itself–is a work in progress and will substantially depend upon the extent to which training programs themselves begin to demonstrate some accountability.

The Cost of Quality

The imperatives imposed on managed behavioral health service-delivery systems by external accreditation systems are increasingly affecting the topology of behavioral health services delivery and, in particular, helping to define both quality and the nature of programs that monitor and improve quality. NCQA and JCAHO have made a concerted effort to collaborate with large payers, consumer groups, state and federal governments, and health plans themselves to chart future directions. At the same time, these two organizations have been subject to legitimate criticism–most notably from the health care industry–for failing to recognize the realities of the health care marketplace. In essence, they have been faulted for creating burdensome, costly systems that contribute to health care inflation without demonstrable evidence that these systems have improved outcomes for consumers. That is, accreditation entities have been requiring organizations to make substantial investments of human and financial resources to demonstrate adherence to–let it be said–essentially unverified standards. The costs of these formal quality management systems are ultimately passed on to payers and consumers. Whether these customers will be willing or able to absorb such costs in the interest of uncertain improvements in quality is a question that remains unanswered.

The Stability of Service Systems

A serious challenge to managing quality in behavioral health care is the pervasive instability of MBHOs throughout the 1990s. Mergers, acquisitions, and insolvency have resulted in constant changes, both for consumers and for providers. For consumers, the consequences of this instability range from the irritating to the burdensome. For example, a merger or insolvency may require patients to change practitioners or to learn anew how to access services through the new managed care organization. For practitioners, instability means adapting to new documentation and reporting requirements, utilization-review guidelines, and expectations about adherence to practice guidelines. It also may require forging new working relationships with the MBHO's utilization-review and case-management staff.

Instability also presents difficult challenges for the MBHOs themselves. Changes in the system—such as outcome measures and reporting requirements—make it more difficult for MBHOs to maintain adequate data-collection strategies and management information systems. Instability makes it difficult for MBHOs to monitor outcomes over an extended period of time, and to promote effective population-based approaches to prevention and to patient education.

The Role of Provider Organizations

MBHOs are increasingly recognizing how important it is, for the purpose of providing quality care, that critical treatment decisions be made as close as possible to the point of the clinical transaction. As a consequence, MBHOs are more often pushing the utilization-management decisions—as well as financial risk—down to the provider (usually provider group) level. At the same time, MBHOs are adding to the burden of those same providers by giving them responsibility for monitoring the quality and outcome of the services they deliver.

To respond to this strategy of devolution, provider organizations are being forced to develop increased expertise in the theory and technology of quality management. For many, it is a formidable burden to find the human and financial resources necessary to respond to the managed care companies. Although MBHOs do often offer technical assistance and support, it is probably unrealistic to expect that this type of external support and consultation will effectively compensate for the historical lack of relevant expertise within provider organizations.

MBHOs' program initiatives to improve the quality of behavioral health services for its members have been highly diverse. They vary in nature, intensity, and consistency of implementation. The impact of this heterogeneous set of interventions varies with the procedures required by the MBHO and with the kind of relationships it maintains with its cooperating networks of providers and facilities. The impact is likely to be greater if an MBHO strives to develop partnerships with its provider network. The impact is also enhanced if the MBHO is seen by its providers as being committed to a collaborative, long-term relationship.

As may be imagined, managed care companies also vary greatly as to how they conceive of any particular quality management task (for example, whether network development is deemed a strategic priority, and how collaboration is operationally defined)—which will itself have an impact on implementation. Also affecting the impact of quality management initiatives are the success of MBHOs in obtaining "buy-in" from providers and provider groups, and the manner in which MBHOs go about the development process. Although many MBHOs have promised true partnerships, few have delivered on that promise.

A Few Paradoxes of Managed Behavioral Health Care

In concluding, we choose to highlight the following discontinuities—or paradoxes—that challenge the field of managed behavioral health care.

1. The quality of behavioral health services has, after decades of neglect, come to be valued by the purchasers and consumers of these services. Nevertheless, the provider community is severely lagging in its operational commitment to quality improvement. The progress made in quality improvement will be slowed to the extent that providers do not embrace quality as an essential target in their everyday professional lives.

2. Payers and purchasers perceive a focus on quality as "value-added." Nevertheless, most have failed up until now to come up with the additional funding required to purchase a value-added product. With few exceptions, MBHOs still face demands for continued cost cutting in behavioral health services. Ultimately, purchasers will pay for additional quality only if it is demonstrably cost-effective for them.

3. Many MBHOs that seek to remain competitive feel as though they have no choice but to become accredited. Nevertheless, the accreditation organizations themselves continue to view the accreditation process as voluntary on the part of the MBHOs.

4. More than 30 years ago the medical cost-offset potential of targeted behavioral health interventions was apparent (Cummings & VandenBos, 1981). Moreover, the environment created by MBHOs–in particular, their emphasis on interprofessional collaboration and their capacity to manage data–may very well provide the necessary basis for realizing the potential of cost offsets. Nevertheless, MBHOs have yet to demonstrate any consistent ability to capture such assets.

5. Although quality and outcome measures have been accorded increasing prominence and significance by purchasers, payers, and consumer groups, professional education and training programs across the health professions have substantially failed to address these issues in a meaningful way. Achieving the requisite changes in professional education and training may be the greatest challenge facing organizations attempting to manage care in the interest of quality improvement.

6. Figuring prominently in professional discourse in health care is the concept of health care as a continuum of services, yet the bulk of behavioral health services remains separate from general health care–carved out and operationally marginalized.

7. Primary behavioral health care still awaits its operational mode. Absent the diffusion of this concept, the discontinuities that mark behavioral health services will continue.

8. Population-based approaches to prevention and health promotion in behavioral health remain rare, even though such approaches might help MHBOs to address problems concerning fragmentation in funding and access to care, and improve the marketability of their services.

The above (quasi) paradoxes are characteristic of any complex institutional setting that is in rapid flux, as is clearly the case for the organization, financing, and provision of behavioral health services in the United States. Fortunately, the fog that has so long obscured the quality landscape in behavioral health care has lifted, and the availability of useful, valid, and reliable mechanisms for the assessment and management of quality has never been greater.

If MBHOs are ever to realize the contribution they are capable of making to behavioral health care, as well as to other health services, then they must aggressively adopt a proactive stance with respect to all aspects of quality—its measurement, its management, and its improvement. We believe that the adoption and maintenance of such a stance will signal the maturity of the field and have a pervasive, beneficial impact on health care and its consumers. Further, despite the checkered history of managed behavioral health care—which ranges from wrong-headed decisions and poor provider and consumer acceptance, at one extreme, to productive system-oriented innovation, at the other—the road through the quality landscape of health care continues to be traveled far more frequently and longer by MBHOs than by any other voyagers. In such difficult and chaotic times, that is a signal accomplishment.

POSTSCRIPT:
ACCOUNTABILITY IN PROFESSIONAL TRAINING

We continue to harbor significant misgivings about the academic training community's lack of enduring commitment to the incorporation of quality imperatives, principles, and mechanisms into professional education and training. The resulting professional attitudes continue to undercut provider-MBHO relationships, impede the development of integrated systems, and hinder progress toward the realization of outcome-focused approaches in behavioral health treatment. Ultimately, of course, these attitudes detract from professionalism in the field and compromise health care itself. Consumers, stakeholders, the public at large, and the provider community are all shortchanged by a disinclination of the behavioral health professions to engage in the serious consideration of training reform. Our misgivings are the greater since the academic community has made signal contributions to the science of practice and has contributed impressively to the foundation for the developing technology of clinical management that, as we have discussed, holds out so much promise for improving both general health and behavioral health services.

The principles of quality improvement tell us that quality management and care is not best achieved by compliance-driven, top-down systems such as accreditation—despite the latter's crucial role in diffusing innovations. Quality management and care must ultimately emerge as a strategic product of professional teams, members of which own both the mission and the development process. And prelicensure professional education and training is where the critical normative base to drive and sustain this endeavor must be induced. Continuing education is too late: at that point the task becomes one of reeducation, which ultimately no more than a stopgap.

Within a broader perspective, the major stumbling block to the emergence of a quality-driven behavioral health profession is the prevailing ethos surrounding what it is to be a professional. There is, for example, an ongoing conflict between individual professional autonomy and interdisciplinary, consultative teamwork. Similarly, behavioral health professionals continue to align themselves with personal health services versus a population-based approach. This professional ethos must be reframed and surmounted if the behavioral health field—in all its diversity—is to identify with public needs, the amelioration of distress and disability, and the promotion of behavioral health at the level of the community and beyond.

The key here is the willingness of the behavioral health professions to claim responsibility—collectively as professional groups and individually as facility staff, trainers, supervisors, and educators. Such responsibility—across all aspects of care planning, delivery, and evaluation—is at the very core of an accountability that must be taught, modeled, and formally assessed.

The challenge confronting the behavioral health professions is daunting, and in this context it is perhaps no surprise that progress has been slow—and disappointing. Nevertheless, behavioral health professionals must find it distressing that quality has been operationalized not so much by the provider community itself, but by proxy—by the MBHOs and accreditation bodies that were forced, in effect, to inject both structure and substance into quality management, an area in which both characteristics had previously been lacking. The behavioral health professions surely need to engage in a pandisciplinary Flexnerian inquiry, which should surely work to the advantage not only of these professions themselves, but of the general public and the wider community of stakeholders in the delivery of behavioral health care.

REFERENCES

Agency for Health Care Policy and Research. (1997). *CAHPS: Health care quality information from the consumer perspective* (AHCPR Publication No. 97-0012). Rockville, MD: Author.

Berwick, D. M. (1989). Continuous improvement as an ideal in health care. *New England Journal of Medicine, 320,* 53–56.

Broskowski, A. T. (1995). The evolution of health care: Implications for the training and careers in psychology. *Professional Psychology: Research and Practice, 26* (2), 156–162.

Cummings, N. A., & VandenBos, G. R. (1981). The twenty years Kaiser-Permanente experience with psychotherapy and medical utilization: Implications for national health policy and national health insurance. *Health Policy Quarterly, 1,* 159–175.

Eddy, D. (1990a). Anatomy of a decision. *Journal of the American Medical Association, 263,* 441–443.

Eddy, D. (1990b). Practice policies: What are they? *Journal of the American Medical Association, 263,* 877–880.

Iglehart, J. K. (1997). The National Committee for Quality Assurance. In J. P. Kassirer & M. Angell (Eds.), *Quality of care: Selections from the New England Journal of Medicine* (pp. 74–75). Waltham, MA: Massachusetts Medical Society,.

Joint Commission on Accreditation of Healthcare Organizations. (1997). *Comprehensive accreditation manual for managed behavioral health care.* Oakbrook Terrace, IL: Author.

Lambert, M. J., Huefner, J. C., & Reisinger, C. W. (2000). Quality improvement: Current research in outcome management. In G. Stricker, W. G. Troy, & S. A. Shueman (Eds.), *Handbook of quality management in behavioral health* (pp. 95–110). New York: Kluwer Academic/Plenum Publishers.

Marquis, M. S., & Long, S. H. (1999). Trends in managed care and managed competition, 1993–1997. *Health Affairs, 18* (6), 75–88.

Meredith, R. L., Bair, S. L., & Ford, G. R. (2000). Information management in clinical decision making: The use of computers in behavioral health. In G. Stricker, W. G. Troy, & S. A. Shueman (Eds.), *Handbook of quality management in behavioral health* (pp. 53–94). New York: Kluwer Academic/Plenum Publishers.

National Committee on Quality Assurance. (1999a). *HEDIS 1999.* Washington, DC: Author.

National Committee on Quality Assurance. (1999b). *Surveyor guidelines for the accreditation of managed behavioral healthcare organizations.* Washington, DC: Author.

Shueman, S. A., & Lane, N. E. (2000). Provider profiling: Assessing provider characteristics, performance, and products. In G. Stricker, W. G. Troy, & S. A. Shueman (Eds.), *Handbook of quality management in behavioral health* (pp. 111–128). New York: Kluwer Academic/Plenum Publishers.

Troy, W. G. (1994). Developing and improving professional competencies. In S. A. Shueman, W. G. Troy, & S. L. Mayhugh (Eds.), *Managed behavioral health care: An industry perspective* (pp. 168–188). Springfield, IL: Charles C Thomas.

Troy, W. G., & Shueman, S. A. (2000). The changing health services environment and its impact on quality management in behavioral health. In G. Stricker, W. G. Troy, & S. A. Shueman (Eds.), *Handbook of quality management in behavioral health* (pp. 3–14). New York: Kluwer Academic/Plenum Publishers.

Chapter 8

ETHICS

James E. Sabin and Norman Daniels

Any useful reflection about the ethics of managed behavioral health care must start by defining the term *managed care* itself. That term has so many meanings, however, that it functions more like a Rorschach inkblot than a technical term. In this chapter we use *managed care* to refer to systems that provide health care to a population within a budget, thereby linking accountability for the quality of care with accountability for the financing of care.

When societies commit themselves to providing health care to individual members of a defined population within the limits of a defined budget, they create an agenda that requires management. The purpose of ethical managed behavioral health care is to provide high quality care to individuals within the constraints of reasonable resource limits. Individuals want and need good care. Purchasers of care want the most bang for their collective buck. Whether the population consists of the Medicaid enrollees of a state, the members of Kaiser Permanente, or the employees of a self-insured company, the central ethical issue for managed behavioral health programs is how best to balance individual and collective interests in the resource allocation process.

Americans are worried about whether they can trust managed care organizations to conduct this balancing process in an ethical manner. When a nationwide survey asked a random sample of adults if they

Note: The authors thank the Greenwall Foundation and Robert Wood Johnson Foundation Medicaid Managed Care Program for their support.

were "worried that your health plan would be more concerned about saving money than about [providing] the best treatment for you if you are sick," 61% enrolled in "heavy managed care" plans, but only 34% of those in "traditional" plans, said they were somewhat or very worried. While 72% of the sample agreed that managed care savings "[help] health insurance companies to earn more profits," only 49% believed that that these savings also "[make] health care more affordable for people like you" (Blendon et al., 1998). David Mechanic–the leading student of trust in the U.S. health care system–and Marsha Rosenthal (1999, p. 283) observed that as of 1999, "managed care organizations are in the midst of firestorm of public outrage over their restrictions on the delivery of care." The *Journal of Health Politics, Policy and Law* devoted an entire 400-page issue in 1999 to "the managed care backlash."

This well-documented backlash is a response to the managed care system in its entirety–not specifically to managed behavioral health care. There is no reason to believe, however, that managed behavioral health is immune to this visceral public reaction. In this chapter we try to present a framework for understanding how managed behavioral health systems can achieve more trust in the midst of societal negativism about the very mention of managed care.

Within the broad definition of managed behavioral health care as a system whose purpose is to provide high quality care to individuals within the constraints of reasonable resource limits, we distinguish three levels at which these systems address resource allocation issues. Each level has its own distinctive ethical challenge.

A. *Purchasers and the question of parity.* Purchasers–primarily Medicare, Medicaid, and employers–must decide how much of the health care dollar to invest in the behavioral sector. This question must be seen as ethical in character because it turns on how much value the payer places on behavioral health care relative to other components of health care. Traditionally, behavioral care has been treated in a discriminatory manner, subjected to different kinds of limits than other sectors. The ultimate ethical question for purchasers is whether to give parity to behavioral care or to continue the long-standing pattern of discrimination.

B. *Setting behavioral health priorities.* Unless the funds available for the population are large enough to pay for any and every potentially beneficial behavioral intervention, choices must be made about priorities. Programs must decide questions like how much of the behavioral health care budget should go to the smaller number of patients with the most serious illnesses, as opposed to the larger number with less serious, but possibly more remediable, concerns. These questions are ultimately ethical ones because they turn on what value we attach to the alternative uses of resources within the behavioral sector. In the U.S. system these questions are largely issues of benefit and program design. Sometimes these questions play out in the contracting process, as when a state identifies the seriously mentally ill as its top priority or when an employer makes worker health and productivity its major concern. Other times the payer leaves the issue of setting priorities to the managed behavioral health program.

C. *Balancing the interests of individuals, the insured population, and other stakeholders.* Finally, within the overall behavioral budget and system of priorities, societies confront ethical questions about balancing the interests of individual patients in achieving maximum possible benefit regardless of cost, with the insured population's interest in making best use of the available resources for the group. This level involves clinical judgments about which interventions are effective and ethical judgments about whether the benefit is worth the cost. In the U.S. system these questions are largely ones about which interventions are judged to be "medically necessary" or "medically appropriate."

These three issues arise for any system that attends not to health care itself, but to finances. The issues are just as pressing for the government-run single-payer system in Canada or the National Health Service in the United Kingdom as they are for the market-driven U.S. approach to managing care. The issues are existential realities, not ethical crimes created by managed care. They reflect the three levels—macro, meso, and micro—at which societies must grapple with the "constructive tension" between *fidelity* to the needs and wishes of individual patients and *stewardship* of the resources made available for the health care of a population.

Over the past 10 to 20 years, we in the United States have turned to a market-based approach to managing care. The policy is intended to control health care costs and improve efficiency through the invisible hand of the market, without requiring divisive public deliberation about values. With the notable exception of Oregon, which fostered extensive public discussion and education about ethical concerns before implementing the Oregon Health Plan, U.S. political leadership has actually pretended that the managed care revolution would perpetuate traditional values and would produce change by value-neutral managerial techniques!

The tremendous backlash against managed care arises in significant measure from what can only be called a national health care strategy founded on make-believe. The public recognizes that insofar as politicians, purchasers, and managed care organizations give assurance that all "medically necessary" treatment is being provided, an evasion is being perpetrated. U.S. political discourse pretends that there is a single objective answer to the question of what constitutes "medical necessity," but as discussed below, the concept of "medical necessity" is ethical as well as clinical.

The public correctly believes that the U.S. managed care system is setting priorities and developing value-laden policies about "medical necessity" and "medical appropriateness," but that purchasers, political leaders, and the managed care industry are not acknowledging what they are doing even though it is exactly what our national policy is asking them to do. Oregon is unique in being explicit about the need for priority setting and hard choices, and in proactively involving the public in creating a framework of values for the process.

In this chapter we try to analyze ethical issues in terms of the practical realities of the U.S. managed care system in ways that can be useful to program managers, behavioral health professionals, policy leaders, and consumer advocates. Section I argues that managed behavioral health programs can attain and sustain legitimacy for their resource allocation role only if they hold themselves accountable for showing the reasonableness of these policies. Section II focuses on the first ("macro") level of resource allocation by arguing that parity for behavioral services is justified on ethical grounds and that managed behavioral health care is crucial for achieving parity. Section III focuses on the third ("micro") level of resource allocation through a consideration of (a) how "medical necessity" can best be defined and (b) the distinction between treatment and enhancement. Section IV considers the contested topics of for-profit behavioral care and the ethics of payment by capitation. Section V touches on the middle ("meso") level of resource allocation in the course of identifying ethical lessons that can be learned from public sector managed behavioral health programs.

The concluding section takes on the larger question of whether the concept of ethical managed behavioral care is an oxymoron. In order for the reasoning presented in sections I–V to be more than a sterile academic exercise, it must provide practical guidance for the future. Section VI shows how accountability for reasonableness can be applied to two ethical issues that will be important in the next decade: (a) the ethics of managing what are promising, but costly, developments in psychopharmacology, and (b) the active debate about whether ethical clinicians can participate in "gatekeeping," or "bedside rationing."

I. THE LEGITIMACY PROBLEM:
MAKING MANAGED BEHAVIORAL HEALTH CARE MORE
ACCOUNTABLE FOR REASONABLENESS

Given that behavioral health care is not the only important social or medical good, resources for behavioral services will inevitably be limited. Hard choices must be made about what conditions and problems should be given priority and how much care individuals will receive. Hard choices cause pain and disappointment. Under what circumstances should patients, families, clinicians, advocates, and the public accept the resource allocation decisions of private, often for-profit, behavioral health organizations as legitimate and fair (Daniels & Sabin, 1997)?

While this question is an important one for all sectors of health care, it is crucial for behavioral services–which, above all, require trust and collaboration. Patients and families who are left bitter and distrustful by the results of the resource allocation process will be more difficult to treat, and clinicians who are bitter and distrustful about the system in which they practice will be less effective clinically.

If individuals purchased health care in a well-functioning market–and consequently selected their insurance with the kinds of information and choices available when they purchase a car or a stereo–the issues of legitimacy and fairness would be less difficult. If individuals did not like the policies of one insurance program, they would be free to choose another. Most of the insured actually have little relevant information available to them, however, and most have only a few insurance choices available (or perhaps only just one). Moreover, 17% of the U.S. population has no insurance at all. As a result, managed care programs can rarely claim legitimacy on the basis of being chosen by informed consumers in a free market.

Similarly, if we had clear, compelling, and widely accepted principles from which we could derive persuasive answers to our resource allocation questions, it would be possible to respond to challenges about legitimacy and fairness within the framework of these shared principles. In a pluralistic society like the United States, however, there is little likelihood that publicly acceptable, principled solutions will emerge in the foreseeable future (Daniels, 1993) to answer questions concerning how to distribute behavioral resources across a population of patients suffering from conditions that range from severe and persistent illness to less serious, but common and clinically meaningful, adjustment disorders, or how to allocate resources among child, adolescent, adult, and elderly patients.

We have argued in detail elsewhere (Daniels & Sabin, 1997) that managed behavioral health programs can best achieve patient, clinician, and public acceptance as legitimate and fair by meeting the following four conditions:

A. Key policies and limit-setting decisions must be publicly accessible. "Gag rules" and proprietary "medical necessity" criteria have largely been eliminated in managed behavioral care. Public wariness about managed care policies, however, appears to continue relatively unabated. Because of this national climate of suspicion, behavioral care programs are well advised to try to ward off unearned negative assessments by presenting policy rationales in an educative manner more like that of a good teacher than a bureaucrat reluctantly disclosing policies in technical jargon and small print.

B. Policies and decisions should be based on a comprehensible and plausible explanation of how they meet the behavioral health needs of the insured population under reasonable resource constraints. The rationale should refer to clinical needs and show how the particular policy choices can be construed as providing the best value for money for the insured population in the light of available resources. If a drug formulary restricts the agents that can be used, clear explanations of the rationale, supported by clinical data and acknowledging relevant trade-offs, should be presented. If treatment goals are limited to acute stabilization and return to baseline functioning, a similar explanatory justification should be provided.

Experience and common sense support this second condition. When people recognize that the basis of their disappointment arises from legitimate considerations, they—and others looking at the situation—are readier to see it as painful, but not as unfair. Thus, when an HMO—in an effort to stay within a set budget, and after extensive consultation with members, clinicians, and payers—reallocated its behavioral health budget to provide unlimited outpatient care to the sickest patients, but at the same time introduced a new copayment for the less sick patients after the eighth outpatient session, virtually no patients and families who had to pay the fee saw the policy as unfair, even though they were not happy about having to pay more (Abrams, 1993).

Ideally, political and clinical leaders would educate the public about the need for trade-offs and hard choices, and about the ethical challenge of providing care within a budget. Unfortunately, anti-managed-care demagoguery has been more common than serious engagement with real issues. Given the absence of educative political and clinical leadership, managed care organizations need to fill the vacuum by taking an educative, as well as managerial, role.

C. There must be a mechanism for dealing with challenges and disputes regarding policies and limit-setting decisions, as well as a process that ensures learning from these challenges, so that policies can be altered in accord with experience. Ethical managed behavioral care needs a quality-improvement approach grounded in what Feldman (1992) describes as a relationship of "constructive tension" between the clinical community and the managed behavioral health organization. Such an approach treats challenges and appeals as opportunities for change (when warranted) and for educating patients, clinicians, and the public about the soundness and shortcomings of allocational policies (Sabin, 1995).

D. There must be either voluntary agreement by managed behavioral health organizations to adhere to the first three conditions, or public regulation to ensure that the conditions are met.

The above process, which we call being "accountable for reasonableness" (Daniels & Sabin, 1998), is analogous to clinical methods familiar to most behavioral health clinicians: explicit presentation of the reasoning upon which clinical recommendations are made; readiness to enter into reflective give-and-take about the treatment plan; and a commitment to learning from experience. Just as skillful clinicians learn to cultivate a therapeutic alliance with their patients, skillful managed behavioral health programs must learn to cultivate a trusting relationship with their members. Good communication and reasonableness in policy and practice are the key organizational skills.

II. MANAGED BEHAVIORAL HEALTH CARE AND THE ETHICAL BASIS FOR PARITY

From the inception of health insurance in the United States more than 60 years ago, behavioral health services have been treated much more restrictively than other health services. Insurance has typically limited hospital and outpatient treatment in ways not applied to other sectors of health care. Sometimes insurance omits behavioral care altogether. This categorical distinction between behavioral and other sectors of health care must be regarded as unethical for both theoretical and empirical reasons, but ethical arguments, no matter how passionate, have not brought about parity. By demonstrating that behavioral health care costs can be predicted and controlled, managed behavioral health care has provided the missing link in the quest for parity.

The theoretical rationale for arguing that behavioral services should compete on equal footing with other sectors of health care within the resource allocation process turns on the moral importance of health care itself, and on the moral grounding for the widely recognized societal obligation to ensure a basic level of health care for all. The distinctive importance of health care comes from its role in protecting and promoting fair equality of opportunity. Effective health care prevents, restores, corrects, or limits the degree to which illness impedes our ability to form and pursue conceptions of the good life (Daniels, 1985). Because health care contributes to fundamental human opportunity in such a significant manner, virtually all societies regard basic health care as a societal obligation. The United States is an outlier in allowing so many citizens to go uninsured.

If there were reasons for considering behavioral health care per se as fundamentally less important to human opportunity than other sectors of health care, there might be justification for placing behavioral services on a lower footing as different in kind from other health services. In fact, mental and substance use disorders cause substantial impairment, equal to or greater than many chronic medical diseases about which there is no controversy regarding insurance coverage (Hays, Wells, Sherbourne, Rogers, & Spritzer, 1995). Similarly, if there were reasons for regarding behavioral treatment as uniquely ineffective, justification would again exist for omitting or uniquely disadvantaging them. In fact, behavioral health care is comparable in effectiveness to most other areas of medical treatment (National Advisory Mental Health Council, 1995).

On the basis of these arguments, Boyle and Callahan (1995, p. x) correctly argue that "mental and physical health should be fully integrated in any priority-setting plan; mental health research and services should not be discriminated against in favor of physical health." A particular managed care program may reasonably decide to give the behavioral health sector more or less priority relative to other sectors. There is no single "right" answer to the question of how much of a total health care budget should be allocated to behavioral health care. It is not ethically defensible, however, to keep the behavioral health sector from competing for resources on a level playing field.

The empirical rationale for regarding the common practice of imposing distinctive limitations on behavioral health services in the resource allocation process as unethical comes from the Oregon Health Plan. Oregon provides the clearest test of what happens in a democratic process when behavioral health conditions compete not as a sector, but as individual disorders, comparable to diabetes, pneumonia, and appendicitis. If the Oregon priority-setting process had systematically ranked mental and substance use disorders below all other medical and surgical conditions, it would have provided evidence that the widespread practice of allocating resources for behavioral health services by coverage rules that uniquely disadvantage the behavioral health sector was at least a reflection of public opinion.

What happened was actually quite different (Sabin & Daniels, 1997). Schizophrenia ranked just behind asthma and respiratory failure in the priority listings. Chemical dependencies ranked just behind treatment of closed hip fracture. Attention deficit disorder ranked just ahead of hypertension. The relatively small number of conditions that fell below the cutoff point for coverage created by the legislatively determined budget included only hypochondriasis, transsexualism, and personality disorders other than borderline or schizotypal.

The final ranking of conditions depended on assessment of the severity of impact of the condition and the effectiveness of treatment (Garland, 1992). Most mental and substance use disorders fell into the groups for which treatment (a) prevents death with full recovery (top priority), (b) prevents death with less than full recovery (third), and (c) improves life span and quality of life (fifth). The few conditions that were not covered were judged to be less responsive to currently available methods and therefore fell into lower-priority groups, for which (d) repetitive (meaning extensive) treatment improves quality of life (thirteenth) or (e) treatment causes minimal or no improvement in quality of life (seventeenth and last). Thus, even the conditions that fell below the cutoff point for funding were seen as significant in terms of the impairment that they produce.

The fact that the citizens of Oregon gave mental and substance use disorders comparable priority with all other medical and surgical disorders supports the theoretical argument that there is no principled basis for selectively disadvantaging behavioral health services at the macro level of resource allocation. A just resource-allocation process will put the behavioral health sector on the same footing as other sectors and will subject it to the same forms of priority setting and management. Oregon shows that this kind of process is actually practicable (Pollack, McFarland, George, & Angell, 1994).

Given that there is no clinical or principled basis for opposing parity, the only argument against parity is affordability. A group of managerial approaches ranging from global budgets to the use of selected networks, combined with guidelines and utilization review, provide substantial evidence for the insurability of generous behavioral health benefits (Goldman, McCulloch, Cuffel, & Kozma, 1999). As a result, critics of managed behavioral health care are caught in a double bind. On whatever grounds they oppose managed behavioral care, they must assimilate the fact that the managed behavioral health care "industry" has provided the most persuasive evidence from U.S. experience that behavioral health care costs can be controlled without arbitrary caps on benefits.

III. MEDICAL NECESSITY AND THE TREATMENT/ENHANCEMENT DISTINCTION

For the past 50 years, the concept of "medical necessity" has been the major tool for deciding what insurance should pay for. Sometimes the concept makes obvious sense and can be applied without controversy. Using clozaril to improve the cognitive capacity of a person whose thinking is impaired by severe schizophrenia is "medically necessary." Using a stimulant to improve the cognitive capacity of an outstanding graduate student who wants to achieve even greater excellence is not "medically necessary." Using cognitive psychotherapy to improve the mood of a patient with severe major depression is "medically necessary." Using psychotherapy to improve the mood of a non-depressed, already happy person who hopes to become "happier than normal" is not.

Often, however, it is not so easy for even fair-minded observers who believe that limits must be applied in health care to agree as to whether a proposed intervention should or should not be covered. When we studied (Sabin & Daniels, 1994) frontline reasoning in a series of contested coverage decisions, we found that many disagreements arose because stakeholders unwittingly applied three different beliefs concerning, or models of, the ultimate goal or purpose for behavioral care. Since "medical necessity" can be determined only in the context of answering the question "medically necessary to achieve what goal?" different views of what behavioral treatment is *for*–if not clarified–can yield an especially intractable form of disagreement about what insurance should pay for. What participants in the controversy often defined as a clash pitting "hard-line" bureaucrats or bean counters against "expansive" bleeding hearts or fee-seeking clinicians was often better understood as disagreement about the purposes for behavioral care.

In each of the three models that we identified, the ultimate goal of behavioral care was defined as helping the patient come as close to equal opportunity in life as possible, but the models answer the ques-

Table 1

MODELS OF MEDICAL NECESSITY

Equal Opportunity (Type)	Target of Clinical Action	Ultimate Goal of Health Care
Normal Function	Medically defined deviation	Decrease impact of disease or disability
Personal Capability	Unchosen constraint of personal capability	Enhance personal capability
Welfare	Unchosen constraint of potential for happiness	Enhance potential for happiness

tion "opportunity for what?" in subtly different ways (see Table 1):

A. According to the "normal function" model, the central purpose of health care is to maintain, restore, or compensate for the restricted opportunity and loss of function caused by disease and disability (Daniels, 1985). Successful behavioral care either restores people to the range of capabilities that they would have had without the pathological condition, or prevents further deterioration.

The normal-function model takes unequal distribution of human capabilities as a fact that health care systems are not ethically obligated to try to change. Some people are socially adept and have many friends. Others are shy and socially maladroit in ways that cause suffering. The normal-function model prescribes compassion for those who are less fortunate in the natural lottery that distributes capabilities, but makes the health sector responsible for correcting only those conditions that, in DSM-IV terms, can be diagnosed as "a manifestation of dysfunction," that is, as a behavioral disorder.

Treating illness and enhancing human capabilities may both be desirable social goals, but they should not be confused with one another. Health care is not the only agent of social responsibility. People suffering from shyness, social maladroitness, and other disadvantages can be ministered to by education, families, friends, religious and community groups, and other social institutions. The normal-function model holds that insurance coverage for behavioral care should be restricted to addressing the disadvantages caused by a diagnosable behavioral disorder unless society explicitly decides to use it to mitigate other forms of disadvantage.

B. The "capability" model prescribes a broader role for health care. It holds that the distribution of personal capabilities like confidence, resilience, and sociability in the natural lottery should not be taken as a given. Behavioral health care should strive to assist those whose diminished capabilities (whatever the cause) put them at a relative disadvantage. The capability model makes no moral distinction between treatment of illness and enhancement of disadvantageous personal capabilities. It makes the relative disadvantage in a person's ability to function the morally relevant characteristic for determining insurance coverage. If psychotherapy or Prozac would give "the introvert the social skills of a salesman" (Kramer, 1993, p. xv), the capability model would hold that health insurance should provide coverage. The capability model makes a single DSM-IV criterion for diagnosing a behavioral disorder–"impairment in one or more areas of functioning"–its central focus, but unlike DSM-IV it does not require that the impairment be the result of an underlying disorder.

C. According to the "welfare" model, if people suffer because of attitudes or behavior patterns that they did not choose to develop and that they are not independently able to alter or overcome, they should be eligible for insurance coverage. This model makes its central focus a different DSM-IV criterion for diagnosing a behavioral disorder–namely, "present distress (e.g., a painful symptom)"–but like the capability model, the welfare model diverges from DSM-IV and the normal-function model in not requiring that the distress be a symptom of a behavioral disorder. Under the welfare model, psychotherapy for "existential unhappiness" or "to help me find myself" without any underlying disorder would be eligible for insurance coverage.

By training and temperament, behavioral health clinicians want to alleviate disadvantage, enhance personal capabilities, and reduce suffering. Offering treatment to a patient whose shyness is a manifestation of chronic depression or social phobia, but not to the person who is simply shy but who may suffer from it just as much, strains their moral commitments. "Expansive" clinicians are attracted to the capability and welfare models because these models allow them to advocate for extending insurance coverage to people whose suffering is not caused by DSM-IV disorders but who may be helped by behavioral interventions. The capability and welfare models provide "expansive" clinicians with a rationale for arguing that one should consider as "medically necessary" the treatment of conditions that DSM-II called "neuroses," that Astrachan and colleagues (1976) described as the "humanistic" tasks of psychiatry, and that DSM-IV includes in the category of "other conditions that may be a focus of clinical attention."

In order to be useful, a model for defining "medical necessity" must pass three tests. Does it make distinctions that the public, patients, and clinicians can regard as fair? Can it be administered in the real world? And does it lead to results that society can afford? We have argued (Sabin & Daniels, 1994)–and insurance practice appears to agree–that the normal-function model meets these three criteria best.

Society needs a publicly acceptable and administrable system for setting the boundaries of behavioral health care. The conception of behavioral disorders embodied in DSM-IV provides a working definition of these boundaries. DSM-IV is not free from error or bias. It is, however, the result of a highly public process open to scientific scrutiny, field testing, and repetitive criticism over time. The alternative to setting the boundaries of behavioral care by the normal-function model and DSM-IV (or its successors) is not a more liberal system governed by the capability or welfare model, but one in which behavioral benefits continue to be arbitrarily capped. Put succinctly–no manageable limits, no parity.

IV. THE ETHICS OF CAPITATION AND FOR-PROFIT BEHAVIORAL HEALTH CARE

It is easy to understand why the very idea of for-profit behavioral health organizations is anathema to so many clinicians and the public. Although fee-for-service practice is a cottage industry form of for-profit enterprise, the owner of the practice was typically an individual health professional presumably guided by professional ethics. By contrast, corporations are impersonal structures whose owners may be mutual-fund investors guided by economic rather than caretaking values. Although managed behavioral health organizations provide substantial information about their performance, patients seem more comfortable assessing the ethics of clinicians by looking them directly in the eye than assessing corporations via data and report cards.

For two reasons, ethical advocacy in its common form of inveighing against market values and for-profit structures (Kassirer, 1995) is neither effective nor informative. First, in purely practical terms, industrialized democracies are increasingly using market mechanisms in health care, so blanket opposition to markets and the profit motive is unlikely to influence national policies. More importantly, as Lazare and colleagues (1975) showed 25 years ago, proper application of the core market concept—customerhood—can lead to improved care and a better ethical orientation towards the patient. Effective advocacy and meaningful ethical assessment of for-profit health care must go beyond sloganeering (Sabin, 1996).

Dividends to shareholders, high administrative costs, and multi-million-dollar salaries for chief executive officers siphon off resources that could—in principle—be used to produce better access and improved care. Attacking these features of for-profit organizations, however, will not persuade legislators or the public to turn against for-profit organizations unless it can be shown that not-for-profit organizations deliver more value per dollar of input. This question is an empirical one, and as of the writing of this chapter, there is essentially no good evidence about the comparative performance of for-profit and not-for-profit organizational forms of behavioral health care. There is, however, early evidence based on the National Committee for Quality Assurance 1997 Health Plan Employer Data and Information Set (HEDIS) that raises concern about for-profit performance in general health care (Himmelstein, Woolhandler, Hellander, & Wolfe, 1999). (Of the 14 quality-of-care indicators on which investor-owned and not-for-profit programs were compared, only 1, outpatient follow-up within 30 days after hospitalization for a behavioral disorder, was from behavioral health.)

Apart from the technical challenges in creating meaningful report cards about health care quality, effective health care requires patient trust. Trust and distrust are important outcome variables in health care. Although the research on the backlash against managed care does not separate out attitudes towards managed behavioral care, it is safe to assume that the behavioral sector has the same mixed record in earning public trust as the general health sector. The early practice, now obsolete, of treating utilization-review criteria as proprietary secrets was unjustifiable on moral and clinical grounds, and public belief that clinicians were subjected to "gag rules" also contributed to distrust.

For-profit behavioral health organizations that aspire to longevity recognize that they operate under a structural disadvantage regarding public perception of trustworthiness. Many of these organizations are actively redesigning themselves to address public and political concern about the integrity of their practices, as by affiliating with academic research programs to use their extensive databases for outcome studies and by developing new ways of giving consumers and families significant influence in the design of programs. Holding themselves accountable for demonstrating the reasonableness of their limit-setting policies will—and should—contribute to potential acceptance as trustworthy. To earn public trust as allocators of behavioral health care in a climate of public wariness about for-profit managed care, for-profit organizations must do more than act honorably; they must show a skeptical public that they are doing so.

As in the case of for-profit corporate structures generally, capitation payment to behavioral health clinicians raises public concerns about financial conflict of interest. Conflict of interest has been defined as excessive influence of a legitimate, but secondary, professional interest (financial considerations) on a clinician's primary interest in patient welfare (Thompson, 1993). Well-managed behavioral health organizations will design capitation programs to "minimize conditions that would cause reasonable persons (patients, colleagues, and citizens) to believe that professional judgment has been improperly influenced, whether it has or not" (Sabin, 1996, p. 1061).

When opponents of managed care criticize capitation for creating financial conflicts of interest, defenders of capitation often respond by citing the fact that fee-for-service practice also creates financial conflicts of interest, albeit by creating an incentive for overtreatment, not undertreatment. This latter statement is true, but fundamentally irrelevant. All payment systems create potential conflicts of interest. The ethical challenge is to assess the intensity of those conflicts and to see whether they can be made small enough to be acceptable.

Although little research has been done on the effects of capitation per se on clinical decision making in behavioral health care, design principles have been proposed to reduce the intensity of conflict of interest and thereby make capitation systems more ethically justifiable (Pearson, Sabin, & Emanuel, 1998). Financial risk or gain for individual clinicians should not be so great as to lead reasonable persons to distrust the integrity of the clinician's judgment. Capitation will create fewer ethical concerns when it is applied to a large population with the risk of financial loss or gain diffused through a sizable group of clinicians. Incentives should be structured to encourage prevention, consumer satisfaction, and clinical outcomes (further discussed in the next section). And in order to avoid penalizing clinicians for caring for more seriously ill persons, capitation payments should be adjusted for clinical risk. Most importantly, however, we need health system research that helps us understand how capitation and other incentive systems influence clinician behavior and clinical outcomes.

In the 1990s, discussions of the ethics of capitation and of the relative merits of for-profit versus not-for-profit systems were too ideological to be useful to policy. The financing schemes that a society chooses are means to an end. For behavioral health care the relevant ends are quality of care, the health of the population, public confidence in the system of care, and the value achieved for the money invested. Behavioral clinicians in fee-for-service practice have long been familiar with the process of negotiating fees with their patients in an open manner that allows fair and mutually understood arrangements. That spirit of collaborative reasoning towards acceptable arrangements is exactly what needs to happen between the major stakeholders–especially purchasers, patient and family representatives, behavioral health organizations, and clinicians–with regard to the ways in which we pay for services and structure incentives.

V. THREE LESSONS FROM PUBLIC-SECTOR MANAGED BEHAVIORAL HEALTH CARE

Although managed behavioral health care largely developed in commercial (employee) accounts before coming to the public sector, public-sector managed behavioral health care can provide crucial ethical lessons for future development of commercial-sector managed behavioral health programs. Public sector programs are required by regulation to be open to public scrutiny and to incorporate various forms of public participation. As a result, the public sector has required behavioral health organizations—whether local not-for-profits or large, national for-profit programs—to interact with key stakeholders much more openly than typically occurs in commercial accounts.

If it is to be viable for the long term as national policy, managed behavioral health care will require ongoing dialogue between the purchasers of care, providers of care, consumers and families, and the public. The rising tide of public concern and the incoherent flailings of state and national legislatures indicate that health care is too vital a public good to have its parameters decided in behind-closed-doors negotiations between employers and managed care organizations. Policies that limit the amount and nature of behavioral care provided to members of an insured population will inevitably create controversy and disappointment. It is not realistic to expect the affected individuals and the public to accept limits as legitimate and fair without an understanding of the rationale for those limits and trust in the integrity of the process through which they were established.

The first key lesson from public sector behavioral health care involves the contracting process. In large measure, the quality of care for patients and families with mental health and substance use disorders, as well as the public's trust in the care system, depends on the quality and trustworthiness of the contracting process between purchasers and managed behavioral health organizations. Although contracts and the financing mechanisms thereby established do not ensure quality, they do "influence conduct directly and indirectly and thus represent two of the health care system's most powerful drivers" (Rosenbaum, Silver, & Wehr, 1997, p. vii). Because it must be conducted openly, public sector contracting offers a key opportunity for society to learn about and influence the ethical dimensions of the dialogue between purchasers, managed care providers, and the public.

Massachusetts has had the nation's first—in operation since 1992—and largest Medicaid behavioral health carve-out contract, with approximately 450,000 recipients. The Massachusetts Division of Medical Assistance applies an activist philosophy of health care purchasing. According to the division's former commissioner, "the prudent purchaser is not a passive buyer who merely selects the best value from among the choices offered [but one] who has a vision of what health care can—and should—be, and who . . . drives the marketplace towards objectives that the purchaser sets" (Bullen, 1998).

In its first negotiations with the current carve-out company, Massachusetts and the vendor struggled over the question of how the state could ensure high quality care and a climate of trust for Medicaid recipients while also allowing the carve-out company to make a reasonable return. The answer the parties came up with was to tie earnings to performance standards rather than to savings in the service budget (Sabin & Daniels, 1999a) and to ensure robust consumer and family participation in developing and monitoring the program (Sabin & Daniels, 1999b). In each contract year, the potential for earnings through not spending funds allotted for services has decreased, and the potential for gain (and loss) associated with meaningful clinical performance standards has increased. Further, consumers and families influence key leverage points of the management structure, including performance standards, clinical guidelines, and quality improvement.

The second key lesson from public sector behavioral health care involves the importance of public deliberation about program objectives—how "medical necessity" should be defined. The large national behavioral health companies drew much of their initial growth from purchaser concern about rapidly rising behavioral health costs. Much of the early gain in cost containment came from rigorous application of "medical necessity" criteria, especially to hospital care. Many programs limited clinical goals to acute stabilization and return to baseline functioning. For employed populations that enjoy a reasonable level of economic advantage and social support, and for patients whose baseline functioning was high, close-to-the-bone definitions of "medical necessity" effectively reduced what many saw as bloated use of the hospital. The public sector provided backup for those who needed more prolonged treatment and rehabilitation.

Public sector clients, however, have fewer economic resources and frequently fewer social supports. The state of Iowa—also among the early leaders in experimenting with public sector managed care—initially encountered severe turmoil when "medical necessity" criteria that may have been appropriate for an employed or commercial behavioral health program were applied to the public sector population. Out of a process of public dialogue involving consumer and family activists, clinicians, government, and the behavioral carve-out company, Iowa clarified its values as a purchaser in the form of a new definition of "medical necessity" (Sabin & Daniels, 2000).

Since the public sector needs to function as a safety net, "medical necessity" was reconceptualized as "psychosocial necessity" to specify the broader goals that the state wanted the program to pursue. Thus, although by strict "medical necessity" criteria an adolescent might not need an acute hospital level of care, the more intense level of care would be judged to be "psychosocially necessary" if a good alternative was not available. In similar fashion, treatment goals were explicitly defined so as to include rehabilitation focused on improving impaired baseline functioning. The important lesson for the future of managed behavioral health care is Iowa's clear recognition that the purchasing process needs to focus on the values and objectives for behavioral care in a publicly explicit manner, and that those values must be reflected in program design and "medical necessity" criteria.

The third key lesson from public sector behavioral health care involves increased public and clinician understanding of what population-based managed behavioral care means and how it can best be conducted. This chapter has identified resource allocation, priority setting, and trade-offs between individual and community or population interests as the central ethical issues for managed behavioral health care. It is easiest to understand and analyze these issues when patient, provider, and the public are all able to specify both numerator (individual patient) and denominator (insured population) in the trade-off equation. When numerator and denominator can both be clearly identified, it becomes ethically and clinically more feasible to deliberate about trade-offs and to give–and accept–"no" for an answer (Daniels, 1986; New, 1999).

Unfortunately, for many patients and clinicians, there is no way to see health care in terms of the triad of patient, population, and budget. Clinicians and patients often have no idea of how savings arising from constrained forms of practice will be used and who is in the population that is served under the budget. It is one thing to accept what feels like early discharge from the hospital and the strain it puts on patient, family, and clinician if it is clear that the savings will be used to promote other health benefits. But in the current U.S. system, patients and clinicians can easily (and perhaps accurately) imagine that the savings are enhancing either the bottom line of a self-insured company hoping to be purchased or the profits of the managed care company, not the aggregate health of the insured population.

As a result, much of the public discussion about managed care has been of the "greed" versus "care" variety, and little has addressed the more difficult questions of trading off one good against another. In principle, not-for-profit HMOs like Kaiser Permanente, with its national membership of more than 8 million, could be the site of this kind of mature ethical reflection. In the absence of societal or political sanction for talking openly about trade-offs and rationing, however, no private organizations are likely to step forward to lead such a discussion.

In these circumstances the public sector—where the budget derives from public funds, applies to defined population, and is set by an open legislative process—provides a unique opportunity for societal learning. The Oregon experience teaches that in a priority-setting process conducted on a level playing field, behavioral health conditions attained high priority. The Massachusetts experience teaches that public values and meaningful consumer and family participation can gain power by being harnessed to the behavioral health care management process. And the Iowa experience teaches that program design and the core ethical concept of "medical necessity" can be shaped to reflect and serve public values through the contracting process. In order for the U.S. system of competing managed care organizations to achieve more public trust, the commercial sector may have to adopt public sector practices that would allow the ethical dimensions of managed behavioral health care to be addressed with more openness and accountability.

VI. CONCLUSION: PLANNING THE ETHICS AGENDA OF THE CURRENT DECADE

If ethics is to be more than a diverting discussion topic or sterile academic exercise, it must be relevant to real world decision making in real time. This chapter has conceptualized the central ethical issues for managed behavioral care as resource allocation, priority setting, and the trade-off process among stakeholder values—or, put differently, as reflecting the tension between *fidelity* to the interests and needs of the individual patient and *stewardship* of collective resources. We proposed heightened accountability for reasonableness as the key area for quality improvement in the ethics of managed behavioral health care. Instead of concluding the chapter with a summary of our analysis, we want to test its usefulness by applying it to two major policy and ethics challenges for the current decade: first, the ethics of managing promising, but costly, developments in psychopharmacology; and second, the active debate about whether ethical clinicians can participate in "gatekeeping," or "bedside rationing."

Pharmacy Management

Pharmacy management will be a turbulent area in the next decade. Scientific advances guarantee that drug development will occur at an ever accelerating pace. Without intervention, costs will continue to escalate. There will be a strong push to control costs by excluding drugs from insurance coverage. Although there is great potential for overuse and misuse, excluding drugs from health insurance coverage makes no more sense than excluding surgery. At the same time, there will also be a strong public counterpressure to cover drugs as prescribed by each individual clinician's judgment, a policy that will be politically popular but wildly unaffordable. Cost control by exclusion and coverage by unfettered clinician judgment are abdications of policymaking, engendered by despair about the possibility of finding an ethical managerial approach.

Treating drugs as a distinctive cost center for managing health budgets is an eminently practical administrative procedure. Prescriptions are filled at pharmacies and can be tracked by well-automated data systems. A subgroup of clinicians is licensed to write prescriptions; their behavior can also be tracked. The public has been using pills and potions for millennia, and understands the category of "drug" and the concept of "drug coverage." In order to address the challenge of developing ethically and clinically sound policies, managed care programs will have to treat drugs as a category of care.

It is important to keep the Oregon precedent in mind. Oregonians decided that considering "behavioral health" as a category was too simple an approach to priority setting. When "behavioral health" was disaggregated into specific conditions, some ranked much higher than others. As with "behavioral health," considering "drugs" as a category is too simple. The relevant metric is clinical outcomes per unit of expenditure. If higher drug costs reduce costs elsewhere, the drug budget need not be a problem.

Ultimately, health systems will deal with priorities in more sophisticated ways and will compare specific drugs for specific conditions to all other interventions, not just to other drugs. Thus, a system might compare clozaril for schizophrenia, cognitive therapy for depression, group psychotherapy for personality disorders, and selective serotonin reuptake inhibitors (SSRIs) for bashful and unhappy, but not clinically depressed, persons. Good managed care management involves careful clinical-program planning, not just squeezing on budget categories like drugs or hospitals. But for practical reasons, most managed care programs will treat drugs as a distinctive cost center in the foreseeable future. Accountability for reasonableness can provide a framework for this approach.

Recent proof that SSRIs improved mood and sociability in normal subjects who had no baseline depression or other psychopathology (Knutson et al., 1998) is just the beginning of an avalanche of new pharmaceuticals that will enhance normal function as well as treat illness. When the same medication (for example, SSRIs) taken in the same way produces improved function in patients suffering from behavioral disorders and in persons with no disorders, making decisions about insurance coverage will require great ethical clarity and also clinical acumen. Unless policymakers educate clinicians, insured populations, and the public about the treatment/enhancement distinction (see section III), it will be impossible to create a coherent and affordable drug-coverage policy.

Whatever specific managerial approach a managed care program takes towards covering clinically important drugs and providing less or no coverage for less important ones, it will be crucial to articulate the reasoning behind the policy. What criteria are being used for determining "importance?" How are pharmaceuticals being assessed relative to other competitors for health dollars? If coverage policies encourage the use of generic medications, what evidence is there to justify that choice? How are decisions made about which priority level a drug goes into?

Evidence-based practice is necessary, but not sufficient, as a management tool. Refusing to cover an ineffective agent poses no ethical problems. But like the SSRIs as enhancers of mood and sociability, many of the new agents will be highly effective, so the coverage question will turn not on effectiveness per se, but on the question of effectiveness for what? As described in Section I, educative leadership will have to present the reasons for the proposed policies clearly, publicly, and recurrently. If drugs are to be covered in an affordable way, leaders will have to present the distinction between treatment and enhancement, and be ready to enter into debate about its application. A process for exceptions and appeals must be structured to provide both a safety valve for patients and a learning opportunity for the system.

The public discussion that followed the introduction of Viagra shows that the public is capable of understanding and accepting cost-benefit reasoning. In systems that elected to cover Viagra, women raised questions about consistency if birth control pills were not covered, showing that the public can discern the logic of a policy and apply it to related situations. Drug coverage can provide a crucial national classroom for learning about how to make reasonable policy in the context of expenditure limits. As with parity, the alternative to a reasonably managed drug-coverage policy is restriction and noncoverage, not free access. If the U.S. population wants insurance coverage for drugs, it will have to learn how to accept clinically informed, ethically justifiable limits. We need to become more accountable for showing the reasonableness of these limits.

Clinical Ethics and Managed Care

Throughout the 1980s and 1990s, U.S. behavioral health professionals have largely maintained consensus that ethical clinicians must advocate for any intervention that they believe will benefit their patients, however costly and however limited the benefit. This consensus holds that the ethical clinician can serve only one master (Levinsky, 1984). To do otherwise is to become an unethical double agent (Angell, 1993). This position derives from a Kantian ethical tradition, which teaches that individuals must be treated as ends in themselves, and from the ancient view of health care as a form of religious calling or vocation.

A minority voice in the debate about clinician ethics has argued that since most health care occurs in a social context—not in a self-enclosed, self-financed dyad of clinician and patient—ethical clinicians must consider societal or population interests, as well as the interests of the individual patient. This view holds that in addition to maintaining fidelity to the needs of the patient, the ethical clinician will also act as a steward of legitimate societal concerns. The position draws on utilitarian and communitarian ethical traditions, and on a public health perspective. Although it is a minority outlook in the United States, it is the dominant view in Canada and the United Kingdom, both of which provide universal coverage within a publicly funded budget. Not surprisingly, those in the United States who have advanced this more communitarian ethic have been based at settings in which–like Canada and the United Kingdom–it is easy to identify the numerator (population) of which the patient is a part (denominator), such as the Veterans Administration (Ubel & Arnold, 1995), the community mental health center (Shore, 1992, 1998), and the older not-for-profit prepaid group practice HMOs (Sabin, 1994).

Caught in a difficult bind are clinicians who believe that if they consider any interests other than those of the individual patient, they become unethical double agents. Although such clinicians are idealists, most are not naïve. They recognize that resources are limited and that health systems must set limits. How can a health system address these limits if clinicians eschew stewardship and commit themselves to advocating for all forms of potentially beneficial care, regardless of cost?

Through the 1980s and 1990s, managed behavioral health care predominantly set limits through various forms of utilization management and third-party review. Clinicians are protected from double agency by restricting their ethical focus qua clinicians to *fidelity* and by making the managed care program responsible for *stewardship*, but new problems are thereby created. At best, clinicians tolerate third-party review, which they joke about in terms such as "1-800-JUST-SAY-NO." At worst (as discussed in Section V of this chapter), when the managed care organization is a for-profit entity and the insured population (denominator) is difficult to identify, clinicians suspect that the wolf of profit maximization is hiding in the clothing of *stewardship*. This perspective is the one that leads to the widely reported cynicism, disillusionment, and despair among clinicians, and to the common assertion that managed care per se is unethical. It also leads to the destructive splitting that can occur when clinicians vent their distress with patients. Indeed, one could predict that a system that makes clinicians responsible for fidelity, and managed care organizations responsible for stewardship, cannot last much longer because of its susceptibility to evoking both intense distrust and splitting.

The next phase of managed care will almost certainly see heightened efforts to manage care by transferring financial responsibility to organized groups of clinicians. These groups will have three basic choices about how to allocate resources and set limits. First, some groups will try to practice "implicit" rationing by shaping their clinical recommendations in the light of financial factors while avoiding open discussion of cost (Mechanic, 1995). When patient trust and clinician integrity are high, the implicit approach may be viable, but in our consumerist culture, the "trust me–doctor knows best" approach is not likely to fly. Second, some groups will choose to keep individual clinicians in the role of pure patient advocates, which will require establishment of a utilization-management process within the group. Clinicians may prefer utilization management conducted by colleagues, but this configuration has the same risk of splitting fidelity from stewardship that our current system has. Finally, some groups will ask themselves to discuss cost factors openly with their patients (Pearson, 2000). This approach is currently unimaginable to most clinicians–but it must also be noted, for example, that openly discussing terminal illness, which was equally unthinkable 35 years ago, is routine practice today.

During the explosive expansion of managed care in the 1990s, clinicians and managed care organizations were often at war over resource allocation. While conflict is inevitable, warfare is not.

In the U.S. system, clinicians and managed care organizations have something in common–they share the middle ground between the purchasers of health insurance and the patients and families who use the insurance to pay for their care. In the 1990s, the "firestorm of public outrage" (Mechanic & Rosenthal, 1999) over limits charred the reputations of managed care organizations. It is naïve to expect that simply transferring responsibility for resource allocation to clinicians will lead the public to accept limits as legitimate and fair. The firestorm will diminish only if clinicians, with their distinctive knowledge of what patients need and want, and managed care organizations, with their distinctive knowledge of what care costs and what purchasers will spend, can orchestrate public deliberation about how to do the job in a reasonable manner. If they are not able to bring fidelity and stewardship into constructive tension, the firestorm will only increase.

REFERENCES

Abrams, H. S. (1993). Harvard Community Health Plan's mental health redesign project: A managerial and clinical partnership. *Psychiatric Quarterly, 64* (1), 13–31.

Angell, M. (1993). The doctor as double agent. *Kennedy Institute of Ethics Journal, 3,* 279–286.

Astrachan, B. M., Levinson, D. J., & Adler, D. A. (1976). The impact of national health insurance on the tasks and practice of psychiatry. *Archives of General Psychiatry, 33,* 785–794.

Blendon, R. J., Brodie, M., Benson, J. M., Altman, D. E., Levitt, L., Hoff, T., & Hugick, L. (1998). Understanding the managed care backlash. *Health Affairs, 17* (4), 80–94.

Boyle, P. J., & Callahan, D. (1995). What price mental health? The ethics and politics of setting priorities. Washington, DC: Georgetown University Press.

Bullen, B. (1998, February). *What is a prudent purchaser?* Keynote address to NASMD/HCFA Medicaid Managed Care Meeting. Available at <http://medicaid.aphsa.org>.

Daniels, N. (1985). *Just health care.* Cambridge, England: Cambridge University Press.

Daniels, N. (1986). Why saying no to patients in the United States is so hard: Cost-containment, justice, and provider autonomy. *New England Journal of Medicine, 314,* 1380–1383.

Daniels, N. (1993). Rationing fairly: Programmatic considerations. *Bioethics, 7,* 224–233

Daniels, N., & Sabin, J. E. (1997). Limits to health care: Fair procedures, democratic deliberation, and the legitimacy problem for insurers. *Philosophy and Public Affairs, 26* (4), 303–350.

Daniels N., & Sabin, J. E. (1998). The ethics of accountability in managed care reform. *Health Affairs, 17* (5), 50–64.

Feldman, S. (1992). Managed mental health services: Ideas and issues. In S. Feldman (Ed.), *Managed mental health services* (pp. 3–26). Springfield, IL: Charles C Thomas.

Garland, M. (1992). Justice, politics, and community: Expanding access and rationing health services in Oregon. *Law, Medicine and Health Care, 20,* 67–82.

Goldman, W., McCulloch, J., Cuffel, B., & Kozma, D. (1999). More evidence for the insurability of managed behavioral health care. *Health Affairs, 18* (5), 172–181.

Hays, R. D., Wells, K. B., Sherbourne, C. D., Rogers, W., & Spritzer, K. (1995). Functioning and well-being outcomes of patients with depression compared with chronic medical diseases. *Archives of General Psychiatry, 52,* 11–19.

Himmelstein, D. U., Woolhandler, S., Hellander, I., & Wolfe, S. L. (1999). Quality of care in investor-owned vs. not-for-profit HMOs. *Journal of the American Medical Association, 282,* 159–163.

Kassirer, J. P. (1995). Managed care and the morality of the marketplace. *New England Journal of Medicine, 333,* 50–52.

Knutson, B., Wolkowitz, O. M., Cole, S. W., Chan, T., Moore, E. A., Johnson, R. C., Terpstra, J., Turner, R. A., & Reus, V. I. (1998). Selective alteration of personality and social behavior by serotonergic intervention. *American Journal of Psychiatry, 155,* 373–379.

Kramer, P. D. (1993). *Listening to Prozac.* New York: Viking.

Lazare, A., Eisenthal, S., & Wasserman, L. (1975). The customer approach to patienthood: Attending to patient requests in a walk-in clinic. *Archives of General Psychiatry, 32,* 553–558.

Levinsky, N. (1984). The doctor's master. *New England Journal of Medicine, 311,* 1573–1575.

The managed care backlash. (1999). *Journal of Health Politics, Policy and Law, 24* (5) [Special issue].

Mechanic, D. (1995). Dilemmas in rationing health care services: The case for implicit rationing. *British Medical Journal, 310,* 1655–1659.

Mechanic, D., & Rosenthal, M. (1999). Responses of HMO medical directors to trust building in managed care. *Milbank Quarterly, 77,* 283–303.

National Advisory Mental Health Council. (1993). Health care reform for Americans with severe mental illnesses. *American Journal of Psychiatry, 150,* 1447–1465.

New, B. (1999). *A good-enough service: Values, trade-offs and the NHS.* London: Institute for Public Policy Research.

Pearson, S. (2000). Caring and cost: The challenge for physician advocacy. *Annals of Internal Medicine, 133,* 148–153.

Pearson, S. D., Sabin, J. E., & Emanuel, E. J. (1998). Ethical guidelines for physician compensation based on capitation. *New England Journal of Medicine, 339,* 689–693.

Pollack, D. A., McFarland, B. H., George, R. A., & Angell, R. H. (1994). Prioritization of mental health services in Oregon. *Milbank Quarterly, 72,* 515–550.

Rosenbaum, S., Silver, K., & Wehr, E. (1997). *An evaluation of contracts between state Medicaid agencies and managed care organizations for the prevention and treatment of mental illness and substance abuse disorders* (Report prepared for the Substance Abuse and Mental Health Services Administration (SAMHSA) Managed Care Technical Assistance Series). Rockville, MD: Substance Abuse and Mental Health Services Administration.

Sabin, J. E. (1994). A credo for ethical managed care in mental health practice. *Hospital and Community Psychiatry, 45,* 859–860.

Sabin, J. E. (1995). Organized psychiatry and managed care: Quality improvement or holy war. *Health Affairs, 14* (3), 32–33.

Sabin, J. E. (1996). What should we advocate for in for-profit mental health care, and how should we do it? *Psychiatric Services, 47,* 1061–1064.

Sabin, J. E., & Daniels, N. (1994). Determining 'medical necessity' in mental health practice. *Hastings Center Report, 24* (6), 5–13.

Sabin, J. E., & Daniels, N. (1997). Setting behavioral health priorities: Good news and crucial lessons from the Oregon Health Plan. *Psychiatric Services, 48,* 883–884, 889.

Sabin, J. E., & Daniels, N. (1999a). Public-sector managed behavioral health care: II. Contracting for Medicaid services–the Massachusetts experience. *Psychiatric Services, 50,* 39–41.

Sabin, J. E., & Daniels, N. (1999b). Public-sector managed behavioral health care: III. Meaningful consumer and family participation. *Psychiatric Services, 50,* 883–885.

Sabin, J. E., & Daniels, N. (2000). Public-sector managed behavioral health care: V. Redefining "medical necessity"–the Iowa experience. *Psychiatric Services, 51,* 445–446, 459.

Shore, M. (1992). Managed care: Reinventing the wheel. *Hospital and Community Psychiatry, 43,* 205.

Shore, M. (1998). On spending other people's money. *Harvard Review of Psychiatry, 6,* 110–113.

Thompson, D. F. (1993). Understanding financial conflicts of interest. *New England Journal of Medicine, 329,* 573–576.

Ubel, P. A., & Arnold, R. M. (1995). The unbearable rightness of bedside rationing: Physician duties in a climate of cost containment. *Archives of Internal Medicine, 155,* 1837–1842.

Chapter 9

THE EMPLOYER'S PERSPECTIVE

Joan M. Pearson

In the late 1980s, double-digit increases in the cost of mental health and chemical dependency (MH/CD) treatment gave birth to managed behavioral health organizations (MBHOs) and managed behavioral health plans. At that time, MH/CD treatment costs were climbing at 15% per year—a rate exceeding that for medical costs in general and well above general inflation. Some companies were determined to explore solutions aside from simply increasing member fees or further restricting the days and visits covered by health plans.

The first employers to introduce managed behavioral health plans were large employers with 5,000 or more employees. These plans, along with pharmacy benefit-management (PBM) plans, were often the employers' initial steps in managing health care. Typically, the implementation of managed behavioral health and PBM plans preceded the implementation of point-of-service medical plans and served as a pilot for broader managed care.

This chapter addresses the following questions relating to the employer's perspective on managed behavioral health plans:

- How do employers select and evaluate MBHOs?
- How have managed behavioral health plans performed financially?
- How have MBHOs explained declining MH/CD treatment costs to employers?
- What are best practices/performance standards for managed behavioral health plans?

219

- What employer trends are likely to shape behavioral health plans in the future?

HOW DO EMPLOYERS SELECT AND EVALUATE MBHOS?

For the most part, despite the mergers in the MBHO industry, large employers have remained with the MBHOs that they selected in the early 1990s. As these employers have gone through their own mergers, however, all benefits–including behavioral health care–have typically been consolidated within a single MBHO, often through the use of a procurement process.

The procurement process usually involves a request for proposal (RFP) to several MBHOs, including the incumbent(s). RFP questionnaires focus on determining if an MBHO can meet the employer's requirements and on identifying differences among the capabilities of the various MBHOs. A summary comparing the proposals serves as the basis for selecting finalists. Often the employer makes a site visit to the finalists before awarding the contract.

The criteria that employers use to select MBHOs vary considerably but most often include:

- clinical research applied to clinical management
- financials (both proposed fees and projected claims)
- industry experience
- integration between the behavioral health plan and the employee assistance program (EAP) (the latter of which provides short-term behavioral health care benefits)
- network match
- references
- Web technology

A few of these criteria need some explanation. The clinical-research criterion focuses on research and its application in order to improve clinical outcomes. There is considerable variability among the major MBHOs in this arena. MBHOs that are centralized and have a large presence in the fully insured market are more likely to be engaged in clinical research.

By way of example, one MBHO explored ways to increase the likelihood of identifying alcohol and drug problems, which are often overlooked by clinicians. Early detection of addictive disorders is critical to successful clinical outcomes. The MBHO experimented with adding an alcohol- and drug-use question to the clinical data routinely requested from network clinicians; the incidence of addictive cases increased from 3% to 6%.

Industry experience is also important, particularly in industries regulated by the Department of Transportation, the Nuclear Regulatory Commission, or the Federal Aviation Administration, all of which have fitness-for-duty and alcohol/drug testing requirements that demand the involvement of the MBHO.

Integration between the EAP and the behavioral health plan basically refers to the use of a single provider network, versus separate networks, for the EAP and behavioral health plan. A detailed discussion of such integration is included below in the section on trends shaping the future.

HOW HAVE MANAGED BEHAVIORAL
HEALTH PLANS PERFORMED FINANCIALLY?

From the employer's financial perspective, managed behavioral health plans have been very successful. Most employers have experienced a steady decline in benefits paid for MH/CD treatment throughout the 1990s. For self-funded plans, the leading MBHOs report that benefits paid per employee were between $100 and $110 per year in the late 1990s. Some employers were paying $500 per employee per year prior to implementing managed behavioral health plans.

The growth in HMO membership contributed significantly to the decline in MH/CD treatment costs. In 1990, there were about 35 million HMO members. By 1998, the figure had risen to 105 million. MH/CD benefit-plan costs (benefits paid plus plan-administration fees) in HMOs are about 60% of the cost of a self-funded plan.

Since 1997, the annual downward trend in general health costs has halted, and costs have begun to increase. As noted above, these increases have not been characteristic of behavioral health care costs, which have continued their downward trend.

Psychiatric-Medication Expense

Although employers have been pleased with the steady decrease in MH/CD benefits paid, two related costs are the focus of growing concern. The first, and most significant, is the increasing cost of prescription drugs for psychiatric conditions. Antidepressant medications, particularly selective serotonin reuptake inhibitors (SSRIs), are among the major categories of drugs fueling the rise in prescription drug costs. Commonly known SSRIs include Prozac, Zoloft, and Luvox. Some employers are reporting that their costs for psychiatric medications equal that for MH/CD treatment. Most employers report one or more SSRIs in their top 10 prescription drugs. Some employers are looking to their MBHOs for help in managing these costs. More will be said later about managing psychiatric-medication costs.

Plan-Administration Fees

A second source of concern is the growing percentage of MH/CD plan costs attributable to plan-administration fees. Administrative fees as a percentage of claims is a commonly used indicator for evaluating financial proposals from managed care companies. Although plan-administration fees have remained fairly flat over the last decade, they have—as treatment expenses have declined—increased as a percentage of total plan costs.

MBHOs have not been very successful in justifying their plan-administration fees. This failure is due, in part, to a lack of understanding either of the differences between administering a general medical versus an MH/CD plan, or of the implications of these differences for the costs of administering managed behavioral health plans.

In a managed behavioral health plan, the MBHO assumes some of the responsibilities of a primary care physician (PCP). In the leading MBHOs, behavioral health clinicians are available on a 24 hour per day, 7 day a week ("24/7") basis for assessment, referral, and triage. The MBHO also performs a gatekeeping function in approving treatment and in directing the care of those whose progress falls below expectations.

MBHOs operate national networks—which, given the current constraints against delegated credentialing, places a substantial cost burden on plan administration. Because between 5% and 7% of plan members access MH/CD treatment, many network providers do not receive even one referral a year. In an MBHO procurement that Towers Perrin conducted for a client in 2000, the three leading MBHOs (with 102 million, or 58%, of the lives covered under behavioral health plans) reported, on average, that 39% of their providers had not received a single referral during the last year. An additional 50% received between one and five referrals. The networks averaged 36,000 providers, and the average annual cost of maintaining a provider in the network was $225.

These large networks are needed to meet the access standards that have been established for the industry. These standards vary by urban, suburban, and rural locations. Network match continues to play a significant role in vendor selections. Maintaining a national network, however—with acceptable access to psychiatrists and other behavioral health clinicians, as well as treatment programs and facilities—is a costly undertaking.

Despite occasional questions about why the administration fees for behavioral health plans have been increasing as a percentage of plan costs, very few employers have chosen to switch plan administrators. Nevertheless, changes have occurred in connection both with mergers and with the desire to consolidate behavioral health plans, EAPs, and, increasingly, work/life programs. Changes have also occurred in response to the growing gap between the capabilities of smaller, regional plan administrators and those of the leading MBHOs.

HOW HAVE MBHOS EXPLAINED DECLINING MH/CD TREATMENT COSTS TO EMPLOYERS?

MBHOs explain the financial performance of managed behavioral health plans by describing the fundamental changes in the delivery of behavioral health treatment over the last decade. The changes include:

- the types of facilities and programs used to treat MH/CD problems
- the advent of more effective medication
- provider discounts
- care management

The biggest single change focuses on the treatment received by the more seriously ill MH/CD patients. The distribution of benefits paid for these patients has shifted away from acute settings and toward outpatient services and alternatives to inpatient treatment.

New Levels of Care

In the early 1990s, three in four MH/CD benefit dollars were paid to inpatient facilities, while the remainder reimbursed outpatient treatment. Today, about one in four benefit dollars is paid for inpatient treatment (26%), while over half (58%) is paid for outpatient visits. The remaining 16% of benefit dollars are paid for alternatives to inpatient treatment, a level of care that did not exist a decade ago. These alternatives, which include residential treatment facilities, partial hospitalization, and intensive outpatient treatment programs, are used in some cases to avoid hospitalization, and in other cases as a means of making the transition from acute settings to outpatient treatment.

While alternative treatment has helped reduce overall MH/CD treatment costs, it has also helped to maintain those with serious psychiatric disorders in their normal, home environments whenever possible. Many such patients do better if they can be maintained at home and are able to fulfill some of their regular responsibilities.

The population most affected by this change in the delivery system is adolescents. In the late 1980s, extended, adolescent inpatient psychiatric stays were the principal driver in the sharp escalation of MH/CD costs. Parents who were frightened by their adolescents' behavior or who feared that the courts would remand their teenagers to juvenile detention centers sought refuge for their children in psychiatric treatment programs. Sometimes these adolescents would be hospitalized for months and even years. Adolescent-treatment facilities sprang up in many parts of the country, abetted by an advertising campaign to recruit patients by preying on worried parents.

Prescription Drugs

New medications for psychiatric disorders have accelerated recovery and allowed some patients with serious psychiatric conditions to be maintained outside structured settings. Examples include such medications as Xanax for the treatment of anxiety, and Clozapine and Risperidone for schizophrenia.

Provider Fees

On average, managed behavioral health plans reimburse network providers about 30% below reasonable and customary retail rates. The consolidation of the MBHO industry–with five companies controlling 69% of the market, or 121 million lives–gives the leading MBHOs tremendous leverage in negotiating favorable discounts. Most providers feel compelled to join one or more networks, in part because the leading MBHOs have the ability to steer many patients to network providers.

A second reason why providers join networks is because there is an oversupply of behavioral health clinicians. According to the June 2000 issue of *Open Minds,* the demand for behavioral health clinicians can support 70 full-time professionals for every 100,000 people. The national average is 176.6 per 100,000.

The managed behavioral health care industry has steadily driven down provider rates over the last decade (see Table 1). This decline is easy to monitor. Four out of five outpatient visits are for 50 minutes of individual psychotherapy–CPT code 90806. Reimbursement for such psychotherapy includes the time required to obtain certification from the MBHO, to arrange for referrals to other providers and community resources, and to submit claims.

Most MBHOs report that visits for HMO members are reimbursed the same as for those enrolled in self-funded managed behav-

Table 1

REIMBURSEMENT RATES FOR PROVIDERS

	1993	1999	Decline
Psychiatrist (M.D.)	$104.43	$90.00	13.8%
Psychologist (Ph.D.)	$82.27	$71.00	13.7%
Master's	$67.07	$61.00	9.1%
Average	$84.59	$74.00	12.5%

Source: Author

ioral health plans. One large MBHO reports, however, that providers are paid 10% to 18% less for HMO members.

Providers have responded to their diminishing revenues in several ways. Many providers decide which referrals to accept based on the fees that they would expect to be paid. Members of plans administered by lower-paying MBHOs wait longer for an appointment or may be told by network providers that they are not taking appointments. In locations where there are not enough providers—child psychiatrists are often in short supply—providers can be even more selective.

The financial pressures are not limited to individual practitioners. Declining admissions and shorter confinements have created severe problems for psychiatric and alcohol/drug treatment facilities and programs. In some parts of the country and in some sizable communities, there is a shortage of acute care, especially for adolescents.

The declining adequacy of acute care is causing some to wonder if declining reimbursement for MH/CD care has gone too far. There may need to be more generous funding arrangements and perhaps new types of 24-hour care to meet the mounting, unmet demand.

Care Management

Managed behavioral health plans use licensed clinicians to oversee MH/CD treatment. Psychiatrists are available on site to consult with care managers and with attending physicians. Most of the activities focus on patients at the highest level of risk—that is, those with serious or chronic conditions. More information about case management is presented in a later section.

WHAT ARE THE BEST PRACTICES/PERFORMANCE STANDARDS FOR MANAGED BEHAVIORAL HEALTH PLANS?

Employers use the best practices, discussed below, in procuring and evaluating behavioral health plan administration services. Some of these best practices also apply to medical plans. Standards that are unique to the administration of behavioral health plans require some comment.

MBHOs are typically asked to place 15% of their administrative fees at risk, with no more than 5% at risk for each standard. Guarantees are most frequently applied to patient satisfaction, to the financial accuracy of claims processing, and to turnaround time. Of these three, only patient satisfaction is discussed below. Industry standards for claims processing are used for all types of health plans.

Performance against these three key standards is mixed. One major MBHO has discontinued the reporting of customer-specific patient-satisfaction data, despite routinely agreeing to provide this information during the vendor selection process. Since there are many customer-specific factors that influence patient satisfaction (for example, plan design and geographic distribution of employees), failure to provide customer-specific data virtually eliminates an employer's ability to evaluate how the plan is performing from the employees' perspective.

MBHO claims-processing performance has historically lagged behind that of medical-plan administrators. This lag results, in part, from problems adapting medical claims systems to behavioral health care, most noticeably in paying and reporting alternative care such as partial hospitalization.

1. TELEPHONE SERVICE: automatic call-distribution system with ability to report standard telephone-service indicators (for example, average speed of answer, abandonment rates). Telephone-service measurement requirements are the same for medical and behavioral health plans. Speed-of-answer standards are much higher for behavioral health plans, however, because the plan administrator is the portal to treatment. In medical plans, the portal to treatment is the primary care physician, who can be selected from printed directories. In managed behavioral health plans, published directories are not available. Instead, the toll-free number is answered by a licensed behavioral health clinician, who does a brief clinical assessment to determine both the urgency with which treatment must be provided and the qualifications of the provider required by the member's presenting problem. For these reasons, the speed-of-answer standard requires that 95% of callers reach a nonrecorded voice within 30 seconds.

2. ASSESSMENT AND REFERRAL: licensed behavioral health clinicians available 24/7 to provide clinical-assessment and referral services. Clinicians answer the toll-free number on a 24/7 basis in order to provide round-the-clock assistance in emergencies and in locating a provider. Medical plans typically staff their phones during normal

business hours.

3. APPOINTMENT WAITING TIME: life-threatening emergencies, immediate; non-life-threatening emergencies, 6 hours; urgent, 48 hours; routine, 10 working days. Standards for the appointment waiting time—which apply to the first encounter—are typically part of the agreement between the MBHO and the providers in the network. Measuring a MBHO's performance on this standard is best done by ensuring that patient-satisfaction surveys contain items pertaining to the acceptability of the time between the call requesting an appointment and the date offered for an appointment. No single, direct measurement of this best practice is reliable and practical.

4. ACCESS TO NETWORK PROVIDERS: urban, 10 miles to practitioners, 25 miles to facilities; suburban, 25 miles to practitioners, 40 miles to facilities; rural, 40 miles to practitioners, 60 miles to facilities. (Network providers will be available if there are at least 100 employees residing in a 5-digit zip code. Otherwise, ad hoc arrangements are made with providers so that maximum benefits are available everywhere.) The nationwide networks of the leading MBHOs were a response, in part, to the needs of large employers. Situations nevertheless arise in which a network provider is not available. For example, some areas may not have a child psychiatrist affiliated with a network. In these situations, ad hoc arrangements are made: an abbreviated credentialing process is undertaken in order to allow the member to receive network benefits.

5. PROVIDER-NETWORK MINIMUM CREDENTIALS: master's degree in licensable behavioral health profession from an accredited educational institution; state license to practice independently; malpractice insurance of $1 million/$1 million for all providers except psychiatrists, who must carry $1 million/$3 million; and primary-source verification on all required credentials. MBHOs that require specific credentials of their network providers must verify these credentials with the entity that issues each particular credential. State licensing departments are contacted for updated license information; institutions of higher education must issue written evidence of program completion; and insurance companies must provide evidence of malpractice coverage.

In the last decade the number of licensed behavioral health clinicians has grown. For example, in the early 1990s, only a handful of states licensed marriage and family therapists, and no states licensed pastoral counselors. Now, most states license the former, and some the latter.

For the sake of simplicity, it is best to define covered providers as any network provider or, out of network, as any licensed behavioral health clinician with a minimum of a master's degree.

6. LEVELS OF CARE: providers are credentialed, and approved for treatment, along the full continuum of care, including residential treatment centers, 23-hour care, group homes, halfway houses, and in-home therapy. A primary reason for the success of managed behavioral health plans is due to the expansion of treatment alternatives between the inpatient and outpatient levels of care. The most common examples include residential treatment, partial hospitalization, structured outpatient treatment programs, and intensive outpatient treatment programs. More recently, in-home assessments, 23-hour care, group homes, and halfway houses have been added.

As long as services are rendered by network providers and approved by the MBHO, the MBHO is in the best position to decide what services should be covered. Alternatives to inpatient treatment should be covered at the discretion of the MBHO. In order to avoid creating a sense of entitlement, however—and also in order to manage care more effectively—the types of alternative care that may be approved should not be explicitly communicated to plan members. Residential treatment centers (RTCs), for example, sometimes hold themselves out as the last hope for adolescents who pose a serious problem for their families or for society. Although RTCs may make an important contribution to treatment when properly credentialed and overseen, they are typically hundreds of miles from the adolescent's home, all but precluding any involvement of the family in treatment. There is often little or no treatment provided in these facilities, and duration of treatment is expected to last months and even years. Nevertheless, when parents perceive that RTCs are available out-of-network, denying treatment can be contentious.

7. CARE MANAGEMENT: licensed behavioral health clinicians oversee all inpatient and alternative care, and selected outpatient cases; care managers have ready access to physician advisers. During the 15-year history of managed behavioral health care, the focus of case management has shifted to the more seriously ill. Oversight typically does not begin until after the 10th session of outpatient treatment. Leading MBHOs have case managers who specialize in seriously and

chronically ill cases.

Clinical research has also focused on the more seriously ill, specifically those who are readmitted within 12 months, as well as those who have been diagnosed with alcohol/drug addiction. About 30% of those admitted to inpatient psychiatric or chemical dependency treatment are readmitted within 12 months. Readmission-related research has studied the factors associated with those who are readmitted versus those who are not. A key finding is that those who are seen as outpatients shortly after discharge from the hospital are much less likely to reenter the hospital. Based on these findings, care management now includes efforts to ensure that the patient has and keeps an outpatient appointment following discharge.

Employees who have addictive disorders such as alcohol or drug dependency have also been studied. These employees—particularly if their jobs involve safety risks—are at risk for more on-the-job accidents, poor attendance, and performance problems. Regular follow-up and aftercare have been found to significantly improve sustained recovery.

8. QUALITY ASSURANCE AND IMPROVEMENT: a quality-assurance and -improvement program should be established with the capacity to:

- collect and analyze data related to quality of care (e.g., readmissions, high-risk patients, patients with serious chronic conditions)
- identify opportunities for improvement
- develop interventions to improve performance
- implement interventions
- measure effectiveness of interventions
- distribute results to practitioners and providers
- detect both over- and underservice, with methods in place to detect both under- and overutilization
- handle denials and appeals in accordance with American Accreditation Healthcare Commission (formerly Utilization Review Accreditation Commission) standards for denying treatment and ensuring timely appeal
- publish and make available to providers the clinical guidelines and protocols for MH/CD treatment
- monitor and rigorously evaluate providers' performance, with referrals made to top-rated providers when feasible and appropriate

9. PATIENT-SATISFACTION SURVEYS: patient-satisfaction data should be collected and, at a minimum, enable the organization to measure patients' satisfaction with access (that is, time to first appointment), provider, and outcome (that is, progress toward resolving problems that led patient to seek treatment), as well as their overall satisfaction. The goal should be to obtain a response rate of at least 25%. A reasonable standard for measuring success is that 85% of the responding patients indicate, on average, satisfaction for all survey items. In practice, it is feasible to expect customer-specific patient-satisfaction data (along with information on the sample size and selection method, and either a copy of the survey instrument or a list questions used) to be made available to customers with over 1,000 employees.

No performance standard is more important for managed behavioral health plans than measuring patient satisfaction. Because the outcomes of behavioral care often cannot be measured objectively in the same way as medical outcomes, patients' perceptions of their treatment experiences remain the most valid indicator of whether the services delivered by the plan were effective.

10. WEB-ENABLED BEHAVIORAL HEALTH CAPABILITY, INCLUDING:

For Members:

- information about behavioral health conditions
- self-assessment tools
- self-development programs for personal problems
- electronic messaging to MBHO clinicians
- ask the expert
- access to provider directories
- behavioral health, EAP, and work/life services

For Providers:

- admissions and continuing-care certification guidelines
- clinical reference information
- benefit designs (by customer)
- claim submission
- claim-payment status inquiries
- requests for authorization of additional treatment

Web-enabled behavioral health services are expanding at a very rapid rate. New capabilities are being implemented every few weeks on the Web sites of the major MBHOs. These sites are consistent with the self-service platforms that are being implemented in the human resources area in order to enable employees to find information, send queries, and enroll in their benefit plans.

Web technology is particularly well suited to behavioral health treatment. Plan members can find information about behavioral health care without having to ask anyone. They can determine whether or not a problem is serious enough to warrant treatment. They can engage in skill development. They can communicate with a clinician electronically. All these capabilities are believed to reduce barriers to treatment and to supplement the treatment process.

WHAT EMPLOYER TRENDS ARE LIKELY TO SHAPE BEHAVIORAL HEALTH PLANS IN THE FUTURE?

Integrated EAP, Behavioral Health, and Work/Life Programs

A growing trend among large employers is to use the same MBHO to administer the EAP, behavioral health plan, and work/life program. The first step was to carve out behavioral health coverage from the medical plan and to assign plan-administration responsibilities to companies that specialized in managing behavioral health care. A few years later, employers began to downsize their workforces and to outsource functions to companies that could deliver the services less expensively. During these organizational restructurings, most companies chose to outsource their internal EAP or to consolidate their external EAP with the same company that administered the behavioral health plan.

EAPs have traditionally offered some services that are also considered part of work/life programs–for example, locating community resources, including child and elder care services. For the most part, EAPs referred callers to community-funded child care information and referral services. For elder care, referrals were made to the local area Council on Aging.

Integration Models

The most common integration model involves the use of the following:

- one vendor
- one toll-free number
- one billing
- one management report
- one Web site

The EAP and the behavioral health plan remain unchanged except that the services listed above are delivered by the same MBHO. Integrated EAP, behavioral health, and work/life programs offer clear advantages from both the employer's and the employee's perspectives.

Integrated EAP and Behavioral Health Plans from the Employee's Point of View

Reduced Confusion

From the employee's perspective, integrating the EAP and behavioral health plan eliminates the confusion of deciding whether to seek help from the EAP or from the behavioral health plan. EAPs are perceived as a resource for relatively minor problems, while the behavioral health plan is perceived as a source of help for more serious problems. Most people cannot determine the seriousness of a psychiatric or alcohol/drug condition. An integrated EAP/behavioral health plan directs the member to providers and resources available to support problem resolution.

Multiple Referrals

An integrated model also offers multiple referral possibilities. For example, in a recent annual EAP report to a large employer, 12.6% of the referrals were to community resources. The MBHO said that community resources—particularly advocacy groups such as the National Alliance for the Mentally Ill and self-help groups such as Alcoholics Anonymous—are playing an increasingly important role in treatment. These resources are recommended to complement treatment.

Continuity of Treatment

Another advantage of integrated EAP/behavioral health plans is the opportunity for employees to remain in treatment with the clinician who performed the EAP assessment. The discontinuity that results from transferring care to another clinician has been the biggest source of complaints from employees about EAP services. For many people, the decision to see a behavioral health clinician or EAP counselor is a difficult hurdle. Once the hurdle is overcome and the first visit is completed, many people would prefer to remain in treatment with the first clinician, rather than having to start over with another one. Since the majority of treatment episodes (80%) are completed in 10 sessions or less, undergoing a second assessment visit delays the completion of treatment and will result in some employees not proceeding with treatment that otherwise could have concluded satisfactorily.

Integrated EAP and Behavioral Health Plans from the Employer's Point of View

Reducing the Number of Vendor Relationships

The trends towards outsourcing and lower head count are consistent with reducing the number of vendors, bills, and reports that require an employer's attention.

Reducing Costs

Integrated EAP/behavioral health plans lower plan costs due to elimination of duplicate services. The integrated model means that the employer does not pay twice for account management, toll-free numbers, 24/7 clinical telephone staffing, management reports, and the initial assessment visit. For an assessment-and-referral EAP (the most commonly used model), 45% of the cost of the EAP can be eliminated. On average, the savings amount to $12 per employee per year.

Fully Integrated EAP/Behavioral Health Plans

A fully integrated EAP/behavioral health plan is essentially a behavioral health plan with EAP features. This model strives to offer comprehensive, seamless delivery of services. The underlying notion is that separate plans for EAP and behavioral health treatment services is akin to offering one health plan for minor medical problems, such as the common cold, and another plan for more serious medical conditions, such as pneumonia. Fully integrated models cover psychiatric disorders as well as personal problems such as marital and family discord. Increasingly, work/life programs are integrated with EAP and behavioral health plans.

Those who have personal problems that they feel unable able to resolve on their own rarely know the seriousness of their conditions. The line between cases that warrant a psychiatric diagnosis and those that do not is often gray and subjective. Trying to draw a line between the two also defeats one of the basic tenets of good behavioral health treatment–namely, early intervention.

Historically, behavioral health plans have not covered relationship problems, most of which are between husband and wife, or between parents and their children. If employees presented a behavioral health plan administrator with these problems, one of several things might have happened. In some cases, the employees would have been refused treatment. In other cases–if they were eligible for an EAP– they would have been referred to one. Finally, either with or without the encouragement of the administrator, they might have been successful in locating a therapist willing to assign one or more family members a psychiatric diagnosis (such as adjustment disorder) in order to obtain coverage for the services.

Employers who seek a more fully integrated EAP/behavioral health plan offer the following program features in addition to those described above:

- *Seamless transition from an EAP clinician to a behavioral health clinician.* A fully integrated EAP/behavioral health plan is most effectively delivered by MBHOs with a single provider network that includes clinicians with expertise in EAP issues (e.g., ability to assess alcohol/drug dependency, work-site conflicts, job-performance problems attributable to MH/CD conditions). All providers have the same basic credentials; some specialize in

EAP issues, just as others specialize in the treatment of marriage and family problems. In most situations, the plan member can continue in treatment with the therapist who conducted the initial assessment. The exceptions are based on the clinical needs of the patient, such as a referral to a psychiatrist for a medication evaluation or to a chemical dependency treatment program.

- *Coverage and management of treatment for personal problems that do not warrant a psychiatric diagnosis.* Most often the problems that do not warrant a psychiatric diagnosis concern marital and family relationships. Typically, the number of covered visits (generally, three) for these types of problems is determined by the EAP. By expanding the coverage to include personal problems without limiting the number of visits for these problems, fully integrated EAP/behavioral health plans encourage members to seek help early, rather than to wait until the problems arc more serious.

  – The leading MBHOs differ with respect to their experience with unlimited coverage for personal problems. The best data available suggests that unlimited coverage for personal problems increases MH/CD benefits paid about 2%, or $2 per employee per year. As noted above, however, about $12 per employee per year in EAP costs can be eliminated, yielding a net saving.

  – MBHOs with extensive experience managing unlimited coverage for personal problems do not report any difficulties with overutilization and abuse. For the most part, episodes of care for personal problems are completed in four sessions.

- *Incorporate the use of community resources into treatment.* Referrals to community resources are an integral part of the assessment and treatment process. In recent years, advocacy groups have formed to provide a forum for people to exchange information and support one another. In some instances, advocacy groups assist their members in navigating the government and private agencies available to help in the care of disabled children. Such groups also lobby and organize in order to make their concerns known to the public. One example is the Million Mothers March, which took place in Washington, DC, on Mother's Day 2000 to promote gun control.

- *Administrative services only (ASO) funding arrangements.* Most EAP services are fully insured or capitated, and typically include:
  - 24/7 clinical telephone assessment and referral
  - network of credentialed providers
  - database on community resources
  - triage for psychiatric emergencies
  - clinical visits with a credentialed clinician
  - legal and financial services
  - consultation services for supervisors who believe that an employee's job performance problems are caused by MH/CD conditions
  - on-site orientation and training
  - critical-incident stress debriefing
  - promotional materials
  - Web-based services

In a fully integrated EAP/behavioral health plan, employers are more likely to negotiate a self-funded financial arrangement and to eliminate one or more of the services listed above. The most common services that are eliminated from the list are on-site training and promotional materials, which can be purchased as needed. Critical-incident stress-debriefing services—which deploy experts in debriefing employees following an accident or death—are also usually purchased as needed.

Work/Life Balance

The Changing Balance between Work and Home

In 1999, the U.S. Department of Labor issued its fourth report on the American workforce. In the preface, work/life balance is identified as one of three key workforce issues:

> The three themes covered in this edition—workplace responses to an increasingly competitive global environment, the central role of improved skills for all participants in the labor market, and the balance of work and family—will be central concerns for policymakers, researchers, and American workers and their families well into the 21st century. (U.S. Department of Labor, 1999, p. iii)

In the report, the Department of Labor cites compelling statistics regarding changes in the workforce and the impact that those changes have had on employees' responsibilities outside work.

- Average weekly hours worked by women have increased steadily (13.6 in 1976, to 19.3 in 1998).
- In the last 30 years, there has been a significant increase in the number of families maintained by a single adult. In 1999, the Council of Economic Advisers reported that the share of families headed by a single parent (usually a woman) rose from 13% of all families in 1969, to 30% in 1996.
- In 1969, 23% of women with children under three were in the labor force. Now, the majority (63%) is working.
- Married couples spent an average of 14 more hours working in 1998 than they did in 1969. Married couples with children under six experienced the largest increase—16 hours a week.

The Urban Institute conducted a National Survey of American Families in 1997 that sampled 44,000 households and reported on the number of hours spent by children under five in nonparental care (see Table 2).

These findings provide a backdrop for the Department of Labor's decision to place work/life balance among its leading three concerns facing employers in the new millennium. The data also lends credence to the growing insistence, particularly among younger workers, upon working for companies that acknowledge and support claims on the employee's time and attention that arise from family commitments and other sources.

Table 2

NONPARENTAL CARE OF CHILDREN UNDER THE AGE OF 5 YEARS

Hours/week of Nonparental Care	Percentage of Families Reporting
35+	41%
15–34	25%
1–14	16%
0	18%

Source: Urban Institute, 1997.

Shift from Pay and Benefits to Total Rewards

The growing challenges for employees trying to balance work and home responsibilities, combined with a tight labor market, have forced employers to reassess their programs for attracting and retaining employees. Historically, employers have relied largely on their income and benefits programs to encourage the right employees to join and remain with a company. Employers are finding, however, that these programs are failing to deliver the rewards that employees are seeking today. In fact, two other categories of rewards are gaining ascendancy in governing how employees choose their employers.

The first category encompasses learning and development opportunities, and includes:

- career development
- learning experiences
- performance management
- succession planning
- training

Today, employees recognize that they are responsible for managing their careers. They also believe that their current employment situations are temporary and unlikely to endure for their entire work careers. Employees are no longer looking to the company to deliver training according to what the company thinks the employee needs to know. Instead, employees are setting their own development goals and looking for the company to provide the experiences–both formal and informal–necessary to accomplish those goals. Because the goals are tied to a work career that is expected to extend beyond the current employment situation, the employer's support for these activities and experiences is increasingly seen as an essential component of the reward structure.

Although this category of total rewards may seem far removed from behavioral health, the resources becoming available on MBHOs' Web sites are closely aligned with some of the key skills associated with a successful work career. More will be said about this alignment below–during the discussion of Web-based resources.

The second emerging category of total rewards is the work environment itself–the culture and leadership of the company, as well as the employer's support for work/life balance. A recent issue of *Benefits Quarterly* (Sladek, 1999; see Table 3) reported on the prevalence of time/work/life programs. With respect to child and elder care, work/life programs have emerged to provide employees with a level of help in locating work/life resources that goes well beyond the level of community resources and referral agencies.

Table 3

PREVALENCE OF TIME/WORK/LIFE PROGRAMS

	1991	1997
Child care	66%	85%
Elder care	13%	33%
Alternative work arrangements	53%	69%
Adoption	12%	26%
EAP	75%	88%

Source: Sladek, 1999 (citing Hewitt Associates SpecSummary™)

The core of work/life programs assists employees in defining the care needs of their dependents–including the type of resource, location, hours of service, availability, cost, and licensure. After these needs are defined, work/life staff members conduct a search to locate the particular resources that meet the employee's requirements.

In addition, work/life programs offer informational and educational resources on topics related to child and elder care (see Table 4). Some employers are also purchasing convenience and concierge services that provide resource information about indoor/outdoor home maintenance, chore services, transportation/travel, automobile, moving/relocation, entertainment, restaurants/food, and security.

Four types of total rewards–income, benefits, learning and development opportunities, and the work environment–are shaping employers' understanding of the programs needed to attract and retain a competitive workforce. While different employees and employee groups value different rewards (which may vary at different stages in employees' lives), the need to redefine the reward structure and to match rewards to various employee groups is capturing employers' attention, particularly those in sectors of the economy where the shortage of employees is acute.

Table 4

TOPICS ON CHILD CARE AND ELDER CARE

Child Care	*Elder Care*
• Prenatal care	• Grandparents as parents
• Adoption	• Welfare-to-work services
• Child development	• Active senior/mature transitions
• Child care	• In-home services for the elderly
• Parenting	• Meals on wheels
• Child wellness and illness	• Transportation
• Loss and grief information	• Assisted living
• Relocation	• Nursing homes
• Temporary/backup care	
• Summer care	
• Share care	
• Teen issues	
• At-risk/high-risk adolescents	
• Special needs	
• Colleges/university/vocational information	
• Academic services	

Disability Management

A third emerging area for behavioral health care is in connection with managing lost time from work due to illness or injury; employers' concern about the cost and management of paid time off for illness has risen steadily during the last decade. The 1998/1999 Staying@Work survey reported that direct costs of disability equaled 6.1% of payroll. Disability costs included workers' compensation (2.0%); sick pay (1.9%); short-term disability (1.1%) (usually defined as including disabilities leading to absences of 2 to 26 weeks), and long-term disability (1.1%). Employers able to track the impact of disability-management programs reported average savings of 19% (Watson Wyatt Worldwide, 1999, pp. 2–3.).

The resolve to manage lost time has been hampered by several factors, the most significant of which is the absence of data about the incidence, magnitude, and cost of lost time. For many employers, paid time off is a payroll practice, not a benefit plan; payroll systems have not historically been able to capture and report paid time off for illness. Another problem is the lack of connection between medical treatment and lost time from work when the disabling condition is unrelated to the work site. Workers' compensation–the program that covers medical treatment and wage replacement for on-the-job injuries–balances the intensity of treatment with an effort to reduce the duration of disability and to return the employee to work. Under workers' compensation, medical costs are likely to be higher than for a lost-time case unrelated to work, but the reduction in wage-replacement costs is expected to result in lower total costs.

Despite these challenges, employers struggling with staffing shortages recognize that they cannot afford to disregard paid time off for illness. Even if employers cannot quantify their costs for lost time, they are increasingly willing to mount initiatives to minimize unnecessary lost time.

As employers have gained experience with managing disability, they are recognizing that psychiatric disabilities are different from other medical disabilities. Some of these same differences contributed to the establishment of the managed behavioral health care industry; employers have enlisted the help of their MBHOs to support the management of psychiatric disabilities.

The capabilities that have been developed by MBHOs include:

- specialty providers
- specialized case management
- rapid assessment
- intense of treatment
- cost-effective treatment
- inclusion of work issues in treatment
- appropriate emphasis on return to work

Psychiatric-disability protocols call for the MBHO to place the disabled employee on a different treatment track than that for plan employees and dependents who are not disabled by psychiatric disorders.

The most important element of the MBHOs' psychiatric-disability management efforts involves changing the focus of treatment from symptom alleviation to maximizing functionality. Nonoccupational medical treatment typically does not take functionality into consideration in formulating a treatment plan. By shifting the treatment focus to functionality, the assessing or treating provider is asked to determine how the employee's ability to carry out his or her responsibilities both at work and at home is affected by the psychiatric disorder. The provider is also asked to develop a treatment plan designed to facilitate return to functionality.

The intensity of treatment for those disabled by psychiatric conditions is also escalated—for example, more frequent therapy sessions, increased likelihood of a referral for a medication evaluation, and regular discussions between the disability-case manager and the treatment provider.

The results for some of the early psychiatric-disability programs are impressive. One study found that duration of psychiatric disabilities decreased from 84 days to 40 over the course of several years. The likelihood of a second episode of psychiatric disability within 12 months also decreased from 22% to 14%.

There is a good deal of work yet to be done concerning psychiatric disability. A major challenge is successful return to work. One MBHO found that 46% of those who filed a claim for a psychiatric disability had a documented performance problem prior to going on disability leave. Performance problems complicate an already awkward return-to-work situation, given the stigma that continues to be attached to psychiatric disorders.

Another opportunity for improvement lies in disabling conditions where a nonpsychiatric diagnosis is considered primary. It has been estimated that 60% of all disabilities have a psychiatric component—most often depression and sometimes alcohol/drug addiction. Musculoskeletal and circulatory conditions are among the leading disabling conditions (along with maternity). Secondary psychiatric conditions frequently accompany these disorders.

Finally, psychiatric-disability management is more difficult when the employee is enrolled in an HMO where the plan design and funding arrangements do not support the increased intensity and functional orientation of treatments that have been found to accelerate return to work.

CONCLUSION

From the employer's perspective, managed behavioral health plans have fulfilled—if not exceeded—the goals that initially led to the establishment of these plans. The cost of care has steadily declined, and without placing limits on necessary treatment. The MBHOs have also accommodated their customers' broader behavioral health needs by offering EAPs, psychiatric-disability management, and work/life and Web-based services. For these reasons, employers are generally pleased with their MBHOs and with the performance of their behavioral health plans.

The future of employer-sponsored managed behavioral health plans will be shaped by broader human-resources priorities, which are shaped, in turn, by economic trends. The booming economy of recent years has shifted human-resources attention toward recruitment and retention. With this shift have come expanded work/life program offerings, as well as opportunities to integrate these offerings with behavioral health services. The migration toward employee self-service and also that toward electronic benefit administration have heightened employers' appetite for Web-based services. In the future, successful MBHOs will be the ones that follow these broader human-resources goals, determine the implications for behavioral health, and develop capabilities that support their customers' abilities to meet their goals.

REFERENCES

Open Minds. (2000, June). Number of U.S. BH professionals increased 14% from 1996 to 1998. *Open Minds,* pp. 6–7.

Sladek, C. M. (1999). Work/life: It's all about time. *Benefits Quarterly, 15* (2), 7–11.

U.S. Department of Labor. (1999). Report on the American workforce 1999. Washington, DC: Author.

Urban Institute. (1997). 1997 national survey of America's families. Washington, DC: Author.

Watson Wyatt Worldwide. (1999). Staying@Work 1998/1999: Third annual survey report. Bethesda, MD: Author.

Chapter 10

LAW

John Petrila

The law affects behavioral health care in a variety of ways. Malpractice litigation may be the most obvious. Although behavioral health practitioners are sued relatively infrequently–particularly compared to many other health care professionals (Montgomery, Cupit, & Wimberley, 1999; Simon, 1998)–practitioners continue to have concerns regarding potential liability. Malpractice is simply one example, however, of the relationship between the law and behavioral health care. Legislation and regulation also play a significant role (Petrila & Levin, 1996). For example, enactment of the Community Mental Health Centers Act in 1963–during the administration of President John Kennedy–had important ramifications for behavioral health policy in the United States. The states also exercise regulatory authority in diverse ways, ranging from practitioner licensing laws, to state regulations on Medicaid, to civil commitment statutes.

The emergence and growth of *managed* behavioral health care has complicated the relationship between law and behavioral health care. When managed health care and managed behavioral health care first developed, "the law" was comparatively unimportant. First, policymakers appeared, in general, to concur that containing costs was an overriding policy goal. Second, many policymakers at both the federal and state levels believed that the most effective way to contain costs was to permit the market to operate with little interference from government. Third, as this chapter indicates, it was initially difficult to apply to managed care the traditional legal and regulatory principles that governed health care and behavioral health care.

Since the mid-1990s, this situation has changed. The reluctance of legislators to impose regulatory requirements on managed care companies has been replaced by efforts to respond both to constituents' complaints regarding denials of care and to practitioners' concerns regarding perceived intrusions into the therapeutic relationship. In addition, courts have begun accommodating claims against managed care companies under a variety of theories. By the fall of 1999, one house of Congress had passed legislation that would ease federal statutory barriers to imposing liability on managed care companies in state courts.

This chapter describes the relationship between law and managed behavioral health care at the turn of the twenty-first century. It focuses on a number of core issues, including: liability of providers, payers, and managed behavioral health organizations; extension of the doctrine of informed consent to the new behavioral health care environment; access of providers to managed behavioral health panels; applicability of antitrust law and principles; and state and federal legislative developments.

As a prefatory note, most of the developments discussed in this chapter apply not only to managed behavioral health, but to managed care, in general. Although the management of behavioral health benefits is often "carved out" from the general health benefit, the legal principles discussed throughout this chapter are typically general in application, not peculiar to managed behavioral health care. Illustrations of particular points are drawn whenever possible from managed behavioral health care. On some issues, however, the examples are drawn of necessity from general managed care. Unless noted specifically to the contrary, the legal principles that apply to managed care, in general, and to managed behavioral health care, in particular, are the same.

LIABILITY

A malpractice lawsuit may be filed against a behavioral health care provider on a number of grounds. Examples include claims of incorrect treatment or incorrect diagnosis; breach of confidentiality; suicide; and failure to take steps to protect a third party from harm threatened by a patient (Montgomery, Cupit, & Wimberley, 1999; Simon, 1998). In bringing a lawsuit alleging negligence on the part of the provider, the person making the claim (the plaintiff) must prove four things (Furrow, Greaney, Johnson, Jost, & Schwartz, 1997, chap. 3). First, the plaintiff must prove that the provider had a duty to the plaintiff. A general duty to the patient most commonly arises when the provider agrees to provide care to the person. In managed care contracts, the provider may assume duties that would not exist ordinarily. For example, a provider may contractually commit to assess any plan beneficiary presenting in his office. Without such a contractual obligation, the provider would have more discretion in deciding not to accept individuals for assessment. The overarching duty owed to the patient is to provide care according to prevailing professional norms. Providers may also owe more specific duties, and sometimes courts create new duties. An example is *Tarasoff v. Regents of University of California* (1976), a case in which the California Supreme Court ruled that a behavioral health care provider had a legal duty to take steps to protect a third party whom a patient had threatened in therapy. This case effectively created a duty where none existed before.

Second, the plaintiff must demonstrate that the provider breached his or her duty. This breach is typically demonstrated through the use of expert witnesses. The standard of care must first be established, after which the plaintiff must show a deviation from that standard. Third, the plaintiff must show that he or she suffered injury, or damages, which may include medical expenses, pain and suffering, wages lost from employment, and other types of damages recognized by law. Fourth, the damages must have been caused by the defendant's breach of duty. These four elements for malpractice are the same whether the case involves general or behavioral health care. In either situation, what gives rise to litigation most frequently in a managed care context is a denial of care.

The legal standards that govern malpractice reify the ethical standards of the health care professions, which require health care professionals to act for the benefit of each individual patient. The American Medical Association, in its Code of Ethics (1999), states that "when physicians are employed or reimbursed by managed care plans that offer financial incentives to limit care, serious potential conflicts are created between the physicians' personal financial interests and the needs of their patients." The Code of Ethics also states that "a physician has a duty to do all that he or she can for the benefit of the individual patient." Courts take these ethical principles very seriously.

In the traditional fee-for-service environment, the core relationship was between provider and patient. Although costs were not unimportant, there were few legal cases in which the absence of financial resources became an issue in either the plaintiff's or defendant's theory of the case. Managed care changed the relationships at the heart of health care. Today, there may be multiple, contractually linked parties, each with their own distinct interests concerning what occurs in treatment. These parties have a variety of relationships, including: the relationship between provider and patient, which is governed by traditional ethical and legal duties; contractual relationships between the payer of health care (for example, an employer) and a managed behavioral health company; contractual relationships between the managed care company and the provider; and contractual relationships (in the form of insurance) between the payer and the enrollee/patient.

The various techniques employed by managed care companies to control costs and access often have the effect of inserting cost concerns squarely into the patient-provider relationship. In addition, contracts between these companies and providers often contain financial incentives designed to affect provider decisions in ways that control costs. These incentives, which are usually not explained to patients (see discussion of informed consent, below), may compromise, or at least appear to compromise, the provider's fiduciary duty to patients. This perceived conflict, combined with complaints over denials of care, lies at the heart of the debate over whether managed care companies should face malpractice liability.

Malpractice litigation against managed care companies, whether general or behavioral health, has developed slowly for a number of reasons. First, malpractice law originated out of efforts to redress injuries caused by a *provider* of care. Managed care companies often administer a benefit but do not provide care directly, making application of malpractice law conceptually difficult. Second, malpractice litigation is brought most frequently in state court, but federal law creates a barrier to such litigation in many circumstances. In particular, the Employee Retirement Security Act of 1974 (ERISA) preempts (that is, supersedes) "any and all state laws insofar as they may now or hereafter relate to any employee benefit plan" (29 U.S.C. §1144(a)).

Most health insurance in the United States is purchased through employers, and most employers, other than small businesses, meet the standards established by ERISA. Consequently, these employers historically have been exempt from litigation, including that for malpractice, in state court (Stone, 1995). One of the reasons that Congress enacted ERISA was to create a uniform national standard to govern employer-sponsored benefit plans. The courts, in response, commonly ruled that litigation against such plans could not be pursued in state court, thus creating a "significant barrier" to negligence claims against ERISA-qualified plans (Blum, 1989). Third, in addition to these legal barriers, courts have been reluctant to shift liability from the provider to a managed care company, reasoning that the fundamental duty to the patient lies with the provider.

Provider Obligations in the Absence of Compensation by a Plan

Several cases involving behavioral health care providers illustrate courts' continuing focus on the fiduciary responsibility of providers, even when cost becomes a concern. Two cases are noted here.

In *Varol v. Blue Cross* (1989) a federal district court addressed a challenge by psychiatrists and other behavioral health providers to a decision by General Motors to contract with a managed care company to manage its behavioral health benefit. The managed care plan required prior approval of treatment and used a closed panel of providers. The plaintiffs argued that the plan violated state law designed to maintain the provider-patient relationship and that the plan would cause them, as providers, to breach their ethical obligations to their patients. The court was unpersuaded and noted that "the purpose of the Pilot Program is to determine in advance whether the GM plan will pay for the proposed treatment. Whether or not the proposed treatment is approved, the physician retains the right *and indeed the ethical and legal obligation* to provide appropriate treatment to the patient" (p. 833, emphasis added). The court also characterized the plaintiffs' argument in the following terms:

> Plaintiffs say, in effect, "Irrespective of any professional obligation I have to my patients and to my profession, my judgment as to what is in the best interests of my patients will not be determined by the exercise of my medical judgment, but by how much I will be paid for my services." . . . In other

words, protect me from my own misconduct. This is strange stuff indeed from which to fashion a legal argument. (p. 833)

Another affirmation of the importance of providers' fiduciary duties came from the North Carolina courts in *Muse v. Charter Hospital* (1995). In *Muse*, an appellate court upheld a multimillion dollar jury verdict against the defendant. The patient, a 16 year old, had been admitted for depression and suicidal thoughts, and had a psychiatric history. His physician ordered laboratory work as part of a diagnostic workup, but the teenager was discharged when his insurance benefits were exhausted–the day before blood results were due. The parents had signed a note promising to pay for additional expenses, but the boy was discharged anyway, with a referral to a state-operated outpatient clinic. The patient committed suicide approximately two weeks later. In affirming the jury award for the patient's parents, the North Carolina appellate court wrote that it was reasonable for a jury to find that the defendant "had a policy or practice which required physicians to discharge patients when their insurance expired and that this policy interfered with the exercise of medical judgment" (432 S.E. 2d, p. 594). The North Carolina Supreme Court affirmed the decision (*Muse v. Charter Hospital*, 1996).

A number of commentators have argued that malpractice law should recognize on behalf of defendants that the availability of economic resources does affect a provider's ability to render care (Hall, 1990; Henderson & Siliciano, 1994; Morreim, 1992). These commentators assert that adjusting the standard of care to take into account the availability of resources would simply acknowledge the reality of today's health care system. Courts to date have rejected such arguments, however, largely because to accept them would further disadvantage patients who lack financial resources.

Given the courts' continued emphasis on the provider's ethical responsibility to the patient, providers must recognize that they will continue to be responsible for caring for patients with significant clinical needs even if delivering appropriate care may disadvantage the provider financially. This problem reinforces the need for providers to take care in negotiating contracts with payers and managed care companies; a badly negotiated contract may lay the groundwork for ethical and legal problems later.

Managed Behavioral Health Company Liability

Early cases against managed care companies did not typically involve ERISA as a defense. Instead of relying on claims of malpractice, a handful of cases sought recovery under the contract defining the patient's benefits. Since breach-of-contract cases are a primary vehicle for litigating claims against insurers, the use of such claims against managed care companies did not represent a stretch of legal doctrine. Courts ruled in various cases involving behavioral health care that utilization review of a claim had to be thorough, and found in favor of the plaintiffs when the review was cursory—especially when the utilization review did not consider all available treatment records. In such cases, the employer will not be found liable if the review process is, in fact, independent of the employer; liability for the benefits that were denied will rest, instead, with the managed care organization. Some of these cases (*Crocco v. Xerox Corp.*, 1997; *Hughes v. Blue Cross of Northern California*, 1988; *Salley v. DuPont*, 1992) in-volved psychiatric care.

Other cases sought recovery under liability theories designed to shift to the managed care company the responsibility that, in malpractice litigation, would ordinarily lie with the provider. The first case to pursue this theory sought judgment against the State of California and its intermediary for the Medi-Cal program (*Wickline v. California*, 1986). The plaintiff, suffering from a leg infection, argued that a failure to authorize reimbursement for the length of hospitalization recommended by her physician led to the eventual partial amputation of her leg. The court found:

> Third-party payors of health care services can be held legally accountable when medically inappropriate decisions result from defects in the design or implementation of cost-containment mechanisms as, for example, when appeals . . . for medical or hospital care are arbitrarily ignored or unreasonably disregarded or overridden. (p. 819)

In this case, however, the court found that the physician's failure to appeal the denial of authorization meant that the plaintiff's case against California would fail. In language much like that of the *Muse* and *Varol* cases, the court emphasized the provider's obligation:

> [T]he physician who complies without protest with the limitations imposed by a third-party payor, when his medical judgment dictates otherwise, cannot avoid his ultimate responsibility for his patient's care. He cannot point to the health care payor as the liability scapegoat. (p. 819)

The next case (also from California) to address the potential liability of a managed care plan under a malpractice theory involved psychiatric care (*Wilson v. Blue Cross of Southern California*, 1990). The managed care company denied authorization for the number of days sought by the treating psychiatrist for a patient who had been admitted as depressed and suicidal. The patient was discharged after the amount of time authorized by the managed care company, and killed himself shortly after. The court found, for the first time, that a managed care company could in some circumstances be liable for the consequences ensuing from denying care:

> In the present case, there is substantial evidence that Western Medical's decision not to approve further hospitalization was a substantial factor in bringing about the decedent's demise. . . . Once the insurance benefits were terminated, there were no other funds to pay for the . . . hospitalization. The sole reason for the discharge . . . was that the decedent had no insurance or money to pay for any further in-patient benefits. (p. 883)

Although this case appeared to presage an era of increased liability against managed care companies, that era did not develop. One reason was the barrier to litigation created by ERISA, as noted above. In addition, ERISA bars monetary recovery for wrongful death, personal injury, or other damages caused by the refusal of an insurer or utilization-review provider to authorize treatment. Therefore, claims against managed care companies administering ERISA-qualified plans were legally difficult to maintain and provided little financial recovery–both of which are significant obstacles to litigation. Indeed, a 1996 study concluded that cases involving claims under ERISA resulted in rulings against patients more than in any other area of law (Hall, Smith, Naughton, & Ebbers, 1996, pp. 1062–1063).

This bar to claims against ERISA-qualified plans has begun to erode, however, in the wake of a 1995 decision by a federal court of appeals (*Dukes v. U.S. Healthcare*, 1995). In this case, two plaintiffs complained of the medical care provided by HMOs organized by U.S. Healthcare. The plaintiffs sought damages in state court on the ground that the HMO should be liable for the conduct of doctors whom the HMO had "held out" as being its competent agents. The defendants removed the case to federal court, claiming that ERISA preempted the state court action.

The federal court of appeals ruled for the plaintiffs, finding that their claims could be litigated in state court. The court noted that the plaintiffs did not claim that the defendant had improperly refused to reimburse for the care provided. Were that the case, ERISA would preempt the lawsuit, which would then be tried in federal court. Instead, the court found that the HMO had played two roles. One role was that of a utilization reviewer—a role that could not be challenged under a malpractice claim in state court. The other role, however, was that of a party arranging through physician contracts to provide the medical care at issue. It was in this role as a participant in the provision of care that the defendant could be tried in state court under a liability theory.

The court's ruling in *Dukes v. U.S. Healthcare* has transformed the terms of the debate over the liability of managed care organizations. Most courts subsequently considering the issue have ruled that a managed care company that involves itself in treatment decisions—and not just utilization or other administrative decisions—may be sued in state court for liability based on the quality of care (Rosenblatt, Law, & Rosenbaum, 1997, 1998). Some of these cases involve behavioral health care. For example, one federal court permitted trial in state court of a claim that an agent of an HMO had negligently advised one of its associated providers to involuntarily commit a patient (*Roessert v. Health Net*, 1996). The court rejected the defendant's argument that it had acted purely in its capacity as administrator of the plan's benefit. In another, more recent case, a federal court considered the claim of a woman whose 68-year-old husband had committed suicide. The decedent had been depressed and was admitted to the psychiatric floor of a general hospital. After being discharged (allegedly over the objections of his physician), the man committed suicide. The defendants, including a number of managed behavioral health companies and intermediaries, sought removal of the case to federal court on the ground that Medicare provided for federal preemption in such cases. The federal court rejected the claim, however, and ruled that it could proceed under liability theories in state court (*Plocica v. NYLCare of Texas*, 1999).

Despite the emergence of cases that permit malpractice claims against ERISA-qualified plans when they are or appear to be involved in treatment, it would be incorrect to infer that courts will always permit liability claims against such plans to proceed: when the managed care company only administers the benefit plan and plays no role in delivering or coordinating care delivery, the case will be removed to federal court, where the managed care company will enjoy substantial defenses to liability. For example, in a 1997 case in which the plaintiff sought damages for the death of her husband, a federal judge dismissed the suit against an insurance company and the managed care company that had administered the behavioral health benefit (*Andrews-Clarke v. Travelers Insurance Co.*, 1997). Although the decedent had serious drinking and substance abuse problems, the defendants authorized only brief hospitalizations and on other occasions denied authorization for inpatient care. The defendants took these actions, moreover, despite an insurance policy stating that each beneficiary was entitled to at least one 30-day inpatient stay. The plaintiff claimed that her husband's death was caused by the defendants' refusal to authorize appropriate medical and psychiatric care.

The court dismissed her case on two grounds. First, the malpractice claims under state law were preempted by ERISA and would be heard in federal court. That forum was appropriate because the plaintiff was not challenging the *quality* of care (which, as noted above, may be tried in state court), but a denial of benefits. Complaints rising from the latter, which challenge the administration of the plan rather than quality of care, must be heard in federal court. Second, since challenges to the manner in which an ERISA-qualified plan is administered cannot result in recovery for wrongful death or personal injury, the plaintiff's claims, which were based on her husband's death, could not be pursued in federal court, either. The court, though bound to follow established law, labeled this result as "absurd" and as an illustration of the "glaring need" for Congress to amend ERISA. Along the same lines, the court commented that cases against managed care companies engaged in the provision of care would be entirely eliminated when those "plans begin to realize that a clear communication to its enrollees that the plan does not directly furnish medical treatment is all that is necessary to avoid liability" (*Andrews-Clarke v. Travelers Insurance Co.*, 1997, p. 55 n.24).

A more recent case illustrates the different disposition of cases filed against managed care plans over the quality of care and those cases filed alleging problems with the administration of the managed care plan. In *Huss v. Green Spring Health Services* (1999), the plaintiff's 16-year-old son committed suicide after suffering from depression. Seeking a psychiatric referral for her son, the mother had called the defendant but was told on two separate occasions that her family was not enrolled in his stepfather's employee benefit plan. This information was in error, and on the day that a representative of one of the defendants told the plaintiff that her family would be reenrolled in the plan, her son killed himself. She brought suit in state court, seeking to recover damages for her son's death. The case was removed to federal court. The court ruled that she could not recover for the cost of the hospital benefits improperly denied her son, because her son had never been hospitalized and therefore no hospital costs had accrued (*Huss v. Green Spring Health Services*, 1998). In a subsequent ruling, another federal court found that the allegation that the defendant wrongfully advised her that her son was not covered by the benefit plan "goes directly to the administration of the benefits plan" (*Huss v. Green Spring Health Services*, 1999). Therefore, the case could not be tried in state court. In addition, no recovery was available under ERISA for other types of damages. As a result, for a variety of legal reasons, the mother could recover nothing. The court noted that there was "sound reason" to alter the law to permit plaintiffs like Huss to recover, but that such a task would have to left to Congress. A similar result was reached in *Danca v. Emerson Hospital* (1998), a case involving psychiatric care and a patient's attempted suicide.

Plans That Are Not ERISA-Qualified

If a managed care plan is not ERISA-qualified, then traditional malpractice principles may apply if the plan is involved in the provision of care or if health care professionals are in its direct employ. Malpractice liability may also apply if the plan contracts with health care professionals to provide care, or if the plan creates the impression through its marketing material that the health care professionals represent the plan. If the managed care company simply provides utilization review, however, it is more likely that a claim will be based on breach of contract rather than malpractice. In contrast to most cases involving ERISA-qualified plans (where certain types of damages are not available), juries may enter very large awards against non-ERISA plans. In a recent case that has generated considerable comment, a jury found Aetna liable for not authorizing out-of-network care and awarded $4.5 million in compensatory damages and $116 million dollars in punitive damages to the wife of a man who had died of stomach cancer (Wojcik, 1999). The verdict and damage award have been appealed. The damages awarded by the jury would not have been available under ERISA, which does not permit either punitive damages or recovery for wrongful death.

Legal theories other than malpractice have also been invoked in state courts. The Wisconsin Supreme Court recently permitted plaintiffs to bring a claim against an HMO for the tort of bad faith. The HMO had authorized out-of-network care for anorexia suffered by one of the plaintiffs, but had withdrawn authorization and insisted that future care be provided in-network even though treating clinicians disagreed with that decision. The court permitted the case to proceed because, in part, of concerns that "the economic model of health care financiers focusing on reducing aggregate costs . . . [fails] to recognize and to protect adequately the medical needs of individual subscribers" (*McEvoy v. Group Health Cooperative of Eau Claire*, 1997, p. 403).

As this summary suggests, the trend from the mid-1990s to the present has been for courts to look for opportunities to permit liability claims to proceed against managed care companies. At the time of writing, a new development is emerging that may dramatically raise the stakes in this type of litigation. Three *class action* lawsuits have been filed—against Aetna in Mississippi, against Humana in Miami, and (most recently) against CareFirst and Green Spring Health Services—by plaintiffs denied authorization for behavioral health services. Each suit alleges fraud in the administration of insurance benefits. The theory underlying these cases is that the defendants use financial incentives that result in the withholding of care, with the result that patients receive benefits of much less value than those promised at the time of enrollment (Berkman, 1999). Each case will be defended in large measure on the ground that ERISA bars recovery. If these cases succeed, however, they could result in substantial damage awards and, because they allege fraud, may erode the credibility of the defendants.

This trend toward increased liability for managed care companies has not occurred without debate. Some commentators fear that the imposition of liability will lead to increased costs, negating the gains made in controlling costs. Others are simply reluctant to extend the reach of litigation to another arena. An important legal development is that the U.S. Supreme Court has agreed to hear a case addressing the application of ERISA to managed care plans. In the case that the Court will hear, a federal court of appeals ruled that financial incentives in a managed care plan were inconsistent with the best interests of patients and violated the fiduciary duties of plan administrators under ERISA (*Herdrich v. Pegram*, 1999). The Supreme Court's decision should shed light on how the judiciary will handle managed care litigation involving ERISA defenses in the future, though that decision will undoubtedly not resolve the debate about the wisdom of extending liability to managed care organizations.

Legislative Activity

In 1997, Texas became the first state to codify liability for managed care entities (Tex. Civ. Prac. and Remedies Code Ann. Chapter 88). The statute provides:

> A health insurance carrier, health maintenance organization, or other managed care entity for a health plan has the duty to exercise ordinary care when making health care treatment decisions and is liable for damages for harm to an insured or enrollee proximately caused by its failure to exercise such ordinary care.

The statute establishes the liability of insurers, HMOs, and managed care entities for damages resulting from the treatment decisions of its employees, agents, ostensible agents, or representatives acting on its behalf. In addition, the statute originally provided that before a case went to court, it had to be reviewed by an independent review organization.

Insurance companies challenged the Texas statute on the ground that it violated ERISA. The court struck down the external review provision because it would impose state-specific requirements on the administration of ERISA-qualified plans. The court upheld, however, the provision permitting the imposition of liability on managed care plans, including ERISA-qualified plans (*Corporate Health Insurance Inc. v. Texas Dept. of Insurance*, 1998). California has adopted similar legislation, imposing liability on managed care organizations that fail to exercise ordinary care in arranging for or denying health care services. Employers are not liable for these decisions, however, and the managed care organization is not liable for the independent negligence of a health care professional (Managed Health Care Insurance Accountability Act of 1999).

Ultimately, resolution of these issues in a uniform way rests with Congress, which has struggled for several years about whether and how to amend ERISA. At the time of this writing, Congress is faced with the task of reconciling two managed care bills–one passed by each chamber. The bill passed by the House of Representatives would permit lawsuits in state courts for a denial of covered benefits that results in death or injury. The Senate bill, however, contains no liability provision. It is therefore uncertain at this point what liability provisions, if any, the final act will include. Regardless of the outcome, however, one may reasonably anticipate continuing efforts to impose liability on managed care companies, as well as continuing debate about the cost and implications of imposing such liability.

INFORMED CONSENT

Informed consent is a key ethical and legal principle. At its core is the idea that people should be autonomous in making decisions concerning their own health care and whether they participate as subjects in research. There are three elements of informed consent (Appelbaum, Lidz, & Meisel, 1987, chap. 3). First, consent must be voluntary, which means that the individual is not under duress in deciding whether to accept treatment. Duress (or coercion) can come from several sources. For example, an individual may feel pressured to make a particular decision regarding treatment at the end of life because of pressure from family (who may have, for example, a financial stake in the ultimate outcome of the decision). Second, consent must be based on adequate information–that is, informed. In general, a person must be informed of the proposed treatment, its benefits and risks, alternative treatments (including their benefits and risks), and the benefits and risks of having no treatment. Third, the person must be mentally competent. Recent research suggests that people with serious mental illnesses are often competent to consent to treatment. Although people with schizophrenia have more often been found incompetent than people with heart disease or people with no significant health problem, the majority of people with mental illness have met the various tests that the law has used for measuring competence to consent to treatment (Appelbaum & Grisso, 1995).

Since the mid-1990s, the principle of informed consent has been stretched to meet two new situations. The first is whether health care professionals must provide the patient with information about their credentials. In *Johnson v. Kokemoore* (1996), the plaintiff argued that the physician should have informed her about his experience with the proposed surgery (clipping an aneurysm in her brain), about the morbidity and mortality rates for patients who underwent that particular type of surgery from the physician and from other physicians, and about the availability of other, more experienced providers. In ruling for the plaintiff, the court found that the provider's credentials were germane to a patient's decision to accept or reject the treatment suggested by the provider, as was information concerning the option of having the treatment provided elsewhere. The court wrote that the information sought by the patient "would have facilitated the patient's awareness of 'all of the viable alternatives' available to her and thereby aided her exercise of informed consent" (p. 498).

The other important development regarding informed consent–"economic informed consent" (Hall, 1997)–is directly related to managed care. It assumes that people enrolled in health and behavioral health plans require information about the plan's economic constraints and limitations that might affect both treatment decisions and, at the threshold, the choice of health plan and provider. This new facet of informed consent derives from the principle of individual autonomy (which underlies informed consent in its more traditional form) in combination with a more recently formulated principle that providers and managed care plans have fiduciary duties to patients and plan enrollees, and that these duties include that of informing patients about incentives and disincentives that might affect the *provider*'s behavior in giving or withholding care.

The idea that people should be informed about their health benefits is not a new one. Insurance companies have long been obligated to provide information to plan enrollees. In addition, the federal government, in its role as payer of general health and behavioral health care, requires disclosure to beneficiaries of information regarding benefits, of rights available if care is denied, and so forth. The issue has become a more contentious one, however, as managed care has grown. In large measure, the resort to informed consent principles stems from the same complexities in the relationship between patient, provider, managed care company, and payer noted above in the discussion of liability. Managed care, in at least some of its forms, appears to strain, if not break, the loyalty that the provider owes to the patient. One perceived antidote is to establish new liability rules; another is to require the disclosure of the economic factors that shape this multiparty relationship.

There are only a few judicial opinions on this topic of economic informed consent, and none of them specifically involves behavioral health care. Since the principles articulated in the opinions are generally applicable, however, the cases merit some attention. Moreover, as the later discussion of legislation will indicate, legislatures are beginning to enact statutes designed to ensure that individuals are informed about the parameters of their health plans and about incentives that might affect their care providers' decisions.

In *Shea v. Esensten* (1997), a federal court of appeals held that an HMO had a legal obligation, based on its fiduciary duty, to reveal to a plan enrollee the financial incentives used by the plan to influence provider behavior. In this case, a 40-year-old man repeated complained to his primary care physician of chest pains, dizziness, and anxiety over these symptoms (which was exacerbated by a family history of heart disease). His physician, who had been his family care doctor before the HMO assumed responsibility for managing the employee benefits that paid for the patient's health care, discouraged the patient from seeing a specialist. The patient subsequently died of a heart attack. His wife brought a lawsuit against the HMO, arguing that it had an obligation to disclose incentives affecting the physician's decision whether to refer to a specialist. These incentives included the withholding of payment to physicians if they made too many specialist referrals. The court of appeals agreed that the plan administrator had a duty to disclose. "When an HMO's financial incentives discourage a treating doctor from providing essential health care referrals for conditions covered under the plan benefit structure, the incentives must be disclosed" (p. 629).

While the *Shea* case was the first of its kind to arise in a managed care setting, it was not–at least in one respect–a departure from existing law; the court imposed a legal duty on the *plan administrator*, the traditional holder of obligations to provide information to enrollees about plan benefits. A subsequent case, however–which was later overturned–imposed an obligation on the *provider* to disclose economic incentives that might have affected his or her decision making. In this 1999 Illinois appellate case, *Neade v. Portes*, a 37-year-old man with an extensive history of treatment for heart disease, including a previous hospitalization, was denied further hospitalization by the defendant, a physician. Although Portes did not examine the patient himself, he nonetheless overturned the recommendations of physicians who worked for him that the patient be hospitalized for an angiogram. After the patient died, his wife brought suit against Portes on two grounds. The first was a traditional malpractice claim alleging a variety of inadequacies in Portes's treatment of the plaintiff's husband. The second sought to establish an independent legal claim that Portes had an obligation to disclose to the patient that the physician's contract with the patient's HMO created incentives to minimize diagnostic tests and specialist referrals.

The trial court had dismissed that part of Neade's complaint seeking to impose a fiduciary duty to disclose the contractual relationship between the defendant physician and the HMO in which the patient was enrolled. The Illinois Appellate Court reversed, however, agreeing that Portes had an obligation to make that disclosure. The plaintiff's theory was that the contract, by rewarding physicians for minimizing referrals to specialists, placed the physician's financial well-being in conflict with the patient's physical well-being. The court noted several Illinois statutory provisions prohibiting a health care provider from referring patients to services in which the provider is an investor, absent disclosure to the patient. The court wrote that "it follows, then, that there is a potential conflict of interest, which the physician should disclose, where, incompatibly with the patient's interest, he has a financial interest in minimizing referrals or tests" (*Neade v. Portes*, 1999, 710 N.E. 2d, pp. 426–427). In support of its ruling, the court also quoted the following language from the Council on Ethical and Judicial Affairs of the American Medical Association:

> Physicians must not deny their patients access to appropriate medical services based upon the promise of personal financial reward, or the avoidance of financial penalties. Because patients must have the necessary information to make informed decisions about their care, physicians have an obligation to assure the disclosure of medically appropriate treatment alternatives, regardless of cost.

In 2000, the Illinois Supreme Court, on review, reversed this ruling and held that the fiduciary duties of physicians do not include the duty imposed by the Appellate Court. Despite this decision, and although "economic informed consent" is a comparatively new construct, one can predict with reasonable certainty that more and more states will impose on managed care plans a duty to disclose to plan enrollees information not only about benefits, but about the incentives that the plan utilizes to influence provider behavior. Approximately one-half of state legislatures have already enacted such statutory provisions (Stauffer & Levy, 1999).

It is less clear that the Illinois Appellate Court's 1999 holding in the *Neade* case–which, though reversed, was the first to hold that the health care *provider* has an independent duty to disclose contractual arrangements that might influence care decisions–will become the prevailing rule of law. It is worth noting, however, that the trend in informed consent law over the last few decades has been toward more, not less, disclosure, and that the ethical opinions of professional organizations provide support for the *Neade* appellate holding. For example, the American Psychiatric Association directs its members that "when a psychiatrist is aware of financial incentives or penalties which limit the provision of appropriate treatment for that patient, the psychiatrist shall inform the patient and/or designated guardian" (American Psychiatric Association, 1997).

Given the complexities of the relationships governing the provision and payment of health care today, it would not be surprising to see other courts in the future adopting the Illinois Appellate Court's reasoning in the *Neade* case. In addition, a bill passed by the U.S. House of Representatives in the fall of 1999 would make available to plan beneficiaries upon request "a general description by category (including salary, fee-for-service, capitation, and such other categories as may be specified in regulations by the Secretary [of the Department of Health and Human Services] of the applicable method by which a specified prospective or treating health care professional is (or would be) compensated in connection with the provision of health care under the plan or coverage" (H.R. 2723, 1999). If this bill becomes a law, it will extend the trend to disclose the financial incentives embedded in the various contractual relationships entered into by health care providers.

PROVIDER ACCESS TO PANELS

In many markets, it may be difficult for providers to gain access to patients unless they are chosen as providers in managed care plans. Therefore, being selected for, or removed from, a panel may have important economic ramifications for a provider.

One of the strategies that managed care companies utilize to contain costs is to control which providers can treat enrollees. It is axiomatic that not all providers, whether in general health or behavioral health care, practice in the same manner; the different levels of resource utilization represented by these varying patterns are of obvious importance to a managed care company in assessing the financial risk in a particular contract. The pattern of practice engaged in by a particular provider has become an explicit part of the calculations of managed care companies (and often of hospitals, as well) in making decisions concerning credentials (or privileges, in the case of hospitals); this type of analysis is often called "economic credentialing" (Taber & King, 1994).

In general, managed care companies have enjoyed broad discretion in deciding which providers to place on provider panels, as well as in deciding whether to remove providers from panels. Some state legislatures have attempted to create access to panels by enacting "any-willing-provider" legislation. Such laws require managed care organizations to include in their network any provider willing to meet plan provisions upon joining (Ettner, 1999; McCarthy, 1997). Some state laws, however, have been overturned by the federal courts on the ground that they violate ERISA–in particular, because they impose state-specific requirements on benefit plans for which Congress intended to create a national standard (*Cigna Healthplan of Louisiana v. State of Louisiana*, 1996).

Even if such state laws are found to be valid, they do not mean that providers who use them to gain access to panels will thereby receive business: managed care organizations enjoy broad discretion in deciding whether to refer a case to a particular provider and whether to remove a provider from a plan. Providers may, for example, risk removal from plans by advocating too aggressively on behalf of their patients (Martin & Bjerknes, 1996). In addition, although little is known about the precise effects of such legislation, some evidence suggests that any-willing-provider statutes may increase costs to managed care companies. Not only are there the additional costs of processing the increased number of physician applications to join panels, but, perhaps more importantly, a managed care organization with a provider panel expanded by such legislation may find it more difficult to negotiate the volume discounts that have accounted for some of the savings associated with managed care (Hellinger, 1995).

Courts have generally been unsympathetic to provider claims

regarding panel access, and some courts (as in *Mateo-Woodburn v. Fresno Community Hospital*, 1990) have also accepted the validity of "no-cause" termination clauses. Nevertheless, courts have occasionally required that managed care plans provide some process if a provider is excluded or removed from a panel (*Delta Dental v. Banasky*, 1994). For example, the New Jersey Psychological Association has been successful to date in persuading a federal court to let it pursue several claims involving the panel decisions of a managed behavioral health company. In *New Jersey Psychological Assoc. v. MCC Behavioral Health* (1997), the plaintiffs alleged that the manner in which the defendant made decisions regarding panel participation, as well as decisions regarding claims for benefits, violated the law in several respects. In particular, the plaintiffs claimed that MCC terminated providers from panels because the providers were "not managed care compatible," and that this judgment was based on the treatment plans recommended by the providers. The plaintiffs claimed that making this type of judgment violated public policy by impinging on the ability of providers to exercise their best professional judgment. They argued that their terminations were, in effect, "for cause" and that the terminations should therefore be subject to review. The defendants countered that the terminations were not for cause and therefore could not be reviewed administratively or judicially. The plaintiffs also asserted that the defendants intentionally concealed their policy of terminating providers who were deemed "not managed care compatible."

Although the court dismissed some of the plaintiffs' claims and ordered that others be arbitrated, it also allowed the plaintiffs to proceed on a number of their core claims, including those to the effect that the defendant's actions violated public policy; violated notions of fundamental fairness, and illegally interfered with the plaintiffs' capacities to pursue their livelihood. This case, as it evolves, may become the first in which a court explores in some detail the manner in which behavioral health care providers are terminated from panels, and whether such practices are illegal. No matter what the courts do, however, there will continue to be legislative efforts to regulate interactions between providers and managed care companies. Whether these judicial and legislative efforts to regulate the relationship between providers and managed care organizations undercut these organizations' efforts to achieve cost-savings is a separate question—and one that will continue to be controversial.

ANTITRUST

Antitrust law has had a significant impact on health care over the last quarter-century. The Sherman Act, the original antitrust law, was enacted early in the twentieth century to address the concentration of market power in the hands of large trusts—in particular, the power accumulated by John D. Rockefeller through Standard Oil. The Sherman Act prohibits "every contract, combination . . . or conspiracy in restraint of trade," as well as monopolization (15 U.S.C. §§1–2). Congress has since enacted additional antitrust legislation, including section 7 of the Clayton Act (prohibiting mergers and acquisitions that "substantially . . . lessen competition") and section 5 of the Federal Trade Commission Act (prohibiting "unfair methods of competition" and "unfair or deceptive acts or practices").

The basic principle underlying antitrust statutes is that free markets depend on consumer choice, and that consumer choice can be diminished by industry practices that reduce competition. Not every action that reduces competition, however, violates antitrust laws. For example, companies can acquire near-monopoly power if they do so legally; at the heart of the federal government's recent lawsuit against Microsoft is a dispute over whether Microsoft acquired the vast market power it enjoys through legal means, or whether it did so through illegal techniques (threatening other competitors, threatening to withhold products, and so on).

Until the 1970s, antitrust law did not apply to health care professionals or other "learned professions." In 1975, however, the U.S. Supreme Court, in a case addressing the applicability of antitrust to an association of attorneys, held that antitrust laws could be enforced against professions such as law (*Goldfarb v. Virginia State Bar*, 1975). The reasoning of this case was quickly extended to health care. In fact, one of the earliest antitrust cases involving health care professionals was a successful lawsuit by psychologists challenging insurance-company billing practices that required a psychiatrist's signature before reimbursement would be made to a psychologist (*Blue Shield of Virginia v. McCready*, 1982). Since these early cases, antitrust law has become a very important shaper of organizational and institutional relationships in health care (Furrow, Greaney, Johnson, Jost, & Schwartz, 1997).

There are two general standards for judging whether certain

actions violate antitrust law (Litwak, 1999). The first is called the "per se" rule. Some activities are considered fundamentally anticompetitive in their effects and are almost always illegal (Glassman, 1996). Price fixing–an agreement among competitors to fix minimum prices–is one such activity. Another is the "group boycott"–an agreement among competitors to refuse to deal with particular providers of goods (or in the context of managed care, to refuse to deal with particular managed care organizations). Yet another is "tying"–a supplier's refusal to permit purchase of a product unless the buyer also purchases a second product. A recent example in behavioral health care occurred with the introduction of Clozaril; the manufacturer initially required buyers to agree to use a particular blood-testing service.

Other activities potentially violating antitrust law are judged by a legal standard called the "rule of reason." For example, if a hospital chain decides to buy hospitals in a particular metropolitan area, that purchase may lead to the creation of a hospital chain so large that consumers in the metropolitan area will be forced to purchase hospital services from that chain; no other realistic competitor will exist after the purchase. The hospital chain's proposed purchase, however, would not be considered illegal automatically (the "per se" test). Instead, if the acquisition is challenged (by one of three parties that can enforce antitrust laws–namely, the federal government, the state government, or one of the parties affected by the acquisition), the "rule of reason" would be the applicable standard. Under this test, the key issue is the effect of the acquisition on the geographic market and the product market. The definition of the relevant geographic market depends on the choices available to purchasers within the particular geographic area, and these choices depend, in turn, on factors affecting the use of hospital services (for example, how far people will go to use a hospital within that area). The second issue that needs to be resolved is the definition of the product market. Just how the product market is defined may change the outcome of the case. For example, in the above example of a hospital chain's acquiring hospitals in a particular geographic region, assume that the hospitals being purchased operate extensive outpatient, as well as inpatient, services. If so, the product in question is not simply "hospital services," but discrete categories of services, including (at a minimum) inpatient and outpatient services. Consequently, the competitors affected by the proposed purchase include hospitals and other providers of ambulatory services.

Defining geographic and product markets is thus critical to the ultimate question in antitrust law: will the proposed action diminish competition in the particular market in a manner that should be barred?

With the emergence of managed care, antitrust authorities recognized that certain activities that might be considered anticompetitive in most industries might be desirable in health care. Accordingly, the Department of Justice and the Federal Trade Commission–the two federal institutions with primary responsibility for enforcement of antitrust laws–issued Statements of Antitrust Enforcement Policy in Health Care (Kopit & Vanderbilt, 1996). These statements seek to provide guidance to the health care industry concerning the conditions under which certain types of activities will not invite antitrust scrutiny. The statements cover nine subjects, including: hospital mergers; hospital joint ventures involving the purchase of expensive equipment or specialized services; providers' collective presentation of information to health care purchasers; providers' mutual exchange of price and cost information; joint purchasing arrangements; physician-network joint ventures; and multiprovider networks. These statements attempt to respond to the changing face of health care by recognizing that some types of behavior that otherwise would violate antitrust laws might have to be permitted in today's health care market. For example, providers seeking to form networks–a common feature of managed care–generally have to exchange certain types of information, specifically related to utilization and price; exchanging such information would, other things equal, come under the per se antitrust prohibition against price fixing. The federal government has attempted to accommodate the creation of such networks, however, by providing vehicles for the exchange of utilization and price information. Moreover, collaborative action to set prices may be permitted when the providers share financial risk; if risk is not shared, then antitrust laws may apply (Litwak, 1999). This distinction reflects a judgment by the federal government that the sharing of financial risk among providers may ameliorate tendencies to act in anticompetitive ways.

Although the federal government has thus made an effort to accommodate providers under the antitrust laws, in the 1990s payers and managed care companies nevertheless enjoyed significant financial leverage in negotiating contracts with general health and behavioral health care providers. Among the many reasons for this disparity in negotiating power was that there are, in many markets, more providers than are needed by managed care companies, which has enabled companies to negotiate rates downward. Antitrust rules may also have played some role in this comparative imbalance in negotiating power. Unless providers decide to share financial risk, they are generally prohibited from agreeing to set their prices at a fixed level (and providers run significant legal risks if they ignore this prohibition). For example, Tennessee's attorney general investigated nonprofit community mental health centers when they jointly negotiated contracts with managed care companies that had contracted with the state to administer the TennCare program (the common way of referring to the state's managed Medicaid program). In the attorney general's view, the community mental health centers violated antitrust laws by agreeing to "fix" their prices as part of their negotiating stance with the managed care companies. The centers agreed to a settlement that included a reimbursement of $150,000 to the agencies that conducted the investigation ("Settlement ends antitrust litigation," 1996).

In a more recent development, behavioral health care providers have begun utilizing antitrust law as a tool. In *Holstein v. Green Spring Health Services* (1998) eleven behavioral health providers and provider associations filed a federal antitrust lawsuit against a number of managed behavioral health companies. The suit alleges that the companies conspired to fix prices paid to behavioral health providers in order to maximize the companies' profits. The suit also claims that because of these practices, providers have suffered enormous financial losses and that patients have not received adequate care with respect to mental health and substance abuse. Although an earlier case making similar claims was dismissed (*Stephens v. CMG Health*, 1998), a court rejected the defendants' motion to dismiss the *Holstein* case ("Fee-fixing claims proceed," 1999). The plaintiffs are asking the court to award billions of dollars in damages. This case may not reach closure for some time, but it does suggest that managed care companies were much more on the defensive as the 1990s came to an end than they were for the first part of the decade.

Finally, there have been recent legislative efforts to give providers more latitude in negotiating jointly. A bill introduced in Congress, the "Quality Health-Care Coalition Act," would allow health care professionals to conduct collective bargaining when negotiating with health maintenance organizations, thus exempting such activity from antitrust prohibitions (Health Law Report (BNA), 1999). In addition,

Texas has enacted legislation designed to allow self-employed physicians to engage in price negotiations as a group (Tex. Ins. Code Ann. Chapter 29). These legislative efforts seek to redress a perceived imbalance in negotiating power between providers and managed care companies, an imbalance some believe is exacerbated by antitrust law. The bill introduced in Congress has been opposed by antitrust enforcement agencies, and it is premature to assess the effect, if any, of the Texas statute. As health care professionals express increasing interest in acting collectively, however–including the possible creation of unions–it seems clear that antitrust statutes will continue to be a focus of attention.

PATIENT-PROTECTION LEGISLATION

According to one estimate, there were in the spring of 1999 more than 80 bills pending in 25 state legislatures that would regulate managed care in some manner ("80 bills," 1999). Several types of proposed or enacted legislation have already been discussed, including: statutes imposing liability on managed care plans in state courts; any-willing-provider legislation; and legislation creating requirements for disclosure of financial incentives. This section discusses a variety of other legislation introduced since the mid-1990s to protect patients.

When managed care emerged, there was little inclination to regulate it; most policymakers were primarily concerned with containing the rate of inflation in health care costs. Legislative interest in regulation increased, however, in response to growing complaints about managed care's impact on access to treatment. Although the amount of legislative activity, particularly at the state level, has increased dramatically, at least three factors have stood in the way of comprehensive legislation. First, there is continuing concern–some philosophical, some financial–about extensively regulating managed care. The 1980s and 1990s witnessed the emergence of a political consensus that government should step back from what many viewed as the regulatory excesses of the late 1960s and the 1970s. This more conservative approach to the role of government was often wedded to a belief that "the market" should be permitted to resolve what in other eras may have been considered "social" issues. In addition, policymakers continued to be concerned that increased regulation would reduce the ability of managed care entities to control costs.

The second barrier to comprehensive legislation is that it has not always been clear what impact the proposed "reforms" would have in practice. For example, as was noted earlier, legislation requiring a managed care plan to place a provider on a panel does not assure that the provider will receive any business from the plan. Moreover, there is not even a consensus that all providers should be entitled to receive such business (Hellinger, 1995). Consequently, ensuring through legislation that providers have access to panels conceivably would not address the underlying concern that gave rise to the legislation in the first place—namely, physicians' lack of access to *patients*.

The third barrier to comprehensive legislation is ERISA, which has been discussed in various contexts throughout this chapter. There has been, to be sure—as indicated in the section on liability—some erosion of the principle that ERISA stands as an absolute barrier to efforts to impose liability on managed care plans, but ERISA is still a significant obstacle, especially at the state level.

As a result of the above three factors, states have tended to enact legislation in a piecemeal fashion. According to a 1999 review by Stauffer and Levy (upon which much of the following discussion is based), some of the major areas of state legislative activity have been: access to providers; access to coverage; disclosure to enrollees of information concerning treatment options; pharmaceutical issues; and due process and liability. States have not singled out managed behavioral health care for particular legislative focus; the legislation discussed below applies in nearly every instance to managed health care, in general.

Access to Providers

In addressing questions concerning patients' access to providers, a number of states have adopted "point-of-service" provisions. Although there is some variety in the precise formulation, point-of-service legislation generally provides a plan beneficiary with the opportunity, usually at an additional cost, to obtain services from a provider not participating in the managed care plan (Brown & Hartung, 1998). Other common legislation provides plan enrollees with direct access to certain types of specialists. These specialists are typically obstetricians and gynecologists, though some states also provide for direct access to dermatologists, chiropractors, and (in at least two states, Montana and Oklahoma) psychologists and clinical social workers.

Legislatures also have attempted to create some rights for providers who have been denied access to, or removed, from panels. Typical legislation, adopted in approximately one-half of the states, requires written notification to the provider if the provider's contract is being terminated or not renewed. Fewer states provide some type of process—for example, a right to administrative review of the decision before it becomes effective.

Access to Care

Another common complaint about managed care has been the denial of reimbursement for services that appear (at least from a political perspective) to be essential. Legislatures have consequently enacted statutes that mandate reimbursement for some types of services. One example is emergency services. In response to reports of utilization reviews denying reimbursement on the ground that the emergency service was not medically necessary, many states now require that emergency room care be reimbursed, at least until the patient is stabilized (at which point ordinary utilization-review principles apply). This legislation reflects a judgment that the clinical welfare of patients, as well as the fiscal health of providers of emergency services, requires a guarantee that bills will be paid. This assurance has obvious importance in behavioral health care. People with acute psychiatric conditions often enter care initially through an emergency service, and courts also may involuntarily commit an individual to an acute care facility (Petrila, 1998). In such circumstances, it seems reasonable to assure that the facility will be reimbursed for an emergency assessment and for stabilizing the patient.

Some states, as well as the federal government (Newborns' and Mothers' Health Protection Act of 1996), also require that reimbursement be made for some period of inpatient care after childbirth. Enactment of such legislation followed complaints regarding the perceived premature discharge of new mothers; plans refused to authorize longer stays. The legislation is an example of the approach that Congress and many states have taken in response to managed care—that is, to adopt discrete remedies for discrete problems, rather than to pursue more comprehensive reform.

Disclosure of Information concerning Treatment Options

One of the most controversial practices of managed care companies has been the use of "gag clauses." Such clauses, included in contracts with providers, barred health care professionals from discussing specifically identified issues with patients—for example, treatments, expensive or otherwise, not available under the plan. Such clauses strike at the heart of the fiduciary responsibility of providers to patients. As indicated in the above discussion of informed consent, providing information to patients and enabling them to make informed decisions are, taken together, a core element of the therapeutic relationship. If providers comply with restrictions on providing such information to patients, they violate their ethical obligations (Picinic, 1997). But if they violate the contract, they risk being removed from the plan and losing part of their livelihood. Many state legislatures have banned such clauses. Most managed care companies, however, appear to have abandoned such clauses before the enactment of legislation.

Another feature of some state and federal legislation is to prohibit financial incentives to providers (for example, in the form of bonuses) for denying care to patients. Nevertheless, the use of financial incentives is critical to the success of many managed care (and traditional indemnity) plans. Legislation to date tends to restrict the use of bonuses or payments in exchange for a specific denial of care, while preserving the legal authority to use more general incentives that do not reward a utilization-review decision in particular cases.

Pharmacies and Formularies

A number of states have enacted legislation requiring plans to make available to beneficiaries information regarding both the plans' use of formularies and the means of obtaining drugs not on the list. At first blush, the relevance of this type of legislation to behavioral health care may not be apparent. With the introduction of a variety of new medications for the treatment of mental illness, however, the issue of what drugs are available in a managed care plan is often of considerable importance to patients (Sclar et al., 1998).

Liability and Process Issues

As was discussed earlier, there has been some movement toward legislation to create a basis for imposing liability on managed care companies. State and federal legislation has also been enacted to require the availability of appeals and grievance procedures when enrollees wish to challenge a denial of benefits or pursue other types of complaints (Lee, 1996). Although such processes are important, patients invoke them relatively infrequently, and the processes have been criticized, in any case, as inadequate, particularly for individuals enrolled in publicly financed plans (Bonnyman & Johnson, 1998).

SUMMARY

The relationship between managed behavioral health care and the law has changed substantially since the mid-1990s. Prior to that period, there was little regulation of managed care, either judicially or legislatively. The lack of oversight reflected philosophical and political judgments about health care and about the role of government, as well as an uncertain search by patient advocates for legal tools that could be applied in a dramatically new health care environment.

Since the mid-1990s, scrutiny of managed health care (both general and behavioral) has become much more searching. There has been a significant move in both courts and legislatures to impose malpractice liability on managed care plans. The willingness of state legislatures and Congress to enact various types of regulation—despite the more conservative political tenor of the 1990s—is an effort to respond to constituents' complaints, especially ones that dramatized problems resulting in the death of, or serious injury to, patients. Perceived intrusions by managed care companies into the clinical relationship, coupled with denials of care, made those companies a much more inviting political target at the end of the 1990s than they had been at the beginning of the decade, when the need for cost control emerged as the core health care issue.

This chapter has suggested that managed behavioral health care has not been singled out in these debates over the appropriate stance of the law toward managed care. Nevertheless, as the trend toward increased regulation of managed care has gained steam, the number of important managed behavioral health care cases has also increased.

The impact of this shift toward increased oversight and regulation has yet to be measured. What is the practical effect of the legislation being enacted today? Will managed care companies' increased liability exposure lead to increased health care costs, and if so, is that cost worth the benefit to patients who may otherwise lack adequate redress for their injuries? Can behavioral health professionals really put aside financial issues when discharging their ethical duty to act in the best interests of their patients? These questions and the law's evolving role in answering them will continue to attract the attention of providers, payers, managed care organizations, patients, and policymakers in the future.

REFERENCES

American Medical Association. (1999). Current opinions of the council on ethical and judicial affairs, Opinion E-2.03.

American Medical Association. (1999). Current opinions of the council on ethical and judicial affairs, Opinion E-8.13.

American Psychiatric Association. (1997). *The principles of medical ethics with annotations especially applicable to psychiatry, addendum 1.* Washington, DC: Author.

Andrews-Clarke v. Travelers Insurance Company, 984 F. Supp. 49 (D. Mass. 1997).

Fee-fixing claims proceed against mental health managed care companies. (1999). *Antitrust Litigation Reporter, 7,* 14.

Appelbaum, P. S., & Grisso, T. (1995). Comparison of standards for assessing patients' capacities to make treatment decisions. *American Journal of Psychiatry, 152,* 1033–1037.

Appelbaum, P. S., Lidz, C. W., & Meisel, A. (1987). *Informed consent: Legal theory and clinical practice.* New York, Oxford University Press.

Berkman, H. (1999, October 18). New suits pre-empt HMO move by house. *National Law Journal,* p. A1.

Blue Shield of Virginia v. McCready, 457 U.S. 465 (1982).

Blum, J. D. (1989). An analysis of legal liability in health care utilization review and case management. *Houston Law Review, 26,* 191–246.

Bonnyman, G., & Johnson, M. M. (1998). Unseen peril: Inadequate enrollee grievance protections in public managed care programs. *Tennessee Law Review, 65,* 359–387.

Brown, V. Y., & Hartung, B. R. (1998). Managed care at the crossroads: Can managed care organizations survive government regulation? *Annals of Health Law, 7,* 25–72.

Cigna Healthplan of Louisiana v. State of Louisiana, 82 F. 3d 642 (5th Cir. 1996).

Corporate Health Insurance Inc. v. Texas Dept. of Insurance, 12 F. Supp. 2d 597 (S.D. Tex. 1998).

Crocco v. Xerox Corporation, 137 F. 3d 105 (2d Cir. 1998).

Danca v. Emerson Hospital, 9 F. Supp. 2d 27 (D. Mass. 1998).

Delta Dental v. Banasky, 27 Cal. App. 4th 1598, 33 Cal. Rptr. 2d 381 (1994).

Dukes v. U.S. Healthcare, Inc., 57 F. 3d 350 (3d Cir. 1995).

80 bills in states would make managed care more accountable. (1999). *National Psychologist, 8,* 1.

Ettner, S. (1999). The relationship between continuity of care and the health behaviors of patients: Does having a usual physician make a difference? *Medical Care, 37,* 547–555.

Furrow, B. R., Greaney, T. L., Johnson, S. H., Jost, T. S., & Schwartz, R. L. (1997). *Health law: Cases, materials, and problems* (3d ed.). St. Paul, MN: West Publishing.

Glassman, M. (1996). Comment: Can HMOs wield market power? Assessing antitrust liability in the imperfect market for health care financing. *American University Law Review, 46,* 91–147.

Goldfarb v. Virginia State Bar, 421 U.S. 773 (1975).

Hall, M. A. (1990). Health care cost containment and the stratification of malpractice law. *Jurimetrics, 30,* 501–508.

Hall, M. A., Smith, T. R., Naughton, M., & Ebbers, A. (1996). Symposium on consumer protection in managed care: Mechanisms of consumer protection–the marketplace and regulation: Judicial protection of managed care consumers: An empirical study of insurance coverage dispute. *Seton Hall Law Review, 26,* 1055–1068.

Health Law Reporter (BNA), 8, 520 (1999) (bill would allow health care professionals to bargain with HMOs, other health insurers).

Hellinger, F. J. (1995). Any-willing-provider and freedom-of-choice laws: An economic assessment. *Health Affairs, 14* (4), 297–302.

Henderson, J. A., & Siciliano, J. A. (1994). Universal health care and the continued reliance on custom in determining medical malpractice. *Cornell Law Review, 79,* 1382–1404.

Herdrich v. Pegram, 178 F. 3d 683 (7th Cir. 1999).

Holstein v. Green Spring Health Services, No. 98-CV-2453 (S.D.N.Y. 1998) (motion to dismiss case rejected by court on June 16, 1999).

Hughes v. Blue Cross, 215 Cal. App. 3d 832, 263 Cal. Rptr. 850 (1989).

Huss v. Green Spring Health Services, 18 F. Supp. 2d 400 (D. Del. 1998).

Huss v. Green Spring Health Services, 1999 U.S. Dist. 10014 (E.D. Pa. 1999).

Johnson v. Kokemoore, 545 N.W. 2d 495 (Wis. 1996).

Kopit, W. G., & Vanderbilt, T. B. (1996). Analysis and perspective [on new federal antitrust guidelines]. *Health Law Reporter, 5,* 36–43.

Lee, P. V. (1996). The promise and perils of managed health care: Consumers' search for a level playing field. *Whittier Law Review, 18,* 3–11.

Litwak, P. (1999). Anti-trust issues in transactions among healthcare providers. *Behavioral Healthcare Tomorrow, 8,* 19–23.

Managed Health Care Insurance Accountability Act of 1999. Cal. Civ. Code S. 3428 (West 2001).

Martin, J. A., & Bjerknes, L. K. (1996). The legal and ethical implications of gag clauses in physician contracts. *American Journal of Law and Medicine, 22,* 433–476.

Mateo-Woodburn v. Fresno Community Hospital, 221 Cal. App. 3d 1169, 270 Cal. Rptr. 894 (1990).

McCarthy, D. (1997). Narrowing provider choice: Any willing provider laws after New York Blue Cross v. Travelers. *American Journal of Law and Medicine, 23,* 97–113.

McEvoy v. Group Health Cooperative of Eau Claire, 570 N.W. 2d 397 (Wis. 1997).

Mental Retardation Facilities and Community Mental Health Centers Construction Act of 1963, Pub. L. No. 88-164, 77 Stat. 282 (1963).

Montgomery, L. M., Cupit, B. E., & Wimberley, T. K. (1999). Complaints, malpractice and risk management: Professional issues and personal experiences. *Professional Psychology, Research and Practice, 30,* 402–410.

Morreim, E. H. (1992). Whodunit? Causal responsibility of utilization review for physicians' decisions, patients' outcomes. *Law, Medicine & Health Care, 20,* 40–56.

Muse v. Charter Hospital, 117 N.C. App. 468, 452 S.E. 2d 589 (1995).

Muse v. Charter Hospital, 342 N.C. 666, 467 S.E. 2d 718 (1996).

Neade v. Portes, 303 Ill. App. 3d 799, 710 N.E. 2d 418 (1999).

Neade v. Portes, 193 Ill. 2d 433, 793 N.E. 2d 496 (2000).

New Jersey Psychological Association v. MCC Behavioral Health, 1997 U.S. Dist. LEXIS 16338 (D.N.J. 1997).

Petrila, J. (1998). Courts as gatekeepers in managed care settings. *Health Affairs, 17* (2), 109–117.

Petrila, J., & Levin, B. L. (1996). Impact of mental disability law on mental health policies and services. In B. L. Levin & J. Petrila (Eds.), *Mental health services: A public health perspective.* New York: Oxford University Press.

Picinic, N. J. (1997). Physicians, bound and gagged: Federal attempts to combat managed care's use of gag clauses. *Seton Hall Legislative Journal, 21,* 567–620.

Plocica v. NYLCare of Texas, 43 F. Supp. 658 (N.D. Tex. 1999).

Roessert v. Health Net, 929 F. Supp. 343 (N.D. Cal. 1996).

Rosenblatt, R. E., Law, S. A., & Rosenbaum, S. (1997). *Law and the American health care system* (1997 Suppl.). Westbury, NY: Foundation Press.

Rosenblatt, R. E., Law, S. A., and Rosenbaum, S. (1998). *Law and the American health care system* (1998 Suppl.). Westbury, NY: Foundation Press.

Salley v. DuPont, 966 F. 2d 1011 (5th Cir. 1992).

Sclar, D. A., Skaer, T. L., Robison, L. M., Galin, R. S., Legg, R. F., & Nemec, N. L. (1998). Economic outcomes with antidepressant pharmacotherapy: A retrospective intent-to-treat analysis. *Journal of Clinical Psychiatry, 59* (Suppl. 2), 13–17.

Settlement ends antitrust investigation of mental health centers. (1996, September 14). *Tennessean,* p. 3B.

Shea v. Esensten, 107 F. 3d 625 (8th Cir. 1997).

Simon, R. I. (1998). *A concise guide to psychiatry and law for clinicians* (2d ed.). Washington, DC: American Psychiatric Press.

Stauffer, M., & Levy, D. R. (1999). *1999 state by state guide to managed care law.* New York: Aspen.

Stephens v. CMG Health, 165 F. 3d 14 (2d Cir. 1998).

Stone, A. (1995). Paradigms, pre-emptions, and stages: Understanding the transformation of American psychiatry by managed care. *International Journal of Law & Psychiatry, 18,* 353–387.

Taber, J. C., & King, J. P. (1994). Caught in the crossfire: Economic credentialing in the health care war. *Detroit College Law Review [1994],* 1179–1214.

Tarasoff v. Regents of University of California, 17 Cal. 3d 425, 551 P. 2d 334 (1976).

Tex. Civ. Prac. and Remedies Code Ann. Chapter 88 (Vernon 2001).

Texas Ins. Code Ann. Chapter 29 (Vernon 2001).

Varol v. Blue Cross, 708 F. Supp. 826 (E.D. Mich. 1989).

Wickline v. California, 239 Cal. Rptr. 810 (Cal. Ct. App. 1986).

Wilson v. Blue Cross of Southern California, 271 Cal. Rptr. 876 (Cal. Ct. App. 1990).

Wojcik, J. (1999, February 1). Aetna verdict shakes up industry. *Business Insurance,* p. 2.

Chapter 11

THE PUBLIC SECTOR

Danna Mauch

This chapter examines the evolution of managed care in the public sector, including the driving forces behind the adoption of managed care technology and the problems that the adopters have sought to solve. The field is at a significant juncture after a decade of implementation of managed care "reforms." The turn of the new century coincided with the publication of the first report of the surgeon general on mental health (Satcher, 1999), the establishment of the first White House Conference on Mental Health, and the commissioning by the Robert Wood Johnson Foundation of an Institute for the Future report, *Health and Health Care 2010: The Forecast and the Challenge* (2000), and its companion report, *Mental Health Care 2010* (2001). In each case there were calls for recognition of mental illnesses as presenting a fundamental public health issue in America, for clarity about the needs of the citizenry for effective prevention and treatment of behavioral disorders, for a commitment to address gaps in the quality and comprehensiveness of care systems; and for the application of research knowledge to drive proposed reforms. Public sector behavioral health care was at a similar juncture 25 years ago–a decade into community mental health reform. Due to the uneven implementation of those reforms, philosophers and pundits alike called for solutions to the inadequacies of care systems. Critics' refrain was strikingly similar to the litany of complaints about managed care reforms, citing problems in procurement of services, design of the essential services, funding of programs, quality of providers, and adequacy of administrative infrastructure (Foley & Sharfstein, 1983).

The chapter reviews current trends and performance expectations, and includes a comparison of private sector to public sector managed behavioral health care. Comparisons are also drawn to earlier system-change initiatives. Case studies illustrate the achievements and failures of both carve-in and carve-out public sector programs. The chapter concludes with an assessment of the key public policy issues to be addressed in the decade ahead, along with the market opportunities that those issues present to organizations able to modify their products and performance.

During the 1990s, managed care practices were broadly implemented for behavioral health services in the public sector. Prior to that, beginning in the mid-1980s, several state and county mental health authorities adopted some managed care tools from the private sector to support community mental health system reforms, including gatekeeping, utilization review, capitation, and case rates (Anderson, D. F. et al., 2001). Results of these initial managed care efforts in the public behavioral health arena were mixed. A retrospective review published in 1989 recommended significant modifications for successful adaptation of what were, after all, applications developed to control medical and surgical costs in the private sector (Mechanic & Aiken, 1989). Nevertheless, more comprehensive adoption of managed care technology was seen as a handy solution to the problems plaguing states in the early 1990s, especially in the face of reduced government revenues: rapidly increasing Medicaid expenditures and difficulties in providing access for Medicaid recipients to mainstream insurers and their network panels (Leadholm & Kerzner, 1994). Little time and effort was spent making the modifications needed to retrofit managed care technology to public sector conditions.

Opportunities to control the cost of public sector care through the use of fiscal and care-management intermediaries were supported by federal Health Care Financing Administration (HCFA) waivers to Medicaid requirements, granted to 44 of the 50 states by 1994 (Robinson & Scallet, 1998). Early on, managed care, like temporary placement in the child welfare world, solved some short-term problems but without therefore appearing to be the best fit for a new, permanent structure for the behavioral health system. As mentioned above, migration of technology and tools from the private sector required more retrofitting and modification than occurred initially–

which led to significant problems and then, in turn, to demands for change both in the operating practices of managed care organizations and in the oversight methods of their government customers. The substantial capital requirements needed to cover technology expenses and insurance reserves for managed care operations demanded a new set of partners for states. In the main, these partners were private, for-profit companies that had little experience with government contracting, provider politics, or consumer stakeholders.

These problems are reminiscent of the limitations that arose in the implementation of community mental health programs as a less expensive and more progressive alternative to state psychiatric hospitals in the mid-1960s. Lacking a community-based continuum of care that would supplant all of the functions of the state hospitals, early community mental health programs could not achieve the goals for which they were designed (Mechanic & Surles, 1992). Moreover, the success of the effort depended on partnership with small nonprofit entities inexperienced with state hospital patients, who needed more than traditional outpatient therapy and whose medications had significant side effects.

STATE AND COUNTY PLANS AND WAIVERS

In order to implement aspects of managed care technology that conflicted with Medicaid regulations, states sought waivers of the rules as permitted under sections 1115 and 1915(b) of Title XIX of the Social Security Act, the Medicaid law. Many of the first HCFA waiver requests (California, Massachusetts, Oregon, and Pennsylvania) were under section 1915(b), permitting states to waive the freedom-of-choice requirement in favor of enrolling recipients in HMOs, and to negotiate flexible provider-reimbursement structures. Section 1115 waivers allowed states to expand the changes cited above to substantially restructure financing, payments, delivery systems, benefits, and eligibility. In numerous states (Florida, Massachusetts, Pennsylvania, Tennessee, Texas, and Utah), section 1115 waivers extended coverage to uninsured and underinsured persons who did not meet Medicaid eligibility requirements. These waivers also permitted states to combine several funding sources for a single population, to manage mental health or children's services on a carve-out basis to all recipients, and to manage all care provided to special-needs populations (Moss, 1998).

GOALS OF MANAGED BEHAVIORAL HEALTH INITIATIVES

The main goal of states' early efforts with managed care was cost savings. This goal was the same whether achieved through a *carve-in* strategy (where behavioral health care was managed in conjunction with primary health care within an HMO), or a *carve-out* strategy (where behavioral health services were managed by a specialty managed behavioral health organization (MBHO)). Massachusetts, citing a 20% annual increase in Medicaid spending on behavioral health services, awarded the first behavioral health carve-out contract in 1991 (Leadholm & Kerzner, 1994). The state Medicaid agency (SMA) took the lead, explicitly wanting to rein in costs and bring predictability to its budget process, which the SMA saw as driven by the Department of Mental Health and its traditional, community mental health center (CMHC) provider system. The State Mental Health Authority (SMHA) and CMHCs were viewed as having been a driving force in Medicaid cost increases—a result of their efforts to maximize federal financial participation in state behavioral health programs. At the other end of the country, Utah, another early adopter of the carve-out strategy, elected to have the SMHA take the lead and to contract with its CMHCs to manage the care under the HCFA waiver (Robinson & Scallet, 1998). Improved access and quality of care were the companion goals in the now proverbial three-legged stool of managed care: access, cost, and quality.

In a reprise of the role that the federal government played with the states in the early years of community mental health, federal funds supported states' cost cutting as long as accompanied by service improvements. In retrospect, greater emphasis might have been placed on determining the adequacy of care systems and resource investments to meet the needs of the eligible service populations. Federal oversight was accompanied by a lack of clarity on the part of state purchasers of managed behavioral care as to whether they were purchasing management of benefits or management of a system of care. Given that the word "system" implies organized, integrated, and functioning elements, several early managed behavioral care initiatives were, ironically, notable for wresting the Medicaid-covered element of the care system away from the SMHA, the traditional system manager, and awarding its management to an inexperienced private company.

Over time, evolving state policies combined with federal waiver requirements to generate broader goals for managing behavioral health programs, including (Stroul, 2000):

- increasing access to timely treatment targeted to fit individual need
- improving the quality of providers and services
- promoting clinical innovation
- strengthening information management and reporting
- ensuring accountability to consumers through appeal and grievance processes
- fostering recovery and consumer satisfaction
- allocating resources in a clinical and cost-efficient manner

One of Massachusetts's former Medicaid managed-care administrators has argued that there are fundamental differences in emphasis and goals when managed care services are procured by "regulators" versus "purchasers": SMHA "regulators" are far more prescriptive and bring stakeholders to the process, whereas SMA "purchasers" are more focused on cost and access outcomes. In any case, SMHAs frequently prefer carve-out programs with a dedicated focus on behavioral health benefits, and SMAs were the early proponents of carve-in programs in which behavioral health benefits were administered to Medicaid recipients within HMO contracts. Carve-in contracts often resulted in major reductions in services provided to mentally ill plan members. Pennsylvania's Health Choices Program Demonstration in five southeastern counties produced audited findings that one HMO spent as little as 25% of the behavioral health premium dollar on behavioral health care. This finding was one of the more salient reasons to support a 1994 decision to carve out behavioral health services in Pennsylvania's statewide implementation of managed health care (Century, 2000). SMHAs promoted the involvement of MBHOs to manage on a carve-in basis with the HMO as their customer, or to manage on a carve-out basis with the government as their customer.

In the main, HMOs were led by persons without significant experience in behavioral health or psychiatric care—which was reflected in their willingness to enter into contracts with SMAs that had inadequate provisions for behavioral care. Leaders of MBHOs' public sector divisions, by contrast, generally held values informed by years of experience in public practice and policy, and believed that improved access must be complemented by early intervention, comprehensive care management, continuity of care, follow-up, collaboration with stakeholders, and creation of new community care to offset inpatient utilization (Feldman, 1992). Those goals, which resonated with SMHAs, were reflected in the proposals and promises made by MBHOs during the contract-procurement processes, but were not consistently sought by the SMAs, which are effectively the customer and the contract agent in the majority of Medicaid managed care programs. In several instances, SMHAs were unable either to develop, or to persuade SMAs to adopt, measures that reflected the SMHAs' extensive public practice experience.

FINANCING CARE AND UNDERWRITING BENEFIT PLANS

Behavioral health services in the public sector is a big business. The National Alliance for the Mentally Ill (NAMI) reports that 5.6 million U.S. citizens have serious mental illnesses, driving an estimated $69 billion in direct treatment costs (Rice & Miller, 1996). The majority of those citizens are served in public care systems. National Institute for Mental Health (NIMH) data estimate that within the adult population at large, 5.4% have serious mental illness, including 0.9%, or 2 million persons, with schizophrenia, and 1%, or 2.3 million persons, with manic-depressive illness (Kessler, Olfson, & Berglund, 1998). In the adult population aged 18 to 54 years, 8%, or 19 million persons, have depression. A high number of children (some studies mention 15%) have, or are at risk for, serious emotional disorders, including depression, bipolar illness, and schizophrenia (Kessler et al.). NIMH estimates that 3% to 5% of children have attention-deficit/hyperactivity disorder (ADHD) and 1 to 2 children per 1,000 in the population have autism. There exists a high co-occurrence of depression and behavioral problems among these latter two groups of children, who are often treated in publicly financed care systems. Although the publicly insured or covered populations vary from state to state, those citizens with the most serious and disabling conditions are typically included in the coverage—which results in higher penetration, utilization, and costs in public sector managed behavioral health plans.

As noted above, the states—operating under HCFA's Medicaid waiver provisions—implemented managed care plans for behavioral health services under several delivery, risk, and financial structures, including:

- carve-in to managed care plan or HMO
- carve-out to managed care organization (MCO) or MBHO
- full risk, where the HMO, MCO, or MBHO is at full risk for the cost of care
- partial risk, where the risk is shared between the MBHO and government
- no risk, administrative services only (ASO), where the MBHO performs select administrative tasks, and government retains both the full risk of the cost of care and, typically, some care-management functions

In addition to relying on Medicaid reimbursement dollars, some states had MCOs manage other pools of federal, state, or local funding that were historically dedicated to behavioral health services. The total funding package administered might include:

- Medicaid waiver funds
- state appropriations for non-Medicaid-eligible or uninsured persons
- federal mental health or substance abuse block-grant funds
- federal McKinney Act (homeless/mentally ill) block-grant funds
- federal Title IV-E funds for mentally ill child welfare clients
- county Medicaid match or uncompensated-care funds
- state or county appropriations for state or county hospitals

Different eligibility and administrative rules cover each of the above funding sources. The MCO might receive Medicaid payments on a capitated basis with a fixed rate per member per month (PM/PM), therefore having a total reimbursement that fluctuates with the number of enrollees. State appropriations for indigent persons who are uninsured or not Medicaid eligible might be a fixed sum of money, with a cap on reimbursement regardless of the number of persons covered. State-hospital operating-budget appropriations are in some contracts a part of the financing package, with an expectation that utilization be managed. State-hospital appropriation dollars are to be spent exclusively on state-hospital admissions, limiting any other use of the funds. Similarly, block-grant funds must be spent on specific allowable services, which do not include, for example, inpatient/detoxification services. While it may be attractive to the government payer to have the MCO manage a fuller purse, the increase in funding (over Medicaid waiver dollars) does not, for the MCO, necessarily either improve flexibility and per capita resources, or limit the risk of the cost of care.

Montana's statewide carve-out for behavioral health services presents a useful example. The state contracted with a MBHO to manage its behavioral health benefits on a full-risk, carve-out basis. The contract included:

- a modest PM/PM for the Medicaid-eligible population
- a fixed-cap sum of dollars to provide benefits to a pool of non-Medicaid-eligible, mentally disabled persons and uninsured persons whose income was up to 250% of the federal poverty level
- a fund for reimbursement of the Montana state hospital, to be spent only on hospital reimbursement or community care for persons who were long-term hospital residents

MCO expenditure of state-hospital appropriations was permitted for both state-hospital admissions and residential programs for discharged patients. Reimbursements to the hospital, however, had to be sufficient to cover hospital operating costs, requiring the MCO to increase reimbursement rates to the state hospital as the census declined–a result of the MCO's efforts to place patients into community residential care. In effect, every hospital patient that was moved out of the hospital ended up costing the MCO for both community care and increased hospital rates. Despite the inherent financial disincentive, the MCO placed most of the patients into community care, leading Montana to raise even further the reimbursement rate for the remaining state-hospital beds (Mauch, 2000).

Capitation rates vary greatly from one state to another. Today, carve-in rates to HMOs for the Medicaid-eligible population can be as low as $1.10 PM/PM, while carve-out rates vary from $6.65 PM/PM in Texas, to $100 PM/PM in Massachusetts (Satcher, 1999). Benefits to be covered by those sums also vary, and supplemental state appropriations may cover some collateral services in the states with lower

PM/PMs. There is not a consistent, proportional relationship, however, between PM/PM rates, intensity of member need, and benefits covered (Holohan, 1998). Despite challenges to the validity of historical cost and utilization data and also to the actuarial soundness of some state plans, the HCFA approved most states' waiver requests and has withdrawn only a handful of approvals.

Variability in capitation rates has been further complicated by the unanticipated and sizable shifts between the Medicaid-eligible and non-eligible/uninsured populations due to welfare reform. The shift in eligible populations occurred after many managed care rates were set, and contracts were executed without provisions to revisit capitation rates or global-cost caps. Other unanticipated events—such as rapid adoption of selective serotonin reuptake inhibitors (SSRIs), a huge rise in pharmacy charges, and more aggressive implementation of early periodic screening and diagnostic testing (EPSDT) benefits led to increases in the cost of care. These increases, combined with unfunded mandates, changes in the covered population, and questionable actuarial soundness of plans, have come to jeopardize program operations in many public sector managed care initiatives (Kronebusch, 2001).

CONTRACTUAL, REGULATORY, AND LEGAL REQUIREMENTS: PRIVATE SECTOR TECHNOLOGY IN A PUBLIC SECTOR CONTEXT

There are numerous respects in which private sector and public sector managed care programs differ. Many of the differences are reflected in contractual, regulatory, and legal requirements placed on MCOs or MBHOs, which include:

- the length, complexity, and cost of state and county procurement processes
- the detail, restrictions, and regulatory requirements of MCO contract provisions
- the nature and extent of contractual performance standards and incentives
- constraints on administrative costs
- insurance regulations and statutory requirements
- impact of state and federal court decisions

Equally salient are substantive differences that exist between the private and public sectors–which affect the success of applying managed care technology in the arena of government-financed behavioral health care. In the face of falling revenues and explicit goals to reduce costs, the public sector's procurement process and its contract terms with private managed care companies often reflect rising expectations and standards. Moreover, MCOs encounter much more complex, lengthy, and costly bureaucratic methods of procurement in the public sector than are generally used for bidding and contracting in the private sector (Surles, 2001). Competitive requests for proposals (RFPs) in the public sector can exceed 1000 pages and require lengthy clinical, administrative, and financial responses within weeks of RFP publication. The review and selection process is typically far longer, and the implementation period shorter, than in the private sector.

One further, important difference encountered by the MCOs is that numerous program objectives and outcomes–which were never attained when government (with more money available) ran these programs–have been imposed through the politicization of the procurement process. In the first several years of Iowa's managed behavioral health program, for example, there were more than 110 clinical, financial, and process outcomes to be tracked and reported on a monthly basis (Verzbhinsky, 2000). These requirements were not dissimilar to those encountered in early community mental health programs, which were regulated with the goal of achieving care standards that exceeded those in the largely unaccredited state hospitals (and also to provide more treatment for less money than paid to the state hospitals).

In addition to the above complexities generated by the procurement process, MCOs faced other complexities that resulted from the inherent difficulties of dealing with and treating the particular citizens who have serious mental illnesses and are eligible for publicly financed care programs. The pathology, morbidity, and mortality of the eligible population is far more diverse than what is characteristic of the privately insured population. In response to the complex needs of these persons, governments created numerous discrete program responses–fragmenting mandates and benefits in the process, and also creating a diversity of stakeholders. For example, there are 11 federal agencies that administer some form of behavioral health program or benefit. At the state or county level, there are at a minimum several public agencies, in addition to the state behavioral health authority, administering pieces of a comprehensive benefit and believing that they are "purchasing stakeholders." Stakeholders also multiply with the addition of consumer-, family-, and legal-advocacy groups, as well as with the multifarious providers who participate in comprehensive care networks.

Another problem that MCOs and MBHOs encounter in the public sector is a result of that sector's often unsophisticated reporting and billing capabilities. The limited capital investment that has limited those capabilities has also impeded development of technology infrastructure in the government agencies that are the purchaser of managed care services.

Despite the complex medical needs of the patient population, the fragmentation of the benefit/funding structure, the multiplicity of stakeholders, and the weak technology infrastructure in the public sector health care system, MCOs and MBHOs were expected to produce results similar to those seen in the private sector. The government purchasers assumed that they would reap significant, if one-time, savings in the conversion to a managed network. Government purchasers also expected ongoing savings from efficiencies in care utilization. Few of the parties involved recognized the extent to which dollars saved on inpatient and emergency care, for example, would have to be invested in behavioral health services reform, including intensive community-based treatment alternatives (Stroul, 2000).

MBHO POLICIES AND PRACTICES
TO MEET PUBLIC SECTOR GOALS

Managing behavioral health care in the public sector is more challenging than in the private sector and also has greater potential for impact if the HMO or MBHO succeeds in addressing historical deficiencies in care access, delivery structure, and service quality. As other states followed Massachusetts, Oregon, and Utah into the managed care arena, some gained from the early adopters' experience and others repeated some of the initial mistakes by failing to modify the private sector technology. By the second half of the 1990s, California, Iowa, Maryland, Tennessee, and Washington, among others, sought modified approaches to implementing managed care—reflecting their recognition of the public sector's distinctive consumer, provider, and system characteristics. The states' desire for customization led to the now-routine characterization of public sector managed care: "if you've seen one public sector managed care program, you've seen one public sector managed care program." The following are examples of some of the better modifications adopted:

- *Membership outreach and enrollment support.* Instead of mailing enrollment materials and member handbooks–as would typically be done with an employed, privately insured population–MBHOs in California, Maryland, Massachusetts, and Tennessee, among others, took steps to recognize the circumstances and needs of their members. These steps included: distributing materials at program locations commonly used by the target population; enlisting consumers/members in reviewing document drafts for "readability" and "user friendliness"; publishing materials in several languages; and holding orientation meetings to assist consumers with enrollment, benefit utilization, and grievances.

- *Consumer and family governance.* In order to avoid the historical disenfranchisement of the consumers of behavioral health services, MBHOs in California, Iowa, Pennsylvania, Tennessee, and Washington took steps to include consumers in all aspects of operations. The steps taken included: appointing governing or advisory boards comprising a majority of consumers and their family members; hiring consumers in staff positions; implementing care-management protocols that required providers to engage consumers in treatment planning and decision making; and engaging consumers and family members in external monitoring of the MBHOs and provider networks.

- *Integrated clinical- and utilization-review protocols.* Review protocols were developed that reflected the more intensive needs of the public sector population and that incorporated clinical research findings for children having serious emotional disturbances, adults with serious mental illness, and persons with co-occurring addictive and mental disorders.

- *Community reinvestment in innovative services.* In Iowa, Massachusetts, Tennessee, and Washington, savings in the cost of care were invested in evidence-based community treatments. Innovations included mobile care teams, assertive community treatment teams, child safety, home-based treatment and fami-

ly-support services, and consumer-operated psychosocial rehabilitation services.

- *Services preauthorization and case rates.* In order to reduce the
administrative burden for providers and to increase access to
timely and individualized treatment, California, Nebraska,
Oregon, Pennsylvania, and Washington, among others, preauthorized as many as 20 outpatient visits for high-risk consumer groups. They also approved case rates for a blend of
case-management/outpatient treatment and inpatient/residen-
tial treatment, to be employed at the discretion of the lead treatment provider.

Coinciding with the adoption of managed care practices, and pursuant to the promotion of evidence-based practices by the MBHOs
and consumer groups, a number of issues too long neglected are now
more often addressed in public care systems. These issues include:

- *Delays in diagnosis and treatment, resulting in disability.* Significant
delays between the onset of mental illness and the diagnosis and
appropriate treatment of behavioral health disorders cause personal suffering and persistent disability. Studies identify an average gap of 11 years between onset and treatment for depression,
3 years for manic-depressive illness, and 2 years for schizophrenia (Kessler, Olfson, & Berglund, 1998). These delays are
expensive individually, socially, and economically.
- *Reduced life expectancy and serious mental illness.* A 1999 cross-sec-
tional mortality linkage study of 43,274 adults served by the
Massachusetts Department of Mental Health (DMH) between
1989 and 1994 found a significantly shorter life span for persons
treated for serious mental illness. On average, these individuals
lived 8.8 years less than their peers without mental illness in the
general population. With a mean loss of 14.1 years for men and
5.7 years for women, the difference between the DMH group
and the general population was consistent across most causes of
death. The notable exception was the differentially high rate of
deaths among the DMH group due to medications and suicide
(Dembling, Chen, & Vachon, 1999).
- *Opportunity for recovery.* Professional education and public attitudes–both of which have historically reflected a belief that
severe mental illness results in lifelong deterioration–have shift-

ed. Programs and practices do not as yet, however, uniformly promote recovery. Consumers, families, and researchers have identified treatment and rehabilitation services that, in addition to providing relief of symptoms, effectively restore role functioning, self-esteem, and identity as productive community members. Promoting recovery is essential to engaging consumers in illness management or "self-managed care"–which ensures stabilization and prevents relapse, according to the surgeon general's report on behavioral health. Those findings imply a significant restructuring of services in most public care systems (Satcher, 1999).

- *Goodness of fit between need and care.* A poor fit between an individual's need for treatment and the care received produces inefficient utilization, unnecessary costs, and ineffective outcomes. Not only do consumers who get the wrong treatment (or too much or too little treatment) typically fail to get better, they get discouraged, fail to comply with treatment regimens, or drop out of care–later returning in crisis, or worse. Children who get stuck for long periods of time in inpatient units or residential treatment centers lose family connections, community ties, and educational opportunities, and fail to achieve normative developmental milestones. Later, in adolescence and adulthood, these children have substantially higher risk of system dependence or incarceration.

- *Risks of homelessness and imprisonment.* Nearly six times more individuals with behavioral illness are in the country's jails than are in our psychiatric hospitals. In 1999, the U.S. Department of Justice estimated that 280,000 persons with serious mental illnesses were in jail or prison, approaching 16% of the total incarcerated population. Among adjudicated juveniles, an estimated 65% to 70% carry psychiatric diagnoses. Among homeless persons, 34% are estimated to have serious mental illnesses. Risks of deadly infectious disease, of inadequate psychiatric treatment, and of personal violence are nearly universal among homeless and incarcerated persons, further exacerbating higher morbidity and mortality among mentally ill persons (Ditton, 1999).

- *Women in treatment with trauma histories and co-occurring disorders.* Beginning with state hospital populations in the 1970s and continuing in CMHCs in the 1990s, studies have confirmed that 80% or more of women receiving care in public care systems have histories of trauma from childhood or of domestic violence. As a consequence, the majority of these women have co-occurring mental and addictive disorders. Despite the research findings and the identified human needs, few of these women have treatment plans that address their simultaneous needs to be treated for trauma, addiction, and psychiatric disorders. Moreover, where multiple treatment needs are cited, women rarely have access to integrated services. Absent integrated and targeted treatment, these women have a high incidence of medical co-morbidity, with higher costs and poorer outcomes than other patients (Fendell & Honig, 2000).

CASE STUDIES ILLUSTRATING KEY ISSUES

There is both utility and risk to implementing managed care in the public sector. Case studies illustrate both features, while underscoring that local context can be a determining factor in the relative success or failure of a particular managed care strategy. The following case studies center on three strategies employed by MBHOs:

- to blend funding and to integrate treatment protocols in order to address co-occurring addictions and psychiatric disorders
- to reduce utilization and to integrate state psychiatric-hospital patients into communities
- to retool poorly fitting managed care initiatives
- to integrate leadership, vision, and resources

Improving the Treatment of Persons with Co-Occurring Addictions and Psychiatric Disorders

Among persons with serious and persistent mental illnesses, co-morbidity with addictions is found in the majority, and services that effectively meet this population's complex needs are uncommon. This population's problems are complicated by the bureaucratic structure of state and county governments, with separate agencies administering mental health and substance abuse services. Despite the availability of evidence-based treatments, such as the PACT (program for assertive community treatment), few states have adopted public policy that would direct state agencies and providers to use them. Massachusetts is a laudable exception.

Persons who have both mental health and substance abuse disorders typically encounter services provided in separate settings, under separate rules, with differently licensed professionals. Among other things, the treatment lacks integration and continuity. In order to address these problems, the Massachusetts DMH collaborated with the Department of Public Health's Bureau of Substance Abuse Services to formulate a new care model, with the input of consumers, families, providers, legislators, and the Substance Abuse and Mental Health Services Administration. The key principles of the continuous, comprehensive, integrated system of care (CCISC) are integration, continuity, comprehensiveness, quality, and implementation. Based on these principles, the parties framed a four-stage approach to treatment—acute stabilization, engagement, active treatment to maintain stabilization, and rehabilitation and recovery—adopted across systems of care, and to be taken into account in every clinical encounter, regardless of level of care or location of service (Minkoff, 2000). In order to implement this commitment, the state departments pledged to undertake a planning process, now under way, to identify

- existing services for individuals with co-occurring psychiatric and substance disorders, including the specification of the role of those services in a CCISC
- existing services that need to be enhanced in order to meet the requirements of a CCISC, including the development of plans for achieving those enhancements
- significant gaps in existing services, including the development of plans for addressing those gaps through new services, programs, or funding

This policy, based on the joint initiative of the commissioners of mental health, medical assistance, and public health, is being implemented by the MBHO that is managing Massachusetts's public insurance benefits in mental health and substance abuse (Sudders, Bullen, & Koh, 1999).

Integrating Patients from a
State Psychiatric Hospital into the Community

Pursuant to federal court orders to close Haverford State Hospital and place its residents in community care settings–the result of a class action lawsuit brought in 1990 under Title II of the Americans with Disabilities Act–officials in Delaware County, Pennsylvania, sought assistance in the placement of 193 patients. This placement effort was undertaken in the wake of implementing the state's Medicaid managed care program, Health Choices. Historically, Haverford State Hospital played a significant role in the Delaware County continuum of care for persons with serious mental illnesses, but long-term patients could not be enrolled in Health Choices; the consent-decree requirements for their community care did not sufficiently correspond to Health Choices' benefit design (Willis, 2000).

The federal court order outlined unique requirements for the assessment, planning, funding, and placement processes involved in integrating the class members into the community. The MBHO had the task of integrating divergent objectives and satisfying the terms both of the Medicaid managed care contract and the consent decree.

The class members all presented complex behavioral, as well as medical and social, problems and needs. The required clinical-assessment process was designed to determine the types of services that they would need in order to live successfully in the various residential placements in the community. Armed with individual patient-assessment data, an RFP was developed and circulated to all current providers in the Delaware County service network. In order to promote the best results for the class members, the Office of Behavioral Health held an applicants' conference attended by all interested providers, as well as by clinical staff involved in the assessment and discharge-planning process. Applicant-providers were able to learn in detail the profiles, needs, and specific range of services that each consumer would need for community placement. The RFP review team included behavioral health consumers, family members, and staff and board members of the Office of Behavioral Health. Awards were made based on the overall programmatic and fiscal quality of the proposal, in addition to the demonstrated capacity of the applicant-provider.

The selected MBHO assisted the Office of Behavioral Health in implementing 26 residential programs with capacity for the Haverford State Hospital residents. In addition to the residential services created through the RFP process, the following services were developed or expanded to provide essential supports to the class members (Willis, 2000):

- intensive case management (ICM) expansion
- site-based psychiatric rehabilitation (socialization)
- mobile assessment stabilization treatment (MAST) team
- community employment/vocational services
- consumer-operated drop-in center expansion
- permanent housing/supported living service expansion
- psychiatric rehabilitation service expansion

This more robust system of care, coupled with the development of individualized programs for the members of the class, enabled the Delaware County Office of Behavioral Health, with the assistance of the MBHO, to comply with the demanding terms of the consent decree.

Capabilities to Contract for and Support Consumer-Directed Services

Clark County, Washington, is the site of the state's initial venture into managed behavioral health care. The MBHO with which the county first contracted in 1996 introduced several care-management innovations in order to improve access to, and quality of, care for children and adults with mental illnesses who were indigent or Medicaid beneficiaries. Most notable was the effort of the MBHO to support and contract with consumer-directed services.

The MBHO in Washington, like its counterparts in California, Iowa, Montana, Pennsylvania, and Tennessee, regularly engaged consumers in discussions and planning with regard to clinical policy, benefit design, system change, and outcome measurement. In addition, the Washington MBHO supported consumer-run enterprises with technical assistance and contract dollars designed to strengthen the organization's foundations and develop its portfolio of programs.

After being nominated by consumers, the MBHO received an industry leadership award for its various efforts behalf of one consumer self-help organization. Among other things, the MBHO helped with the establishment of a "warm line" for consumer peer support, with a plan for a consumer-run drop-in center, with fundraising and financial-management systems, and with program infrastructure to attract state contracts for providing employment services to consumers. In addition to producing a reported 15% increase in consumer satisfaction with the MBHO, the leadership award for the joint MBHO-consumer initiatives was a source of satisfaction and commitment both for the organization and for the individuals involved in the projects (Anderson, K., 2000).

Retooling Managed Care Initiatives

The Iowa Department of Human Services (IDHS) implemented the Mental Health Access Plan (MHAP) under a section 1915(b) Medicaid waiver. Behavioral health coverage was provided to most of Iowa's Medicaid recipients; others, but not all, were phased in over the first two years of the program. Traditional behavioral health services were covered, including inpatient, outpatient, inpatient alternatives (that is, partial hospitalization and day treatment), transportation, medication management, and psychiatric services. Additionally, the MBHO was required to develop and utilize a broader range of community-based services and supports such as mobile crisis counseling, in-home therapy, and assertive community treatment. The MBHO performed under a fully capitated, risk-based contract to develop and deliver all necessary behavioral health services for eligible enrollees (Verzbhinsky, 2000).

There were numerous and vocal objections—by providers, families, consumers, and advocates—to the state's plan to contract for managed behavioral health services, and the criticisms continued unabated through the implementation period of the MBHO contract. Competitors of the selected MBHO even sued the state of Iowa over the decision to award the contract to that particular organization.

In view of the MBHO's inexperience, the brief time allowed for the implementation of a complex program, and the numerous and ambitious standards to be met (110 performance objectives were specified in the contract), it is little surprise that there were certain deficiencies during the first year of the program. Problems arose, for example, with information systems, claims adjudication, and provider payment. Although IDHS contemplated terminating the MBHO's contract at the end of the first year, IDHS had a vision of what the MHAP should be. This vision was described in the state's original RFP as follows (see Verzbhinski, 2000):

> The Mental Health Access Plan (MHAP) will enhance the opportunity for Iowans to obtain mental health services, which they need to help them live full and productive lives. This plan will help people maintain their mental health through education, prevention, early intervention and appropriate treatment. By offering a flexible array of community-based services and supports, the MHAP program will allow people to receive mental health care while they continue to live and work in their communities.

This vision was one that was shared by the MBHO, and both IDHS and the MBHO wanted to make that vision into a reality. Consequently, rather than abandoning a flawed work in progress, IDHS leadership decided that the program could be retooled effectively if the MBHO and IDHS forged a strong partnership. IDHS leadership also believed that retooling, coupled with a strong partnership and mutual commitments, would be a shorter path to success than contract termination and rebidding. This partnership was built over time as problems arose, and came to include consumers, family members, and providers in the planning and implementation of solutions.

Iowa's MHAP succeeded in the end because (Verzbhinsky, 2000) it

- had a clear vision; strong, experienced government leadership; and an open decision-making process that incorporated stakeholders' views
- provided coverage for all traditional behavioral health services, including inpatient, outpatient, inpatient alternatives (that is, partial hospitalization and day treatment), transportation, medication management, and psychiatric services
- covered most of Iowa's Medicaid recipients, elders, medically needy, and otherwise ineligible persons who were seriously disabled
- incorporated most funding streams
- required the MBHO to develop and utilize a broad range of community-based services and supports, such as mobile crisis counseling, in-home therapy, and assertive community treatment

According to an industry analysis (Nardini, 1999), several factors were essential to the retooling effort that enabled the MHAP and

MBHO to overcome the problems of the first year:

- *Joint treatment planning.* Case-by-case planning between the MBHO, care managers, provider programs, and advocates had the effect of reducing disputes, of focusing attention, and of bringing diverse resources (including those of managed care) to bear on problems.
- *Performance indicators.* The original 110 performance indicators were reduced in number to 60, shaped by stakeholder input that reflected what the people of Iowa wanted from managed behavioral care. The indicators were also effectively prioritized, with 8 being subject to performance bonuses, and 10 subject to performance penalties.
- *Community reinvestment.* As much as $2 million from savings on administration and care delivery were spent on new services that strengthened the system's clinical and recovery capabilities.

Integrating Leadership, Vision, and Resources

Under the terms of the rollout of Pennsylvania's managed Medicaid program, Health Choices, different counties were permitted to act as their own managed behavioral health agents—in effect, to form their own MBHOs—or to contract with licensed MBHOs. There were threshold requirements for counties to satisfy if they elected to act as their own managed care agents—among which were requirements for capital reserves as reinsurance. Only Philadelphia County elected to act as its own MBHO by creating a quasi-public, not-for-profit MBHO, Community Behavioral Health. Philadelphia and its health and human services administration undertook this complex task because, they believed, Health Choices had brought together three factors that were key to behavioral health reform: leadership, vision, and access to adequate financial and human resources.

For 30 years, the city's public service administration participated in numerous state, foundation, and local reforms. It saw the Health Choices option as an opportunity to create "one unified behavioral health system out of many parts" (Century, 2000). For the first time, the city would control, with more flexible rules, the largest part of the behavioral health budget, Medicaid. And it planned to do so according to the values and vision that guided earlier phases of reform, particularly the closure of Philadelphia State Hospital. The investments in the community care system that resulted from the hospital's closure were considered by the city's health commissioner to be too new to tamper with. By running the managed care operation itself (with the commissioner becoming head of the MBHO, known as Community Behavioral Health), the commissioner's office could continue to take a strong leadership role and would be able to blend funding from city, state, federal, and foundation funds in a manner that was consistent with the reforms that were already under way. The reported results include:

- assisting providers to develop managed care infrastructure
- emphasizing training for all care managers and providers on the frontlines of managed care
- extensive consumer involvement in policy, planning, and operations
- conservation of savings, to be used for reinvestment in community services, thus safeguarding the future of the care system
- investing in housing and special supports to aid homeless and mentally ill persons
- investing in the needs of multicultural populations previously underserved
- grants to providers, enabling them to assist public schools
- rapid reimbursement of providers
- increased community tenure and satisfaction among consumers

WHAT WORKS, AND WHAT ENABLES GOALS TO BE ACHIEVED?

Managed care initiatives are associated with positive developments in various facets of public behavioral health systems: access; accountability; innovation; quality of care; utilization and distribution of resources supporting care; and use of technology in care systems.

- *Access to care.* Borrowing from standards established in commercial insurance contracts, public sector managed care programs have imposed standards requiring providers and care managers to comply with policies and practices that represent major improvements over those encountered by most public sector patients:

- *timeliness:* access to crisis services within hours of a call for help, commencement of outpatient care within days of request or referral, and, upon admission for inpatient services, immediate initiation of discharge planning
- *geographic proximity:* access to all services within a narrow radius of members' homes, whether rural or urban
- *network capacity:* inclusion in the provider network of a broader range of services, including ones oriented toward recovery, self-help, and community support

• *Consumer accountability.* Public sector managed care programs more commonly adopt the best practices of public and private care systems:
  - *governance:* consumers invited to be part of MBHOs' governing, advisory, or executive boards
  - *service operations:* consumers employed in various clinical or operational-staff positions, thus–through the direct input of persons who have experience as users of care–increasing both the sensitivity of staff and the responsiveness of programs
  - *program outcomes:* outcome measures specifically intended to reflect the perspective of persons who are users of care

• *Services innovation.* Public sector managed care programs have regularly employed knowledge derived from clinical research and from management reports in order to design and operate more effective services:
  - *care protocols:* evidence-based practices used to produce the best clinical and most cost-effective results
  - *network enhancement:* excellent practitioners brought into network, effective service programs made available, and incentives established to develop more progressive services
  - *prevention/recovery:* services introduced or expanded that prevent illness, relapse, and disability, while promoting recovery from mental illnesses

• *Quality improvement.* Public sector managed care programs have raised provider standards beyond professional licensing, and have incorporated experience, practice environment, and consumer accountability. From the provider side, the programs have promoted the measuring and reporting of treatment outcomes, thus promoting, in turn, an orientation toward results.

From the patient side, the programs have helped to define, formalize, and implement roles for consumers in the operation and oversight of care-management services.

- *Resource utilization and distribution.* Public sector managed care programs have effected a more flexible allocation of care resources through direct contracting with providers and use of management information to guide distribution.
  - *case-rate reimbursement schedules:* combined reimbursement for two or more levels of care, enabling providers to meet client needs in the most clinically and cost-effective manner
  - *allocation of premium dollars between direct care and plan administration:* ratio of expenditures optimized to maximize investment in patient care
  - *reinvestment of savings:* savings in hospital expenditures (whether associated with full or partial inpatient care) used to expand the range of community-service alternatives
- *Information systems.* Public sector managed care programs have used clinical and financial information systems—including e-commerce innovations, electronic-record integration, and data-based decision analysis—to help integrate behavioral care across multiple providers and crisscrossing benefit arrangements.

WHAT FAILS, AND WHAT UNDERMINES REFORM?

Despite the achievements cited above, there remain considerable gaps in the provision of well-managed, comprehensive, evidence-based, and recovery-oriented behavioral health care. As with the earlier CMHC reform, flaws in procurement methods, benefit design, financing structures, and system infrastructure pose threats to success. Among the most salient issues are the following:

- *Public procurement process.* Most public procurement processes are designed to avoid historical problems in the award of government business and are effective at protecting against arbitrary or unaccountable awards to the highest bidder. The processes are not often designed, however, to be efficient in ensuring that the highest quality award is made. There is a high cost of participation for prospective bidders due to the timetables for submissions and the complexity of the responses required. Because the processes often are open, the bid development is subject to multiple reviews and stakeholder input—which, in an effort to satisfy too many interests, can affect customer clarity about objectives. In this atmosphere, the inflation of expectations is common and, ironically, accompanied by resource deflation. Providers' interests can, in the process, become politically polarized from the government payer and from consumers. Once the contract is settled, parties are typically determined to avoid the process again for as long as possible, leading them to avoid any flexibility in, or amendment to, the contract—which might require reopening the process.

- *Benefit design and actuarial comparability.* Although it is at the core of the care-management equation and the financial model in managed care, the benefit design is often inadequate. SMAs and SMHAs do not often have sufficiently rich data to make the predictions required to determine the structure and scope of benefits; the historical utilization data that are used in benefit design and actuarial analysis are rarely complete and reflective of changes in the population and service environment. Changes in mandates, expansion of coverage for special needs, and unintended consequences of parallel social-policy reform contribute to unsound actuarial analysis. As a result, plans often end up with underfunded benefits and mandates. The significant factors that affect public sector managed care planning include: increased unit costs and order frequency of prescription drugs; expanding mandates in children's services; changing technology in addictions treatment; and impact of hospital closures on ambulatory-service utilization. When such changes occur, MBHOs that operate on a risk basis lose money, and consumers lose access to needed care.

- *Payer and provider readiness.* Payers are not always prepared to turn some or all of the administration of public insurance programs over to a private entity. Although the executive or legislative branch may direct the managed care initiative on a policy or political basis, that initiative may not be consistently embraced by the discrete agencies within government that are charged with implementation and administration. In such a situation, the administering agency may lack the technical or staff infrastructure that would enable it to manage the contract, or it may be overweening in its control of MBHO operations. Similarly, providers are often both disinclined to embrace the changes that managed care initiatives represent, and lacking in the management infrastructure that would facilitate the reporting and claims submission required by the MBHO.

- *Pitfalls in MBHO operations.* MBHOs are vulnerable to the same problems that plague all health care companies today. The pitfalls include poor financial planning and controls—which start with the incorrect actuarial assumptions (noted above in relation to the public procurement process) that drive unrealistic pricing models, and which spiral into cash-management problems that affect medical-cost management and provider payments. Deficiencies in administration may affect customer service, information-technology effectiveness, and claims-processing capacity. Undue complexity pervades many operations, whether driven by government-contract requirements or internal failure to simplify or abandon old, dysfunctional systems.

CONCLUSIONS AND FORECASTS

Behavioral health care is at a critical juncture in its evolution. The possibility of "radical reform" is raised by key commentators in the field (Surles, 2001). In addition, more than a decade of managed care experience—on top of 30 years of state and federal reforms in public care systems—provides us the information that we need in order to identify clinical, organizational, and financing practices that work. Lest the past be the prologue to a half-implemented future, transformational leadership is required in order to capitalize on the hard-earned knowledge of the national research agenda, on the decade (and more) of experience in managed care, and on the consumer-empowerment movement. A redefined partnership between MBHOs and government will enable both sides to respond effectively to the expanding call for careful management of public resources.

With such a redefined MBHO-government partnership, there will be new opportunities for MBHOs to expand their business with government customers. Areas that have an emerging growth potential include:

- integration of multiple financing streams to address eroding government revenues
- expansion of coverage to uninsured persons, while remaining within current expenditure levels–which demands skill in benefit redesign, resource integration, and care management
- privatization initiatives in the child welfare, criminal justice, and juvenile justice arenas
- diagnostic, assessment, and treatment innovations
- implementation of organized delivery systems (ODSs)
- adoption of lower-cost e-health technology that complies with the federal Health Insurance Portability and Accountability Act of 1996 and frees administrative dollars for other uses
- evolving risk arrangements
- more effective administration concerning patient rights, privacy protection, and consumer benefits

If the above opportunities are to be realized in the public sector, the stakeholders, including government and the MBHOs, need to revisit the core elements of success in the public health arena. As noted in the 1997 Presidential Address to the American Public Health Association, these elements are "values, vision and leadership" (Levy, 1998). Conflict in, and lack of clarity about, values have confused the implementation and clouded the success of managed care initiatives. The introduction of managed care has, indeed, often disrupted and fragmented the vision of behavioral health leaders for a defined and integrated system of care, particularly where the focus is exclusively on the Medicaid program and is administered by a state's Medicaid authority. There consequently continues to be a pressing need for creative and assertive leadership. Fortunately, the opportunities are as great as the need; successful leadership–which needs to be nurtured–will generate both more progress and further consolidation of the field of managed behavioral health care.

REFERENCES

Anderson, D. F., Berlant, J. L., Mauch, D. D., Sternbach, K. O., Maloney, W. R., Widdington, H. G., & Goens, T. (2001). Managed behavioral health care and chemical dependency services. In P. Kongstvedt (Ed.), *The Managed Health Care Handbook* (4th ed., pp. 451–479). Gaithersburg, MD: Aspen.

Anderson, K. (2000). United Behavioral Health's Public Mental Health Partnership in Clark County, Washington. *Behavioral Health Management, 20* (5) (Suppl.), 9–11.

Century, K. (2000). Innovations in American government: Outlook. Philadelphia: Mayor's Office of Communications.

Dembling, B. P., Chen, D. T., & Vachon, L. (1999). Life expectancy and causes of death in a population treated for serious mental illness. *Psychiatric Services, 50* (8), 1036–1042.

Ditton, P. M. (1999). *Mental health and treatment of inmates and probationers* (Report No. NCJ-174463). Washington, DC: Bureau of Justice Statistics.

Feldman, S. (1992). Managed mental health services: Ideas and issues. In S. Feldman (Ed.), *Managed mental health services* (pp. 3–26). Springfield, IL: Charles C Thomas.

Foley, H. A., & Sharfstein, S. S. (1983). *Madness and government: Who cares for the mentally ill?* Washington, DC: American Psychiatric Press.

Honig, J., & Fendell, S. (2000). Meeting the needs of female trauma survivors: The effectiveness of the Massachusetts mental health managed care system. *Advisor, 50,* 9–33.

Institute for the Future. (2000). *Health and health care 2010: The forecast, the challenge.* Princeton, NJ: Robert Wood Johnson Foundation.

Institute for the Future. (2001). *Mental health care 2010.* Princeton, NJ: Robert Wood Johnson Foundation.

Kessler, R. C., Olfson, M., & Berglund, P. A. (1998). Patterns and predictors of treatment contact after first onset of psychiatric disorders. *American Journal of Psychiatry, 155* (1), 62–69.

Kronebusch, K. (2001). Medicaid for children: Federal mandates, welfare reform and policy backsliding. *Health Affairs, 20* (1), 97–111.

Leadholm, B., & Kerzner, J. (1994). Public managed care: Developing comprehensive community support systems in Massachusetts. *Managed Care Quarterly, 2* (2), 25–30.

Mauch, D. (2000). *Montana case study.* Magellan Public Solutions Group.

Mechanic, D., & Aiken, L. (1989). *Paying for services: Promises and pitfalls of capitation.* San Francisco: Jossey-Bass.

Minkoff, K. (2000). An integrated model for the management of co-occurring psychiatric and substance disorders in managed care systems. *Disease Management & Health Outcomes, 8,* 250–257.

Moss, S. (1998). *Contracting for managed substance abuse and mental health services: A guide for public purchasers.* Rockville, MD: U.S. Department of Health and Human Services.

Nardini, C. (May 1999). *Keys to successful implementation of public managed mental health programs: Iowa program success borne of 'hands on' learning* (available from Open Minds, 10 York Street, Gettysburg, PA 17325).

Rice, D. P., & Miller, L. S. (1996). The economic burden of schizophrenia: Conceptual and methodological issues, and cost estimates. In M. Mosscarelli, A. Rupp, & N. Sartorious (Eds.), *Handbook of mental health economics and health policy: Vol. 1. Schizophrenia* (pp. 321–324). New York: John Wiley and Sons.

Robinson, G. K., & Scallet, L. (1998). *State profiles on public sector managed behavioral health care and other reforms.* Rockville, MD: U.S. Department of Health and Human Services.

Satcher, D. (1999). *Mental health: A report of the surgeon general.* Rockville, MD: National Institute of Mental Health.

Stroul, B. A. (2000). *Health care reform tracking project: 1999 impact analysis.* Miami: Florida Mental Health Institute.

Sudders, M., Bullen, B., & Koh, H. (1999). Consensus principles for the treatment of individuals with co-occurring mental illness and substance use disorder. Boston: Massachusetts Department of Mental Health.

Surles, R. (2001). *Publicly financed managed behavioral healthcare: Can it survive?* Center for Health Strategies.

Verzbhinsky, M. (2000). *Iowa case study.* Magellan Public Solutions Group.

Willis, K. (2000). *Haverford state hospital case study.* Magellan Public Solutions Group.

Chapter 12

THE INTERNET

Richard D. Flanagan and Susan L. Needham

Managed care has brought about major changes in the health care delivery system. In its relatively short lifetime, managed care has left few, if any, participants with neutral feelings about its role. The industry has lowered the cost of treatment, while alienating providers with reduced fees; made treatment more understandable and accessible through referral services and care management, while creating barriers to care by acting as a gatekeeper; organized providers into networks and panels, and forced the adoption of better business practices, while being seen as the cause of reduced provider income; and championed the cause of provider accountability through outcomes-based and empirically driven treatment models, while creating reams of paperwork and administrative hassles for providers. To some, managed care is the reason that behavioral health benefits are still so widely offered, given that the initial reaction of many insurers and employers to rising behavioral health costs was to eliminate coverage; whereas others contend that the advent of managed care has caused a systematic reduction in care.

The explosive growth of the Internet has itself stimulated a new round of major changes in the health care industry. Consumers are taking on more and more responsibilities for their own care. Employers, who are seeking ways to reduce escalating health benefit costs, are asking employees to manage their own health insurance coverage, as evidenced by the movement toward defined-contribution benefit plans. Companies in the e-health industry are rapidly introducing new technologies to eliminate clinical and administrative inefficiencies in the health care delivery system. The question to be answered is whether the Internet will be a tool that helps meet these challenges and leads to a new wave of positive innovation in the industry or, as some predict, will be the next new thing not to fix the ailing U.S. health care delivery system (Goldsmith, 2000; Kleinke, 2000).

This chapter will discuss the current (and ever changing) state of health care and the Internet, then focus on the current status of behavioral health care and the Internet, and, finally, look at the future opportunities, challenges, and obstacles for managed behavioral health care in an Internet-connected world.

HEALTH CARE AND THE INTERNET

The Internet offers enormous potential as a vehicle for change, but in the area of health care, it is not clear if or when that potential will be realized. There are formidable barriers, technological and otherwise, to such change.

The World Wide Web has emerged as the first new mass medium in a generation, arguably the fastest-growing new technology in history. The polling company Louis Harris and Associates estimates the current number of American adults using the Internet at home, work, or school at 114 million, or 56% of the adult population (Harris, 2000). Overall, 70% of the public uses computers, with 84% of those using the Internet. One of the most common motivations for people to use the Internet is to locate health care information and services; Harris polls indicate that about 86% of adults who accessed the Internet sought information about health care or about medical topics such as depression or cancer. Finally, the Pew study of Internet use for health-related purposes found that 92% of "health seekers" say the online information that they found was useful (Fox, 2000).

The Internet has transformed many areas of industry and commerce. The financial-services sector is an example of an industry that has rapidly embraced the use of Internet technologies to streamline almost every aspect of how it operates, including banking, investing, and money management. From almost anywhere in the world, one can use the Internet to deposit, withdraw, borrow, and transfer money, to buy and sell stocks, and to conduct almost any other financial transaction. In manufacturing, the Internet has taken "just-in-time" ordering of components, parts, raw materials, and supplies to new levels, allowing even for real-time bidding among vendors. Cisco Corporation, as one example, estimates that its online customer-care solutions saved the company $270 million and increased customer satisfaction by 25% (Cisco Systems, 2000). Ninety percent of its orders are placed online—with a 99% accuracy rate the first time they are entered, and an estimated annual savings of $60 million (compared to an estimated 90% accuracy rate for provider-payer communications by phone or mail, and a 67% accuracy rate for health insurance claims (Clulow, Frisch, & Phillippe, 2000)). In a recent year, implementing a virtual supply chain reduced inventory levels by 45%, reduced time to market, and saved Cisco $175 million in annual operating costs. Finally, and perhaps more directly relevant for the subject of this chapter, all of Cisco's sales and technical staff participate in online training, a program that has reduced the company's training expenses by 60%, not counting savings from decreased time spent away from work (Cisco Systems, 2000).

Not all industries have been transformed, however. Retail companies on the Internet, for example, have met with very mixed levels of success. All but a few that were not previously part of strong traditional businesses have yet to demonstrate they are capable of making money. In particular, most of the Internet companies that have relied on online advertising as their primary source of revenue have been unsuccessful; viable advertising models for reaching customers on the Internet have yet to be demonstrated. The recent plunge in Internet stocks has left a trail of dead and dying dot-com companies, with many more still searching for viable business models.

So how has the Internet affected the health care industry? There has been significant optimism and speculation that a major transformation could occur in the health care services industry, which, at $1.2 trillion, represents the largest market segment in the United States economy. The industry has seemed ripe for change—in part due to complex and inefficient delivery systems that create an estimated $400 billion in annual administrative costs alone (Clulow et al., 2000; Lutz, 2000; Pew, 2000). Participants in the system—consumers, payers, providers, vendors, facilities, pharmacies, and laboratories, among others—have functioned in independent and often disconnected ways. Consolidated records and standardized modes of communication are

uncommon, and the sharing of information is slow and labor intensive, at best. Records are still frequently handwritten or, if electronic,
usually require entry into multiple systems. Costs are high and continue to escalate. There have been pressures for greater efficiency,
improved care, and cost savings on all fronts (Martinez, 2000), which
led, among other things, to the passage of the federal Health Insurance
Portability and Accountability Act (HIPAA). The law, which will be
returned to later in this chapter, includes requirements to create uniform standards for the transmission of all electronic medical information.

To date, both the development and adoption of Internet solutions
in the health care industry have been relatively slow and not particularly successful. The health care delivery system is not only vast, but
exceedingly complex. Many electronic systems are already in place,
but their functioning has been suboptimal or worse. Corporate cost-
benefit analyses have only recently justified the move to what will likely be the broad replacement of paper and existing information systems
with Web-based solutions.

Propelled by consumer demand for health care information and
services on the Internet, health care providers, payers, and vendors
have gradually been adopting Internet strategies and tools. Initially,
they have focused on providing information and marketing materials,
with some attempts at administration, service delivery, and even treatment. A number of independent companies–including large firms
such as McKesson HBOC and Healtheon/WebMD, and small ones
such as NaviMedix, RealMed, Trizetto, and Xcare.net–are focusing on
developing Internet-connectivity solutions to streamline the transactions and communications between providers and payers. These
efforts have focused primarily on eligibility and benefit verification;
claims submission, inquiry, and appeal; referral, authorization, and
reauthorization; scheduling; care management; communication
between patients, providers, payers, vendors, and facilities; care delivery and disease management; and practice management.

Despite the many early predictions of rapid transformation,
change seems to be unfolding gradually. At this point the industry
leader, Healtheon/WebMD, has been unsuccessful at broadly attracting providers to its system. The smaller connectivity vendors are for
the most part concentrating on local and regional connectivity, with
individual health plans primarily focusing on claims and claims-relat-

ed transactions such as eligibility and referrals. Internet health care innovators are finding that in health care, as in any other system, the existing business processes and solutions, while often inefficient, are familiar and entrenched.

Although the behavioral health care delivery system suffers from many of the same problems as the rest of health care, it may actually be a better candidate for Internet transformation. Behavioral health services are frequently carved out from insurance plans to either independent (for example, APS Healthcare, Compsych, Integra, and Magellan Behavioral Health) or captive (for example, Cigna Behavioral Health, MHN, Pacificare Behavioral Health, and United Behavioral Health) managed behavioral health organizations (MBHOs). Compared to the rest of health care, a relatively small number of national managed-care companies control much of the referral, authorization, care management, and payment for services. According to the consulting firm Open Minds (Fox, Oss, & Jardine, 2000), over 80% of the market is controlled by the 10 largest MBHOs (Table 1). As a result, the possibility and desirability of developing a broad, national Internet approach is compelling and could become a

Table 1

ORGANIZATIONS WITH LARGEST MANAGED BEHAVIORAL HEALTH PROGRAM ENROLLMENT, 2000/2001

Organization	Enrollment	Market Share
Magellan Health Services	55,158,000	34.87%
ValueOptions	19,123,710	12.09%
United Behavioral Health	18,530,000	11.71%
CIGNA Behavioral Health	9,694,220	6.13%
First Health Services of Tennessee	6,039,748	3.82%
MHN, Inc.	5,332,670	3.37%
APS Healthcare, Inc.	5,200,000	3.29%
PacifiCare Behavioral Health	3,861,518	2.44%
Behavioral Health Services Employee Assistance Program	3,820,000	2.41%
Integra, Inc.	2,957,778	1.87%
Total	**129,717,644**	**82.0%**

Source: Fox, Oss, & Jardine, 2000.

model for the rest of health care. In addition, most behavioral health services require authorization, reauthorization, and care management, which introduces an additional level of interaction that could be simplified and streamlined using Internet technologies to allow payer-specific expert systems to handle much of the decision making.

On the provider side of the equation, behavioral health care itself is delivered primarily by specialty providers, who include psychiatrists, psychologists, social workers, nurses, and counselors—frequently working at specialized treatment facilities. These providers have been much slower than their general medical counterparts in adopting technology; there is consequently less technology, at least on the provider side, to be replaced. Moreover, while face-to-face contact with patients is certainly desirable, the primary medium of treatment, psychotherapy, requires no direct physical contact; many assessment and treatment services could potentially be delivered, at least in part, over the Internet.

BEHAVIORAL HEALTH CARE AND THE INTERNET: CURRENT STATUS

As of the time of this writing (the middle of 2001), many of the participants in behavioral heath care—consumers, providers, and payers—are using, or exploring the possibility of using, the Internet as a means of meeting their needs. The reasons for this effort are clear and compelling. The Internet is ubiquitous, inexpensive to use, easy to access, and beginning to provide applications that can be updated quickly and easily. This section will look at the tools and applications currently available for each of these stakeholders, and the next section will look at where the industry is likely to move in the future.

Consumers

For many consumers, as previously indicated, the Internet has already become the communication and information-gathering medium of choice. At any of hundreds of Web sites (for example, nimh. gov, nih.gov, athealth.com, apa.org, about.com, Epotec.com, lifescape.com, mentalhelp.net, and webmd.com), consumers can find information and statistics regarding behavioral health concerns, learn about treatment options, and find support in chat rooms and bulletin boards. Information about providers, medications, disorders, support groups, treatment centers, and self-help are readily available, as is information about health plans and benefits. Consumers can search online databases to find providers for face-to-face therapy (both health-plan sponsored and independent), and in some cases request authorization or schedule services. Despite many controversies surrounding the provision of online therapy, consumers are able to find licensed, and for that matter unlicensed, professionals offering therapy or support groups online.

Providers

Behavioral health professionals, though generally thought to be slow to adopt new technology, are using the Internet to improve their knowledge bases, business practices, clinical skills, and outcomes. The Internet provides easy and often free access to clinical and research information that previously would have been tedious, expensive, or even impossible to collect in a timely manner. For example, sites such as @Health.com and those for the National Guideline Clearinghouse (http://www.guideline.gov), Journal of Medical Internet Research, National Institute of Mental Health, American Psychiatric Association, and American Psychological Association offer information regarding best practices, diagnostic and treatment updates, research studies, references, and patient handouts. Through email, online communities, and list serves, professionals are networking with colleagues around the world and often providing or receiving consultation and supervision.

The Internet offers a new avenue for providers to market themselves. Providers are setting up personal Web sites in order to promote their practices and provide consumers with previously unavailable information about their backgrounds, theoretical orientations, approaches to treatment, specialties, and credentials. Email, chat, and audio/video conferencing provide means for some to communicate with patients in between, or in some cases in place of, face-to-face sessions.

Despite the lack of research about, and training to provide, online clinical services, some providers have jumped at the chance to provide therapy online, and there are a number of Web sites offering providers ways to market and conduct online practices. Many professionals remain skeptical, however. Concerns over privacy and security top the list of reasons that many providers are shying away from the Internet as a medium for therapy. Most consumers and professionals guard behavioral health information even more closely than general health data. To be comfortable with online behavioral health communications, they want assurances that privacy and confidentiality will be safeguarded. Higher-level encryption technologies permit greater protection, but—in the view of many—not enough at this point.

Assuming privacy and security concerns can be adequately addressed through technology and the development of appropriate procedures, there remain great concerns about whether online therapy is as safe or effective as more traditional face-to-face methods. There is not yet an adequate body of published research to guide professionals in knowing for whom online therapy is or is not appropriate. Most therapists, trained to pay close attention to sensory cues and nonverbal communications, have received little or no training in understanding the differences between a face-to-face encounter and a text-based or a teleconferenced communication. Although some of the behavioral health professions have developed guidelines for the ethical provision of services via teleconference or the Internet (for example, the American Counseling Association, American Medical Association, American Psychological Association, and National Association of Social Workers), the legal issues regarding provision of services across state lines have yet to be resolved and continue to provoke controversy in provider forums and list serves. The safest procedure to date appears to be that of restricting online therapy practice to clients living within the state or states in which the provider is licensed.

Online continuing education would seem a very likely candidate for early provider acceptance and adoption. Online education enables professionals to meet licensure requirements and to keep current with the latest developments in the field without the additional time and expense of travel. What's more, it can be accomplished on the professional's own schedule. Many state licensing boards accept credits awarded for completing online courses as satisfying at least part of the continuing education requirement for license renewal. Such services—offered by Internet start-ups (for example, Continued Learning

Online, @health.com, and PsyBC.com), as well as by managed care organizations, hospital systems, and pharmaceutical companies–are new to the market, and their penetration and use are unclear at this point.

On the computerized practice-management front, many behavioral health systems (for example, Creative Sociomedic, CMHC Systems, PsychConsult, Therapist Helper, and Anasazi) are offering so-called Web-enabled front ends to their programs. These systems basically put a browser-based user interface on a traditional program to allow data entry through the Internet. Application Service Provider (ASP) models using completely Web-based systems are beginning to emerge (for example, Centromine), and promise new flexibility for managing practices from multiple locations, submitting claims online, using wireless transmission from hand-held computers, and making real-time upgrades and repairs. ASP companies host and manage Internet applications for multiple users from a central facility with expert staff and state-of-the-art equipment. These companies offer their services through contracted leasing arrangements and provide secure, reliable, and up-to-date service. By outsourcing their data processing and portions of their IT management, ASP subscribers can control and reduce their technology and IT costs.

A number of commercial Web sites have emerged offering therapists tools and even online offices to conduct their practices online. As mentioned earlier, secure communications with clients are essential but require more technology know-how than the average provider wants to, or is equipped to, handle. Several companies (for example, Virtual Couch, Here2Listen, and eTherapy.com) offer secure private chat rooms or encrypted email services, and even act as therapy matchmakers by providing referrals. Some have gone so far as to offer "virtual" offices with built-in scheduling and billing packages (for example, e-therapy.com, HelpHorizons.com, and WellPlace.com). As of this writing, the business model for such companies is far from proven, and most are experiencing economic hard times.

Payers

Payers in the behavioral health system, such as MBHOs, HMOs, and health plans, have experienced great success in the past decade at reining in the cost of behavioral health treatment. While providers have railed against managed care and seen their earning power decline (Psychotherapy Finances, 2000), access to treatment has arguably become easier, cheaper, and more widely available. There has also been increased focus on outcomes and provider accountability. In the process of industrializing the delivery system, the managed behavioral health system has also added many administrative hurdles and inefficiencies to the delivery system, with a multitude of complex and difficult-to-administer requirements and systems for referral, eligibility, benefits, authorization, reporting, and claims submission.

In order to grasp the level of complexity involved, one need only look at the steps associated with submitting and processing a typical health insurance claim. For every claim, the following questions, and sometimes others, must all be answered, submitted, and entered correctly into one or more claims-payment systems to determine whether the claim will be paid, to whom, and for how much:

- Is the subscriber a current member of the plan?
- Is the patient covered under the subscriber?
- Is it a covered service?
- Where was the service delivered?
- Is there other insurance that should cover the service?
- How much should the other insurance cover?
- Is the service covered under workers' comp, disability, or liability?
- Was the service authorized?
- Is the submitting provider a member of the correct network?
- Is the submitting provider eligible for reimbursement?
- What is the provider's reimbursement rate for this service?
- What is the patient's deductible and copayment?
- Who is being reimbursed: patient, provider, or facility?
- Does the diagnosis require parity consideration?

Unfortunately, even prior to claims submission, a number of time-consuming and labor-intensive steps must occur. In general, in order to have any chance of being reimbursed for services to be rendered, a provider or her staff must call to confirm eligibility, determine level of benefits, and obtain authorization to provide services. This process is extremely costly for both the payer and provider. The American Medical Association estimates the cost of processing paper claims at $6 to $12 per claim in labor and overhead, which is really just the tip of the iceberg. When one considers the estimated 33% error rate that results in denials and often multiple resubmissions, as well as the significant number of transactions involved in claims-status inquiries, the cost becomes enormous.

Payers are now feeling the squeeze of shrinking health care dollars and are seeking new ways to improve services and outcomes, to achieve greater efficiencies in care delivery and administration, and, of course, to reduce costs and improve their bottom lines. Early efforts have merged to develop smart systems and interactive-voice-response (IVR) approaches using clinical algorithms to streamline the entire care-management process. Most managed care companies have developed Web sites for providing information to providers and subscribers on such matters as policies, panels, forms, and processes. The sophistication of these efforts varies from company to company, depending on the quality of internal or outsourced technology resources. In terms of care management and delivery, efforts to date have focused primarily on offering collateral information and self-help programs, with very little effort devoted to the delivery of direct services. There are basically no processes in place even to reimburse providers for Web-based services.

The Internet offers great possibilities for reducing myriad business and administrative inefficiencies, but early pioneers have found the level of complexity of the business processes more daunting than even the technical process of connecting to a variety of legacy systems. As of this writing, efforts to use the Internet for connectivity are just beginning, with a number of companies (for example, Epotec, Lifescape, and MedUnite) proposing a single-portal model for providers to connect to multiple payers. For the most part, these companies are focusing on the so called "RACER" issues–that is, referrals, authorizations, claims, eligibility, and reporting–which will be discussed in the next section.

MANAGED BEHAVIORAL HEALTH CARE AND THE INTERNET: THE FUTURE

The Possibilities

The Internet offers many opportunities for improving the behavioral health care industry and reducing hassles for all participants.

Consumers seem eager for new tools and vehicles of service, assuming that they are safe, confidential, and secure. Providers are desperate to simplify the administrative hassles of their practices, to boost their earning power, and to get paid more quickly and reliably. Payers are desperate to control costs, reduce their overhead, and maintain or improve their market share. Because of their financial strength, MBHOs have the leverage to be at the center of this change and are beginning to take steps both to reduce inefficiencies and to create a new way of conducting the business and providing the service of behavioral health care.

The future of managed behavioral health care rests heavily on the ability of the industry to adopt and share common platforms for conducting administrative, care-delivery, and provider-relations functions. Although the establishment of proprietary systems of communication once made sense, the Internet has changed everything. Because of the need for information to be shared and exchanged among providers, hospitals, pharmacies, labs, health plans, and managed care companies, proprietary solutions become impractical, dysfunctional, and a prescription for failure. Companies that lead the way in developing a common platform will reap the rewards of customer loyalty and enhanced efficiencies.

Of course, the savings from enhanced efficiencies will not be immediate. Companies that participate in the early development of a common platform will incur significant costs—in both time and money. Nonetheless, these early adopters will earn the right to define the course of development, a move which could pay dividends down the line. The key is bringing about the transformation in logical stages. Initial efforts are likely to be kept narrow and aimed at proof of concept. Success at this stage will pave the way for a broad roll-out that leverages the benefits and savings over the industry's national networks.

A View of the Future

So what will this transformation look like for each of the constituents in behavioral health care? First, clinical records will be more broadly under the control of the patient, who will have the ability to assign rights and privileges to this personal information (McGoldrick & O'Dell, 2000). Although there is currently considerable provider resistance to this concept, it is the only model that works in the connected world of the future. The economics of "owning" a patient by virtue of owning her records will gradually become an exception, as will this method of valuing a practice.

Second, the concept of a single portal for connectivity will be adopted, allowing providers to communicate and do business with multiple payers from one Internet location—a single point of access for connecting providers to multiple payers and utility functions. An Internet-connected system brings together multiple participants so that data can be verified and information can be shared from common databases, with effective exchanges between health care organizations, providers, and consumers. Going separately to each payer's site makes little sense if all of the common elements can be handled through one portal that has adequate security for consumers, providers, and payers. This piece is absolutely essential. Any other model offers little help to the majority of providers, most of whom, according to Open Minds, work with about 12 payers. To be sure, this level of cooperation may be difficult to achieve among competing payers, but if payers are not ultimately successful in meeting the needs of providers, their Internet business model will likely not be accepted and will lead to failure.

Third, broadband access to the Internet will be the norm, with availability through public kiosks, schools, and libraries for those without a computer or other Internet-connected communication device. Though some may disagree with this claim, consider the Asian experience. Singapore is now wiring every home, office, and factory to a broadband cable network, with 98% of citizens having access. Those without computers will have access at public facilities. South Korea boasts a third of its population having Internet access, with 3.5 million homes having high-speed access—double the number only five months before.

In the United States, the time is coming when computer-based video cameras will be available at each user's discretion, and improved voice-recognition software will be widely used to input information. Digital phones will function as personal assistants (or perhaps vice versa), allowing wireless connectivity between providers, patients, and payers. When the patient's name is entered into a provider's practice-management system, and whenever the name is on a provider's schedule, the patient's benefits, eligibility, and claims status will be automatically checked. If authorizations are needed for treatment, a

Web form will be provided for completion, and sessions will often be automatically authorized. At the same time, the system will indicate when there is a problem with a claim or when there may be a delay in payment. Clicking on the patient's name on the scheduler of a Web-based practice-management system will offer a menu of options such as transferring diagnosis-specific or treatment-related content to the patient's secure message box, and sending a specific self-help or educational program, or audio or video file. Do not be too surprised if sophisticated iris scanners and fingerprint readers become common and help overcome many confidentiality and security concerns of consumers.

A key to this portrayal of the future is the broader question of what behavioral care delivery or therapy will look like in an Internet-connected world. Treatment will become far more multidimensional with a mix of face-to-face, telephonic, email, audio, and video communications employed to fit each patient's needs and problems. The practice of psychotherapy has been fundamentally Procrustean in nature—not only in forcing patients into a provider's particular theoretical approach, but also typically requiring one-on-one, 45- to 60-minute sessions for most problems. Most therapists agree that education is a primary component of healing. Aside from the tutoring implicit in therapy, however, they have had little to offer other than bibliotherapy. In the future, increasingly elegant online multimedia educational and self-help vehicles will be incorporated into treatment. Many of these will be developed and provided by payer organizations seeking to enhance value in the delivery of care, including the prevention of disorders. Obviously, there will be challenges in how to compensate for such a broad range of delivery mechanisms. The current model of weekly, hour-long therapy sessions—a model based less on treatment needs than on therapists' scheduling needs—will certainly shift. As new models emerge, there will most likely be significant increases in capitated and case-rate reimbursement structures. Payers will also become far more collaborative with providers and offer many of the continuing and ongoing educational opportunities.

Challenges and Obstacles

While the Internet presents diverse and important opportunities to improve access, care delivery, practice management, payment, and administration, there are also serious challenges and obstacles. Perhaps the greatest challenges noted by consumers, providers, and payers are those of security, privacy, and confidentiality. The importance of these issues to the success of online behavioral health care practice should not be underestimated. The administrative simplification provisions of the Health Insurance Portability and Accountability Act of 1996 (HIPAA) mandated that Congress or the secretary of health and human services create standards governing the privacy, security, and transmission of health-related data. Of the eight rules proposed under these provisions, two–Standards for Electronic Transactions (Health Insurance Reform, 2000) and Standards for Privacy of Individually Identifiable Health Information (2000)–have been finalized as of this writing. The rule on security is expected to be finalized by mid-2001. These rules provide guidance regarding minimum standards for protecting the confidentiality of personally identifiable health information while it is either stored in any form or transmitted electronically. Health care providers, plans, and clearinghouses are considered covered entities under these rules and face considerable challenges in understanding and implementing the requirements of each new rule. The full potential of the Internet to transform behavioral health care will not be realized until the issues of security and privacy can be addressed to the satisfaction of all participants.

The second greatest challenge to using the Internet in behavioral health care involves the multitude of options available to everyone concerned. Consumers are faced with what seem like limitless amounts of information and misinformation, with little idea of how to tell the difference. They may be unaware of the limitations of online therapy or of the differences among providers (that is, social workers, counselors, psychologists, psychotherapists, psychiatrists, and others, as well as unlicensed "coaches"), approaches, and standards. A number of organizations and Web sites offer guidance to consumers in evaluating behavioral health information and services on the Internet, but concerns remain that the majority of consumers who seek such information or services over the Internet may not know how to evaluate the quality of what they obtain.

Many providers, particularly those new to the Internet, face a similar challenge when it comes to judging the quality of the various Web sites that they encounter. They face an array of online therapy companies and tools, as well as a host of practice-management companies.

In addition, behavioral health care providers as a group tend to be less computer-savvy and slower to adopt new technology. Those who already have adopted some back-office technology and processes are reluctant to convert, due to the investment of time needed for learning the new systems. Internet-based systems are especially troubling to providers who have only a passing level of proficiency with the personal computer or who are completely unfamiliar with how the Internet works. Consequently, companies and health plans wishing to draw providers to their online products and services find that recruiting providers and then supporting them are expensive endeavors.

For payers, the challenges lie in determining Web strategy—including budgeting for developing and maintaining Internet capabilities, deciding whether to develop online services alone or to join forces, and selecting the right partners, solution, or portal. For MBHOs, another major challenge lies in determining how to integrate Internet-based applications with existing legacy systems. Many MBHOs have, through mergers and acquisitions, acquired multiple information systems, most of which contain inaccurate or obsolete data. Cleaning up the data in these disparate systems and finding ways to integrate them (within the business and also within Web systems) is a major undertaking. Nevertheless, Internet transformation is moving forward rapidly, and the eventual benefits are becoming clear to the leaders in the industry.

A Sample of the Future

How, then might things look ill describe how things might look a few steps down the Internet-connected road? To make the abstract more concrete, meet our fictional patient, Fred, as he uses the tools of the future.

It's 2 A.M. and Fred lies in bed, dead tired but wide awake—again. His worries gnaw at him: work has gone flat, and so has everything else. Even his wife and kids—the joy and center of his life—can't seem to revive him. The other day, he forgot to pick up his son from soccer practice. For the first time in his life, Fred feels powerless and hopeless.

"That's it," he thinks. "I've got to do something." In the glow of his digital clock, he tells his video communication device to wake up and go to his employer's Internet home page, specifically its self-help area. With so many interactive programs to choose from, Fred lets the system suggest his path. His answers to questions about his life and health prompt feedback recommending programs on depression, anxiety, and insomnia, as well as offering him ways to request professional assistance.

Choosing the program on depression, Fred soon responds that he's been feeling hopeless for some time–a sign of serious depression. A message tells him he needs more help than a computer program can provide, and asks him if he would like to reach his managed health care organization. Fred decides to send a secure electronic message describing his situation. Fred's information swiftly reaches the message queue of an intake professional who, spotting alarming content, calls Fred immediately. After the intake professional determines that Fred is not in crisis, she offers the names of several counselors as referral options, and sends information about each one to Fred's confidential message box. Fred selects the names of several counselors, examines their backgrounds, training, and clinical orientations, selects one, schedules an appointment, and decides what information in his clinical record he would like the counselor to be able to access. A message is sent to the counselor through the online practice-management system. Later that day, after the counselor confirms the appointment, everything relating to Fred–the message he sent the night before, the intake professional's notes, and an authorization for an initial evaluation and treatment–is sent electronically to the counselor's account.

The counselor concludes during her first appointment with Fred that he needs treatment for depression. Finding that Fred might benefit from medication, she sends an online request for a psychiatric assessment, which is automatically referred and authorized by the smart referral system. Fred is able to choose a psychiatrist online, and the online system again processes the data on Fred, including the case notes and claims information. Fred's counselor schedules another session and assigns a nine-part, online self-help program on depression to supplement Fred's treatment. Fred's psychiatrist enters his prescription in the system, with periodic email forms to monitor Fred's progress. Automatic refills will be available, if necessary, as determined by the smart medication system.

In his own confidential online account, Fred starts working through his assigned self-help program, periodically receiving messages reminding him of his appointments. He submits homework at the completion of each online session, which generates timely feedback from a coach. For three months, Fred benefits from a combined course of counseling; online self-help; medication; private chat sessions with his therapist; form-driven, online, automatic medication checks; and an online depression support group to learn the skills needed to overcome his depression. After each session—face to face, online, or videoconferenced—Fred, his therapist, and his psychiatrist complete a brief online questionnaire to measure progress and to suggest possible alternative approaches. Each week (or even daily or hourly if necessary), Fred receives online educational materials targeted to his specific diagnosis and presenting problems.

Using such a comprehensive system, everyone wins. Fred quickly gets high-quality help from multiple sources, while his counselor avoids burdensome phone calls and paperwork. Fred's insurer makes it all possible with efficient, well-coordinated treatment—along with greatly reduced management and administrative costs. By the way, Fred's eligibility and benefits are checked automatically whenever his name is on his therapist's schedule; claims are automatically generated when the brief assessment is completed by the therapist; and payment is made directly to the therapist's account almost immediately.

Best of all, Fred's feeling a lot better. His energy is coming back. He told his son so—on the way home from soccer practice.

REFERENCES

American Counseling Association. (1999). Ethical standards for Internet on-line counseling. Available at <http://www.counseling.org/gc/cybertx.htm>.

American Psychological Association. (1997). Services by telephone, teleconferencing, and Internet: A statement by the Ethics Committee of the American Psychological Association. Available at <http://www.apa.org/ethics/stmnt01.html>.

Cisco Systems, Inc. (2000). 2000 Annual report: Discover all that's possible on the Internet from the company that can show you how. San Jose, CA: Author.

Clulow, M. D., Frisch, A., & Phillippe, J. E. (2000). The future of e-health. New York: UBS Warburg Global Equity Research.

Fox, A., Oss, M., & Jardine, E. (2000). Open Minds yearbook of managed behavioral health market share in the United States, 2000–2001. Gettysburg, PA: Open Minds.

Fox, S. (2000). The online health care revolution: How the Web helps Americans take better care of themselves. Available at <http://www.pewinternet.org>.

Goldsmith, J. (2000). The Internet and managed care: A new wave of innovation. *Health Affairs, 19* (6), 42–56.

Health Insurance Portability and Accountability Act of 1996, Pub. L. No. 104-191, 110 Stat. 1936 (1996) (codified at 26 U.S.C. §§ 9801–9806 and scattered sections of 18 U.S.C., 26 U.S.C., 29 U.S.C., and 42 U.S.C.).

Health Insurance Reform: Standards for Electronic Transactions; Announcement of Designated Standard Maintenance Organizations; Final Rule and Notice, 65 Fed. Reg. 50312–50372 (2000) (to be codified at 45 C.F.R. pts. 160 & 162).

Harris Interactive. (2000, October 11). Internet access continues to grow but at a slower pace. Harris Poll No. 60.

Kleinke, J. D. (2000). Vaporware.com: The failed promise of the health care Internet. *Health Affairs, 19* (6), 57–71.

Lutz, S. (2000, October). E-connectivity producing measurable results. *HealthCast 2010* (Price-WaterhouseCoopers).

Martinez, L. (2000). How health plans are using the Internet to reach customers: A survey of payor Web sites. Cap Gemini Ernst &Young.

McGoldrick, C., & O'Dell, S. (2000). Where will the road to e-health lead? *First Reports* (First Consulting Group).

National Board for Certified Counselors, Inc. (1997). Standards for the ethical practice of Web counseling. Available at <http://www.nbcc.org/ethics/wcstandards.htm>.

Psychotherapy Finances. (2000). Survey of fees and practice issues [Special issue]. *Psychotherapy Finances, 26* (10).

Standards for Privacy of Individually Identifiable Health Information; Final Rule, 65 Fed. Reg. 82462–82510 (2000) (to be codified at 45 C.F.R. pts. 160 & 164).

Winker, M. A., Flanagin, A., Chi-Lum, B., White, J., Andrews, K., Kennett, R. L., DeAngelis, C. D., & Musacchio, R. A. (2000). Guidelines for medical and health information sites on the Internet: Principles governing AMA Web sites. *Journal of the American Medical Association, 283,* 1600–1606.

Chapter 13

INFORMATION SYSTEMS

Tom Trabin and William Maloney

Information systems have become the bedrock upon which managed behavioral health care is built. Various complex systems have evolved from innovations to basic routines: for example, computer-based tracking of enrollment and associated benefits; provider-referral systems with specialty credentialing and geographic mapping to facilitate referral decisions; care-management systems with authorizations and clinical-decision support; and claims adjudication. Increasingly demanding reporting requirements from purchaser, accreditation, and regulatory organizations have stimulated more sophisticated use of advanced database technologies. At the frontiers of electronic communication are increased efficiencies for, and enhancements in the care provided by, managed behavioral health organizations (MBHOs).

THE CONTEXT

The Evolution of Information Systems for Health Care Insurers and for Providers

The design of information systems for managed behavioral health care is set within the context of the evolving functional requirements of MBHOs and also within the broader requirements of the health care industry's insurance and provider segments.

The health care system has been divided historically between organizations that delivered health care services–that is, providers–and organizations that financed the services–that is, insurers. Information systems companies and the products they developed for these two groups were also separate and distinct. Health maintenance organizations (HMOs)–especially the staff-model plans–and some integrated delivery systems were, and continue to be, exceptions to this rule because they finance and deliver care within a single entity.

The first behavioral health information systems, as in the field of general health care, were accounting and financial systems. The products developed for providers tracked the services rendered and then created bills that could be sent to patients and insurers for payment. The products created for the insurance industry were essentially the inverse; they tracked the claims received from providers and then generated a payment. Since insurers bore the major financial risk, their systems also tracked the premiums collected against the claims paid. The market allowed steady increases in premiums to match the rising costs of medical care. In that pre-cost-conscious environment, insurers did little to monitor or influence treatment decisions. In the 1970s and 1980s, however, the situation changed dramatically: costs went out of control–to the point of impeding American business competitiveness in the global marketplace. At that point, insurers, employers, and the government began to take action. The financial pressure caused the two sides–insurers and providers–to begin moving more closely together, and insurers became increasingly focused on clinical decision making. Indeed, both sides began to take on some of the functions that had traditionally belonged only to the other. Frequently, the implementation of a function by one side did not remove it from the other. Instead, both sides ended up performing some of the same or similar functions.

Software companies, which were following this trend, began to develop new information systems for insurers–ones that could do more than pay fee-for-service claims. The most obvious additional function was utilization review: general-health or behavioral-health insurers were thereby enabled to track cases, keep clinical utilization review notes, elevate cases to increasingly higher levels of review when necessary, review cases against level-of-care criteria, track authorizations for care, and match the authorizations to claims within the adjudication process. Other functions included: increasingly complicated provider-contracting systems; provider accreditation; call-center software for handling member-service issues and referring new cases; provider-search functions; capitation systems; and systems to manage clinical-care protocols. None of these functions replaced anything that the provider organizations were already doing. In fact, provider organizations claim that the additional protocols and forms required by insurers' review processes add significantly to the time that providers must spend on administrative tasks, ultimately making service delivery more inefficient.

Much the same thing happened on the provider side. The software companies selling to providers began to incorporate more of the insurance functions into their systems. Today, the best practice-management systems preadjudicate insurance claims before they are sent to insurers; the goal is to never send a claim that the insurer would reject. In order to achieve this goal, provider systems must incorporate a large part of each insurer's claims-adjudication logic into their billing systems. If a provider has clients from more than one insurer, as most do, this process can become more complicated than the payment process used by the insurers. Providers' claim preadjudication has not stopped insurers from performing basically the same function, however. Although insurers may save time (since fewer claims are rejected), the basic redundancy remains, and when either side changes its rules, the claims start being rejecting again. New provider software includes the ability to manage capitation, to pay fee-for-service to subcontracted providers, and to manage contracts with a variety of payers. Capitated provider organizations have the most complicated job in this new environment. In addition to providing, managing, and paying for treatment services covered by diverse and complex benefit plans that they did not design, these organizations must also closely monitor financial data and treatment quality.

Growth of MBHOs

MBHOs are characterized by (Trabin & Freeman, 1995):

1. management teams devoted exclusively to mental health and chemical dependency issues
2. case-management personnel who are specialty credentialed under the supervision of psychiatrists
3. use of specifically developed mental health and chemical dependency criteria that address medical necessity, medical

    appropriateness, and level-of-care determinations
4. specialty behavioral group practice, staff-model, and PPO networks with a continuum of care, access to a full range of disciplines, and negotiated discounts

Managing care for patients with behavioral health disorders often requires specialized knowledge and skills different from those needed to manage general medical care. The software used by MBHOs and their specialty provider networks also differs from that used in general managed care in that the software is, by necessity, specially designed to meet the demands of behavioral health care delivery. Diagnostic modules support the most recent version of the *Diagnostic and Statistical Manual of Mental Disorders* (DSM-IVR); credentialing modules usually specify behavioral health subspecialties; clinical-decision support modules focus upon behavioral health problems, goals, and interventions; and outcome measures target behavioral health symptoms and functioning. MBHOs that purchase software for general managed health care must undertake significant customization in order to obtain the behavioral health specificity necessary to meet industry operating and reporting standards.

CORE COMPONENTS

Information systems components for MBHOs have been described in earlier publications (Maloney & Hill, 1997; Oehm, 1991), but advances in technology and in external reporting requirements have stimulated considerable change. This section describes the main features of a modern, comprehensive, managed behavioral health information system (see Figure 1). Depending on the particular circumstances of each MBHO, some of the systems and functions described below may be reduced or eliminated. For many large MBHOs, however, all of the described functions are necessary for some part of their business or provider network. MBHOs use several systems to accomplish all of the tasks described below, and many MBHOs have more than one system that performs the same tasks for different client companies or geographic locations. As noted later in this chapter, this multiplicity of systems is typically the result of acquisitions; the acquired firms already have systems in place that continue to serve their customer bases after the acquisition. The functions required by a managed care system include those related to group setup and membership; claims from providers; care management; providers; accounting; and reporting.

Figure 1

MANAGED CARE BEHAVIORAL HEALTH CARE
INFORMATION SYSTEM FUNCTIONS

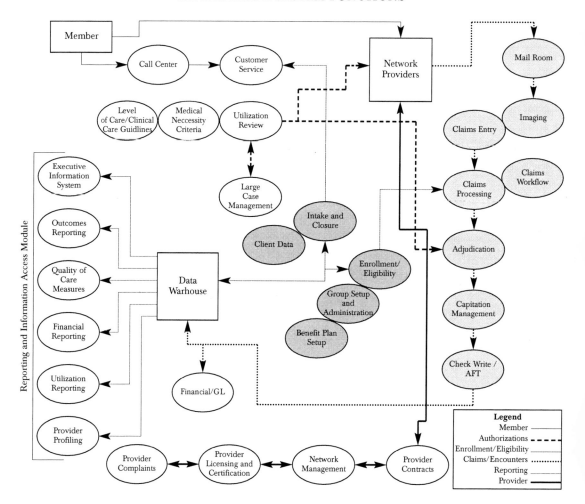

Group Setup and Membership

Among the most basic and essential functions of a managed behavioral health information system are the entry and maintenance of new client companies, their benefit plans, employees, and dependents. Once an employer group is set up in the system, the claims-payment and eligibility functions will always reference the group's benefit and membership data in order to determine how to pay providers' claims. Typical modules in this system include ones for enrollment, benefit plans, eligibility, member services, and registration.

Enrollment

The enrollment module enables a group's employees and dependents to be added to the plan. Historically, these tasks have been accomplished by each employee's completing a form that includes information on the plan chosen by the employee, as well as information on each enrolled dependent. The data on these forms is then entered by the general health plan and passed, in turn, to the MBHO. This enrollment function was one of the first ones to move to the Internet; Web-based enrollment modules began showing up as early as 1995. Internet-based enrollment had a very slow early adoption period but is gaining wider acceptance. Although it may not be the most prevalent form of enrollment for several more years, there is little question that it will become the predominant method for group-insurance enrollment.

An important link in the chain of completing behavioral health care enrollment is the ability to transmit eligibility information from the enrollment application or the contracted health plans to the MBHO. This process is often more difficult for a subcontracted specialty vendor (such as an MBHO) than it appears, especially if the vendor has contracted with many health plans. Each plan may have different formats, media, and timing for sending its enrollment information. Since behavioral health care vendors often have little leverage in negotiating enrollment feeds, they may accept enrollment information on paper, by tape, by modem link to a health plan's files, or by some other means dictated by the prime contractor (fully insured health plan, self-insured PPO, and so on). Access to a complete enrollment file—updated in near-real time and accessible over the Internet—is still more concept than reality for MBHOs.

Benefit Plans

The module for setting up the benefit plan and any associated rules performs an extremely important function for MBHOs, which are often contracted to many employers and many types of health plans. The largest MBHOs may have hundreds of benefit plans they must serve. Unlike the employer or health plan that typically has considerable input into the development of the benefit plan, the MBHO often receives the plans long after the benefits have been set. Consequently, one of the most basic requirements for the benefit-information module is the flexibility to accommodate wide variations in benefit designs.

Eligibility

The eligibility module provides the lookup capabilities that providers and client-service representatives require in order to check the status of an individual member's eligibility. The eligibility module can also feed the enrollment information to the registration module (described below) upon successful verification of eligibility when a member enters treatment.

Member Services

Today, member-services systems can be included within the broader category of customer-relationship management (CRM). Although the historical focus of typical CRM systems has been the MBHO's client customers, rather than individual members, many of the functions are the same whether the focus is the corporate customer, a contracted provider, or an individual plan member. CRM systems track all contacts with such customers, categorize these contacts, track follow-ups and referrals, and provide analyses and reports. These systems integrate information from direct person-to-person contacts, call-center contacts, and the customer's use of the company's Web site. The call-center functions are especially important. The best member-service systems include complete call-center management, with telecommunications functions such as call routing and computer-telephony integration (CTI). The purpose of this module is to provide member-service or provider-relations representatives with all of the information that they will need to service each client inquiry quickly and effectively. The best member-service systems have a complete history of each member's calls, as well as links to the claims and authorization modules to facilitate quick access to the member's claim and authorization status. Since CTI links the phone to the computer system, various trigger mechanisms (for example, the 800 number that the member uses or a code that the member enters upon calling) enable the computer to present appropriate screens to member-service representatives before they get on the line with callers. It is important to note that although CTI is the norm in many call centers, it is still rare in behavioral health care.

Registration

The registration process applies only to eligible members who are receiving services. In addition to designating the person as an active recipient of services, the process collects additional information related to those services—information that would not be applicable to a person who was merely eligible but not receiving services. In staff-model MBHOs, which integrate the managed care and provider functions, this information will include relatively detailed clinical data. In most cases, however, the information simply includes items such as payments received, additional insurance coverage identified, provider information, referrals, and so on. Since only a small percentage of the total eligibles receive behavioral health services, the number of registered members in an MBHO is much smaller than the number of eligible members. Although some type of registration process is a feature of many managed care information systems, just how this registration module is used will vary, depending on the nature of the managed behavioral care system. For example, network-model MBHOs that require all services to be preauthorized will usually register a member at intake, when the initial authorization is made. If preauthorization is not required, the network-model MBHO may not be able to register the member utilizing treatment services until the first claim is received. For a staff-model MBHO, the registration process is performed when the member enters the clinic for treatment, and no services are performed until the member is registered in the system.

Claims from Providers

The functions related to claims from providers are the major "backroom" activities of managed care. The ability to pay providers promptly and accurately is the foundation on which both the integrity of the provider network and the financial stability of the MBHO rest. These functions are also the ones that have historically been the most dependent on computer systems. Modules included in this area are those for imaging, workflow, electronic claims, electronic funds transfer, adjudication, capitation, and check paying.

Imaging

Electronic imaging software was developed to rid the claims office of paper claims. Images are taken in the mail room of the paper claim and of any supporting documentation–before they reach the claims examiners. These images are indexed to the electronic claim record in the managed care system. The best systems will use optical character recognition (OCR) software to create the electronic record from the image, in which case the data-entry function is largely eliminated; only fields not interpretable by the OCR software need to be entered by hand. This technology is rarely embraced by MBHOs because its inaccuracy rate requires a degree of double-checking that prevents the technology from being cost-effective. In any case, as records of claims and encounters become increasingly transmitted electronically, the need for imaging software will diminish.

Workflow

Workflow software was a natural outgrowth of the imaging process. Once the claim and its attachments are rendered paperless, the resulting electronic image can be sorted and queued in whatever manner is required for efficient processing. If, for example, the claim is missing a provider number, the software can detect this deficiency and route the claim to the appropriate staff in order to supply the missing information. The claims supervisor is provided with a management console that shows, among other functions, the speed of each staff member and where the largest processing backlogs are. The supervisor can redirect claims electronically to another processor when necessary. In this way the management of workflow is greatly improved.

Electronic Claims

The best solution to claims-payment problems is to never let the claim be created on paper in the first place. This solution has been slow to develop because it requires the participation of providers. Larger providers, especially hospital systems, moved to electronic claims early on. The smaller providers, especially in behavioral health, continue to lag behind in this respect. Electronic claims systems require that providers adopt a client-software package. This application is either integrated into their practice-management systems or runs as a stand-alone PC product. The software allows providers to enter all of the necessary billing (claims) information and then typically uses a dial-up connection to send the completed billing information directly to the payer or to an intermediary (claims clearinghouse), which will forward it to the correct payer. The newest applications have moved away from traditional electronic data interchange (EDI) and have begun to use thin-client (browser) technology that enables providers to create and send the claims transactions over the Internet. Either way, the paper is eliminated, and the claim arrives at the MBHO as an electronic transaction.

Electronic Funds Transfer

Electronic Funds Transfer (EFT) is another important backroom electronic function. EFT speeds up the payment process and eliminates the need for creating and mailing paper checks to providers. The banking system is well ahead of health care in the adoption of new data-processing technologies, including EFT. An electronic link can be established between the payer's bank account and the providers' bank accounts. Once the payer's claim system determines the correct amount to pay each provider, the funds can be electronically deducted from the payer's account and credited to the provider's account. The transfer occurs much faster than mailing a check and, of course, with much less paper.

Adjudication

A centrally important function of the managed care system is the adjudication of provider claims. In the adjudication process, each claim is run through an electronic decision tree that incorporates all of the benefit plan's coverage rules, exclusions, limits, and other payment rules. The greater the degree to which this decision tree can incorporate all of the millions of possible claims scenarios, the higher the auto-adjudication rate, and therefore the higher the speed and productivity of the claims shop. Auto-adjudication rates in health care have historically been as high as 80 to 90% with a well-established, comprehensive adjudication system. Behavioral health has typically lagged behind these higher percentages for a number of reasons, including: less-developed information systems; larger numbers of benefits plans on the same information system; integration issues with medical/surgical claims systems; the more chronic nature of behavioral health problems; and the greater difficulty in determining what constitutes appropriate care.

Capitation

Prior to the advent of managed care, claims systems were developed to pay only fee-for-service (FFS) claims. Managed care introduced the practice of making capitation payments to provider organizations, and information systems had to respond in kind. The capitation module manages the setup of risk pools and the debiting of these funds upon delivery of capitated services to the eligible population. Depending on the exact structure of the capitation arrangements, information systems may be tracking only encounter information–essentially a claim without the payment. Capitation payments are typically made monthly and are based on an agreed rate per covered member per month. Depending on where an organization sits in the hierarchy of health care organizations serving a population, it may be receiving a capitation payment, making a capitation payment, or both. In the last case, the capitation module would have to manage both incoming and outgoing capitation payments. To further complicate matters, it is not unusual for some services to be FFS while others are capitated. Similarly, individual providers may work part of the time on capitated services or within a capitated clinic, and at other times or locations on a FFS basis. Because of such complications, claims systems that began as pure FFS systems have often had a difficult time incorporating an effective capitation module.

Check Writing

The check-writing module of the claims system actually prints the completed, adjudicated checks. Although claims are adjudicated daily, MBHOs will typically print checks on a biweekly or monthly basis. The adjudicated claims are batch processed through the check-writing module and them mailed to providers. As described above, electronic means of payment are slowly rendering this module obsolete.

Care Management

The care-management functions are another addition that managed care brought to traditional FFS claims systems. This area is also one in which behavioral systems differ somewhat from their medical/surgical counterparts. Due to the longer-term nature of behavioral health treatment, authorizations for care may spread over periods of many months. It is not uncommon, for example, in outpatient behavioral health treatment to provide an authorization that could include six outpatient visits to be provided over a period not to exceed three months. Further, the provider may request additional visits prior to the exhaustion of the six visits authorized initially. In this case, the original authorization would need to be amended, or another overlapping authorization created, for the next set of visits. Behavioral health authorization systems need to handle these conditions while making certain that when the claim arrives months later, it is matched to the correct authorizations. By contrast, authorizations for medical and surgical issues tend to be much more precise (both substantively and temporally), making accounting for them much easier. Modules for care management include those for authorization and for clinical guidelines.

Authorization

This system must allow the care manager to create an authorization for care, communicate it to the provider (via letter generation), track it against the benefit plan, and communicate it to the claims systems through the adjudication process. In addition, this system must maintain the care manager's notes and provide a system for escalating the case to a higher level of review should that become necessary. The system also needs to manage the provider-referral process (sometimes via a separate module), providing authorizations for each referral.

Clinical Guidelines

Care guidelines (level of care, care pathways, best practices, and so on) are a fairly recent addition to managed care systems. The simplest form of a guideline or protocol involves level-of-care criteria. At the other end of the spectrum—the most complex—are clinical pathways where precise treatment steps are defined in the protocols. The best of these systems includes not only the guidelines, but the literature that supports each treatment and protocol. The systems also have a method for tracking provider performance against the guidelines, so that both the deviations from the best practice and the associated clinical results can be compared in order to determine how the guidelines or provider behavior should be adjusted in the future.

Providers

The information system modules related to the provider function are those concerning contracts, search routines, credentialing, and profiling.

Contracts

The contract-management function, like the capitation module described above, has become quite complex in recent years. As in the case of the capitation module, many behavioral health organizations today find that they must manage contracts in both directions. Organizations must "manage up" in order to maximize reimbursement with insurance organizations (which may be paying them through a complex mix of capitated and noncapitated arrangements), and they must also "manage down" to providers (who may be receiving payments from them through a similar maze of capitated, case-rate, and fee-for-service arrangements). The purpose of the contracts module is to set up the contract terms, assure that payments abide by these terms, and maximize each contract's advantages. The management of provider contracts, in particular, must also both take into account the many possible roles (primary care manager, FFS provider, member of a clinic that is capitated for certain procedures, and so on) that a single provider may have, and pay each claim correctly based on both the appropriate role and the rules that govern each claim.

Search Routines

The search-routine module maintains the name, affiliation, location(s), billing, identification number(s), degree and licensure level, and specialty information for each provider. The location data is usually linked to geographic-search routines that are able to calculate distances in either miles or travel time, and to use this information to select providers in close proximity to the prospective consumer. The specialty information may include the disorders, age groups, languages, religious affiliations, ethnic, cultural, and racial groups, and other areas for which particular providers might have special capabilities or sensitivities that would aid in patient care. These data are also linked to search routines that enable an intake coordinator to refer the prospective consumer to a clinician with an appropriate skill set to address that consumer's needs and presenting problems.

Credentialing

Many MBHOs no longer do their own credentialing work. In cases where this function has been outsourced, however, the managed-care information system still must include some type of flag to indicate whether each provider has been credentialed. Credentialing software has developed largely independently of comprehensive managed care systems; MBHOs that choose to do their own credentialing will therefore typically purchase a stand-alone product. Credentialing packages include letter-generation routines for communicating with providers, as well as other programmed routines specifically designed to track the collection and verification of each of the necessary credentialing documents.

Profiling

Provider profiling is essentially a reporting function. Statistics are gathered on each provider over time and compared to norms developed from the entire group of providers. Statistics from the claims data typically include utilization and cost figures. Other information (such as statistics on member satisfaction and access) may also be collected and included in a profile. The best systems will provide more sophisticated comparisons–for example, comparing providers against members of their specialty (based on case mix adjusted by claims data). If the organization has begun to collect outcome data (as discussed later in this chapter), that information can also be included in the profile. Some MBHOs provide financial incentives that are derived from profile information. In this manner, income is being tied to performance across a broader array of measures than just volume.

Accounting

Accounting functions include the general ledger, accounts payable and receivable, premium billing, and other related functions. Managed behavioral health information systems generally do not include accounting functions. Instead, since there are many good accounting packages available in the market, vendors of managed care software will typically recommend an accounting system that interfaces well with their own software. Many of the larger MBHOs–especially those that are part of larger health systems encompassing the entire range of health care services–have come to use particular accounting systems that are independent of their behavioral health software packages. Given these realities, accounting functions have not been a major focus of behavioral health information systems. The primary accounting focus of most managed behavioral health software systems is to provide an interface with at least one commercial accounting package in order to allow for the easy transfer of necessary information.

Reporting

Several important categories of reports are listed below. The executive information system typically presents a high-level view of the entire enterprise–a view derived from reports from each of the other reporting categories. Similarly, the provider profiles described previously are developed by combining reports across several categories to develop a picture of each provider's performance.

Executive Information Systems

The Executive Information System (EIS) is a subset of reports from all categories that is designed to give top executives a quick picture of the overall health and performance of the MBHO. The best systems allow these reports to be run in real time whenever requested by the executive. The results are presented on the screen for quick viewing and may also be printed.

Financial

As with the accounting function discussed previously, the financial reports tend to resemble those of other businesses. These reports include the balance sheet and income statement. Other reports specific to health care will include items such as the incurred but not reported claims, capitation risk pools, high-cost claimants, and profitability of specific contracts.

Utilization

Utilization reports are historically one of the main methods by which managed care firms perform their jobs. Utilization is tracked across individual clinicians, treatment programs, and treatment facilities. It is also tracked across each of the contracted employer groups, and by type of client (for example, age, sex, and diagnosis). Based on these utilization patterns, decisions are made regarding premium increases or decreases, and how the delivery of care could be better managed.

Quality

Quality reports are relative newcomers to the field. These reports include many of the HEDIS measurements such as client satisfaction, access to care, follow-up appointments, and so on, as well as the provider profiles described above. These reports and the issues surrounding them are described in greater detail in the next section of this chapter.

Episodes of Care

Episodes-of-care reports, a relatively recent addition, were developed because MBHOs recognized that managing care on a claim-by-claim basis was relatively inefficient. It was important, instead, to understand the entire treatment cycle for a given condition and member—which required that all of a member's claims for a given ailment be consolidated and reviewed as a whole. The claims, grouped together into "episodes of care," provide significantly better insights into the cost and effectiveness of different treatment approaches.

Many of the above reporting functions are as applicable to general health plan information systems as they are to information systems specifically oriented toward behavioral health care. Nevertheless, there are many unique aspects that distinguish behavioral health information systems, with respect both to the data that are captured and to some of the required functions. For example, an information system designed specifically for behavioral health will include DSM diagnostic codes and be able to handle the additional axes associated with such coding. The information system should also automatically correlate these codes with ICD codes. It will include all of the distinct treatment and treatment-setting designations, including behavioral-health testing designations, residential-care and partial-hospitalization settings, nontraditional treatment alternatives, and so on.

As noted in the authorization section above, behavioral health care often involves longer-term treatment. Behavioral health systems therefore need to manage multiple and extended authorizations efficiently for all levels of care and for all lengths of treatment episodes.

INVESTMENT IN MANAGED BEHAVIORAL HEALTH INFORMATION TECHNOLOGY

If MBHOs are to expand beyond the functional components of the information systems described in the preceding section, they must be prepared for significant new expenditures. The following sections set forth the types of expansion most likely to attract and justify such expenditures. Many of these undertakings require significant capital investments in new hardware and software, as well as significant increases in annual expenses for personnel to install, operate, maintain, and customize the new or refined information-systems components. The money for such investments must come from the revenues MBHOs obtain contractually from purchasers.

The percentage of MBHOs' total revenues spent on their information technology (IT) departments remains low. The coauthors conducted interviews with information systems executives from seven MBHOs (Trabin & Maloney, 1999) and found their information systems budget allocations to be relatively consistent at approximately 2.5% (total annual budget of the IT department, including its staff, capital depreciation of hardware and software, and so on, compared to the total revenue of the organization). Some MBHOs that are in the middle of a large systems-development or -implementation project reported higher figures (in the 3 to 4% range). On average, MBHOs spend less than their medical/surgical counterparts. The most recent Gartner Group survey shows general medical/surgical health care IT spending at 4.23% of revenues on average (Guptill, Stewart, Marcoccio, Potter, & Claps, 1999).

IT spending by health care organizations and especially by MBHOs is substantially less than by many industries, such as 12.12% by banking (Guptill, Stewart, Marcoccio, Potter, & Claps, 1999). This lower level of spending is especially important since the job that behavioral health care IT must perform in managed care is quite large. In fact, since the managed care companies do not usually provide the actual treatment, nearly all of their functions (for example, capitation, provider payments, utilization review, claims payment) are highly dependent upon the management of information. Other industries that are so dependent (such as banking) spend considerably more on their information systems.

MBHOs' already high administration costs make it difficult for them to spend more on their information systems. Although MBHOs need to provide nearly all of the same administrative functions as their health plan counterparts, MBHOs are working with a much smaller percentage of the premium. If they only receive 3 to 4% of the overall premium dollar but still have the fixed costs associated with paying claims, provider relations, member services, and utilization review, it stands to reason that the percentage of premium allocated to administrative services will be higher than for general health care. In this environment, behavioral health plans are already pressed to reduce administrative expenses. Although increased IT expenditures can be shown to have a positive long-term impact on administrative costs, the fiscal picture may look rather bleak for the year in which software development or implementation is occurring—or may occur. This threshold problem will continue to influence MBHOs in the future.

DATA AND THE QUALITY OF CARE

MBHOs are generally required to adhere to specific organizational-performance standards. These standards span such performance domains as service access, appropriateness of care, consumer satisfaction with services, and treatment outcomes. Standards and measurements addressing these performance domains are emerging from regulatory agencies, accreditation organizations, and employee-benefit purchasers in both the public and private sectors. Many of the standards and measurements require extensive data tracking, analysis, and reporting. Without sophisticated information systems, it is simply not possible for MBHOs to meet these market and regulatory requirements.

The methods, technology, and incentives of managed behavioral health care have transformed what was once a fragmented cottage industry into multiple organized-care systems capable of coordinating patient care across a complete continuum of services. At the foundation of this coordination are information systems that track patients throughout the course of treatment. Because the databases produced by these functions are sizable, they have the potential to generate valuable new knowledge regarding the most efficient and effective treatment services and treatment providers for diverse types of patients. This potential is largely untapped, however, and its realization depends upon significant new monetary investment. At the time of this writing, most purchasers of behavioral health services do not seem inclined to finance this work; new strides in quality-related measurement consequently remain very gradual. As public concern mounts regarding the quality of managed care, however, the priorities of, and rewards for, MBHOs are likely to change.

Measurements of Organizational Performance

Both accreditation and regulatory organizations shifted their accountability requirements for managed care during the latter half of the 1990s. One shift was from an exclusive focus on structure (for example, whether a provider network is sufficient relative to existing standards for specialties, geographic distance, and so on) and process variables (for example, whether responses to incoming calls were timely within specified standards) to an additional focus on outcomes (for example, whether there has been a significant reduction in treated symptoms, an improvement in functioning, and so on). Another shift, perhaps more profound, is from an exclusive focus on dichotomous standards (for example, whether the organization does or does not document a quality-management plan) to the addition of performance indicators with continuous variables (for example, what percentage of patients discharged from 24-hour care receive ambulatory care follow-up visits within seven days). Although many regulatory and accreditation standards can be met without the aid of computers, efficient and effective responses to performance-measurement reporting requirements necessitate reliance upon a substantially computerized information system.

The process by which performance-measurement requirements are developed and implemented on a systemwide level results in a mutually reinforcing spiral of improvements. Through an increase in measurement requirements, regulatory and accreditation organizations prompt MBHOs to build a larger information systems infrastructure. And once that infrastructure is in place, with its increased measurement capability, regulatory and accreditation organizations then require still more performance measurements. This is not to imply that accreditation and regulatory organizations make frivolous demands or that MBHOs do not care about quality. More to the point, the constructive tension between MBHOs and those organizations, as well as MBHOs' "go slow" approach, is due to the tremendous expense of expanding the information systems infrastructure in order to implement and satisfy newly imposed performance-measurement reporting requirements.

The purposes and extent of performance measurements vary with the organization requiring the reporting. In order to aid purchasers' and consumers' selection decisions, such measurements may be required for inclusion in public report cards that provide comparative information across multiple organizations of similar types. In order to aid each participating organization in its quality improvement and its marketing efforts, such measurements may be included on a voluntary basis in health care coalitions' confidential report cards that provide each organization's performance report compared against the aggregate norm. In order to judge performance against minimum standards, purchasers and regulatory and accreditation organizations may also require performance measurements periodically.

Some of the larger purchasers and purchasing coalitions have quite sophisticated reporting requirements for MBHOs. As purchasers of managed care services, federal, state, and county mental health agencies are requiring increasingly extensive performance-measurement reports. The most widely used mental health reporting set for the public sector at the time of this writing is the Mental Health Statistics Improvement Program (MHSIP) Consumer-Oriented Report Card (MHSIP Task Force on a Consumer-Oriented Mental Health Report Card, 1996). All accrediting organizations are moving towards at least recommending, if not requiring, some form of performance-measurement reporting. The primary accrediting organizations for MBHOs–the National Committee for Quality Assurance (NCQA) and the Joint Commission for the Accreditation of Health Care Organizations (JCAHO)–both require performance measurement (NCQA, 1999; JCAHO, 1997). At the time of this writing, NCQA's requirements are the most prescriptive and detailed. Even the MBHOs themselves have developed and piloted a performance-measurement set (AMBHA, 1998). To ease the burden and confusion of so many measurement requirements, the American College of Mental Health Administration launched a significant initiative to synthesize all these measurement sets into a set of core measurements (ACMHA, 1997).

Examples from a nationwide study (Kramer, Trabin, Daniels, Theriot, Freeman, & Williams, 1997) of performance measurements used most commonly by MBHOs include (with associated data sources in parentheses):

Access Indicators:

1. Percentage of consumers satisfied with access to care (consumer survey)
2. Telephone response time by staff answering calls (automated call-distribution-machine data)

3. Waiting time for scheduling routine office visits (administrative data entered by intake at first call, and encounter data from claims)

4. Waiting time for scheduling emergency visits (administrative data entered by intake at first call, and encounter data from claims)

5. Acute inpatient days/1,000 members (encounter data from claims, and enrollment data)

6. Acute inpatient average length of stay (encounter data from claims)

7. Outpatient visits/1,000 members (encounter data from claims, and enrollment data)

8. Outpatient average number of sessions (encounter data from claims)

9. Intensive outpatient average length of stay (encounter data from claims)

10. Partial hospitalization average length of stay (encounter data from claims)

11. Telephone call abandonment rate (automated call-distribution-machine data)

Clinical Appropriateness Indicators:

1. Percentage of inpatient cases reviewed with medical director for medical necessity (administrative data)

2. Percentage of patients reporting overall satisfaction with quality of care (consumer survey)

3. Indicators of service quality

4. Percentage of claims paid within specified period (claims data)

5. Percentage of providers recredentialed (administrative data)

6. Indicators of treatment outcome

7. Percentage of patients readmitted after specified period (encounter data)

8. Percentage of patients with adverse outcomes (medical record data)

9. Percentage of patients having improved functioning after treatment (outcome-measurement instrument and patient-survey data)

More recent studies suggest an increased use of consumer-perception surveys to assess the satisfactoriness and effectiveness of services with respect to access, appropriateness, quality, and outcomes. The same studies also suggest an increasing use of performance measurements—in particular, the two NCQA HEDIS measurements—to determine the percentage of cases that adhered to clinical practice guidelines:

1. Percentage of patients receiving an ambulatory follow-up visit within seven days of discharge from inpatient hospitalization (encounter data)
2. Percentage of patients with depressive-disorder diagnoses and receiving antidepressant medication whose psychopharmacological treatment conforms to specific guidelines (encounter and pharmacy data)

Measurements of Treatment Outcomes

Treatment outcomes are potentially the definitive measurements of treatment quality and effectiveness. Commercial-sector purchasers are extremely interested in functional outcomes such as reduced absenteeism and increased productivity at work. Public-sector purchasers, responsible to a consumer population with more serious and longer-term disorders, are also interested in quality-of-life measurements such as readmission rates, morale, arrest rates, and housing. Purchasers in both sectors are becoming more interested in whether effective behavioral health interventions can reduce medical utilization.

The most common outcome measurements, which focus upon a combination of symptom reduction, improved functioning, and improved quality of life, are derived from self-reported questionnaires. Technologically, these questionnaires involve the use of the following: scannable paper-and-pencil survey instruments; questionnaires administered over the telephone through interactive voice response (IVR), with automated entry into the patient's computer-based record; or direct computer entry at clinicians' offices, with data uploaded through the Internet to patients' MBHO records (Strosahl, 1998). The administrative and IT challenge is in streamlining the process of accurately transmitting patients' responses—initially completed in their homes or in their clinicians' offices—and entering the data into patients' computer-based records. Once the data are entered, the technical processes of scoring, aggregating, analyzing, and interpreting them are much easier.

Many of the outcome measurements that focus on patient functioning require administrative data from organizations distinct from the MBHO (for example, from employers concerning absenteeism and work productivity, from schools concerning absenteeism and grades, from health plans on medical cost offsets, from the criminal justice system on involvement with the legal system, and so on). Although these data–once acquired–can appear more reliable and valid than self-reported data, they are notoriously difficult to collect. Because of the administrative burden, and also because of concerns about the privacy of the data, the organizations that must supply such data are generally disinclined to cooperate.

Most MBHO executives will agree about the importance of outcome-measurement data for quality management and accountability. The sheer cost, however–both in labor and in dollars–of administering the outcome measurements has thus far prevented widespread implementation. Moreover, consumers are beginning to ask for something in return for being asked to complete outcome-measurement questionnaires periodically: either the scored results of their own, completed questionnaires, or aggregated reports comparing organizations (like *Consumer Reports*)–which would enable them to make more informed selection decisions in the future. Similarly, providers want something from MBHOs in return for their part in administering the questionnaires–either higher reimbursement rates or feedback on their results. Consequently, for MBHOs to undertake outcome measurement on a broad scale, they must find ways both to minimize the administrative burden and to elicit cooperation from providers and consumers (Moran, 1998). Even so, to bear the additional costs of administering these outcome questionnaires, MBHOs will need to know there is a competitive advantage in doing so, or that purchasers that require such data are also willing to pay more for it. Most purchasers, however, while expressing great interest in outcome data, have thus far stopped short of signaling their willingness to pay extra for it.

A cost-effective method of collecting and analyzing large amounts of data without additional compensation from purchasers is through partnerships between MBHOs and academic research centers (Goldman, Sturm, & McCulloch, 1997). Several MBHOs are developing such partnership centers, including Magellan, Value Options, United Behavioral Health, and Integra. In these partnerships, MBHOs are usually the primary suppliers both of the data and of the knowledge of managed care systems. The academic researchers are the primary data analysts and writers for publication. These researchers are also the lead grant writers and can help the MBHOs obtain federal funds for data collection and analysis that they would not otherwise have been able to afford. The projects these centers undertake can substantially influence the data collected routinely by MBHOs, the data fields in the information system, and the configuration of the databases to support specific analyses.

Clinical-Decision Support

In the early 1990s, managed health care companies were under pressure from many stakeholder groups to document the level-of-care criteria upon which they based their care-management decision making. Requests for this information from purchasers first became routine and then were elevated to requirements by state regulatory agencies and by accreditation organizations such as the Utilization Review Accreditation Commission. Some MBHOs computerized these criteria to provide decision support for their care managers.

A small number of MBHOs went further. They asked their high-volume providers to administer outcome measurements to their patients on a periodic basis and to send the data for scoring and analysis to the MBHO (Brown & Kornmayer, 1996; Sperry, Brill, Howard, & Grissom, 1996). Algorithms were developed to provide an estimation of degree of change over time, and to "red flag" for care-management intervention those cases in which the expected changes were not occurring. Because of the expense in labor and technology–and the inconvenience experienced by patients and providers in completing numerous forms–this approach to clinical-decision support remains uncommon.

A new approach to decision support in MBHOs is based upon practice guidelines–an approach that promises to develop rapidly. NCQA now requires MBHOs to have practice guidelines that emphasize evidence-based treatments, to disseminate those guidelines to their provider networks, and to monitor adherence to those guidelines in treatment (NCQA, 1997). These requirements have presented difficulties, however, since the behavioral health care field has no standardized method for coding types of treatment interventions. The current state of the art is for providers to identify their general treatment (for example, psychodynamic, cognitive-behavioral, and so on) on a treatment-plan form. This method of tracking treatment interventions is too global to capture adherence to practice guidelines, and too subject to "gaming" for the purpose of passing tests of reliability and validity. Consequently, the determination of adherence to practice guidelines is currently accomplished by sampling and reviewing charts. At the same time, efforts are under way to develop more granular taxonomies of treatment that would enable computerized tracking of treatment interventions.

CURRENT CHALLENGES:
A SURVEY OF INFORMATION SYSTEMS EXECUTIVES
IN MANAGED BEHAVIORAL HEALTH CARE

To obtain the most up-to-date information possible for this chapter on information systems trends in MBHOs, we developed a structured survey questionnaire for interviews with the information systems executives of six major MBHOs and one HMO. We conducted the interviews during the summer of 1999. For ease of reference, we will refer to all the companies responding as MBHOs, with the understanding that one is an HMO providing information on how its information systems developments pertain to its behavioral health services.

The survey questions were designed to address:

1. changing priorities of IT departments within managed behavioral health care
2. main challenges that IT departments currently face
3. prospects for integration of behavioral health and general health care data
4. extent of the organization's expenditures on information systems
5. extent to which organizations communicate with their provider networks electronically, and with respect to which business and clinical functions
6. extent to which organization use their information systems to meet quality-focused measurement requirements from purchasers, accreditors, and regulators
7. manner in which MBHOs are conducting provider credentialing (in-house, through outsourcing, and so on)

Changing Priorities

The ongoing migration of function has been from back office, retrospective systems to frontline, real-time systems. The back-office functions have not disappeared in this process; such functions as accounting and claims payment remain central. System functions have been added, however, that support the work of employees–in customer service, case management, and related service and medical-management areas–who deal more directly with customers and providers.

Today, MBHOs are participating in the next evolution of information systems functions. The systems functions that formerly assisted only the MBHO staff are being made available, through various Web and telephone-based applications, directly to clients and providers. Some of these applications, especially IVR, have been available for a number of years. Many of the newer Web-based systems have also been available at least since 1998 in a few of the MBHOs. The immediate future will bring a widespread acceptance of Internet applications (on PCs, kiosks, and various handheld devices). These applications include: enrollment; provider search and selection; appointments and reminders; health-risk assessments; health and benefits information; clinical advice; pharmacy applications that include drug information and refills; and various applications to support Internet communities built around specific health-related topics.

Current Challenges

The main information systems issues facing MBHOs today include a wide variety of items from end-user training to implementing new Web-based technologies. In addition to financing IT, which is a major challenge for MBHOs (as it is throughout health care), the following issues were of central concern to the major MBHOs:

1. The year 2000 (Y2K) issue was the primary concern for most MBHOs when this survey was conducted. Many firms indicated they dedicated up to 60% of their IT budgets to this area in 1999. Some of this expense was devoted to remediation of existing systems, while some was spent on implementing new systems. The expense for new systems would have been incurred in future years regardless of the Y2K issue, but was moved for-

ward to take advantage of the fact that the new systems were Y2K compliant. MBHOs also indicated that for liability reasons, they incurred substantial expenses in order to document their Y2K preparations.

2. Firms that had acquired other behavioral companies were immersed in efforts to integrate, rationalize, and streamline internal systems. This process leads to conversion projects as the companies standardize on fewer platforms and as they match acquired systems to the specific market segments for which they are best suited (for example, public versus private sector).

3. For all MBHOs, large and small, a central goal was electronic connectivity to business partners and providers. The concern was not necessarily to add new automated functions, but to improve administrative efficiency through the reduction of manual interfaces and overly complex system infrastructures. All respondents agreed that there is a wide gap between their own organization's interest and readiness to move ahead, on the one hand, and their provider network's reluctance to adopt the requisite new technologies, on the other.

4. Retention of employees was a major concern. Not only have labor markets been tight in recent years, but the IT market is one of the tightest. In addition, managed behavioral care firms would ideally like to hire IT staff with at least some knowledge of health care–and preferably, of behavioral health care. IT professionals with this type of specialized knowledge are, however, very difficult to find, recruit, and retain (Anderson & Van Eik, 1999).

Data Integration with General Health Care Organizations

There are some demands being placed on MBHOs to integrate with medical/surgical systems and providers (Coke, 1996; Docherty, 1996). These demands vary widely across the organizations surveyed, however. For the majority of carved-out behavioral health vendors, integration with medical/surgical systems typically involves partial data integration that is accomplished on the back end through integrated data reporting. Several of the firms use third-party vendors (hired either by themselves or their clients) who accept data from both the health plan and the behavioral health organization and then produce integrated reports. Excepted from this demand for increased integration are staff-model HMOs in which the behavioral health staff are already integrated into the delivery model. These HMOs report data from all services without the need for back-end data integration.

Investment in Information Technology

Executives were asked several questions about their companies' investments and expenditures in IT-related areas, and their responses are summarized in an earlier section of this chapter that is devoted specifically to those issues. As noted there, companies spend, on average, 2.5% of their revenues on IT-related expenses (including capital depreciation). Readers may also want to consult a previous study by the Workgroup for the Computerization of Behavioral Health and Human Services (1995), which focused on overall dollar expenditures on IT rather than on the percentage of revenue.

Electronic Transmission of Data between MBHOs and Providers

Survey statistics regarding the use of various electronic means of data communication reflect the low acceptance level of various technologies among clinical providers. We found, on average, that use of the Internet for electronic data communication of any form (for example, client and provider inquiries, or claims submissions) was less than 10%. For most MBHOs, standard EDI for claims payment still constituted the highest volume of electronic transactions. The other electronic-communication technologies that are used–but much less extensively–are IVR and fax machines. All respondents agreed that they could not require the electronic transmission of forms (particularly via the Internet) because too few providers have the necessary skills and equipment to comply. This situation is expected to change within a very few years.

Quality-Focused Measurement Requirements

The majority of MBHOs are compliant with respect to accreditation requirements, quality measurements, and outcome measurements. Since many of these measures are also required under client contracts, the way that the measures are implemented typically relates directly to the specific requirements of particular clients.

Most of the MBHOs have developed or are currently developing a data-warehouse and decision-support system to facilitate compliance with current and future reporting requirements. MBHOs vary as to how these data are collected; the more technologically innovative collection methods include scannable forms, client applications with dial-up connectivity, and the use of the Internet.

The leading-edge organizations have also developed methods to distribute quality-focused performance information to providers, typically in the form of a "report card" that compares the provider's quality scores against norms for the company, for the provider's peer group, and for providers in the geographic area. A very small number of organizations go further and give clinicians feedback on some of their patients' progress midway through treatment. The evaluation of progress is based upon the periodic administration to those patients of an outcome measurement that is scored and then compared to their previous scores.

Provider Credentialing

Several firms have outsourced their provider-credentialing work to credential-verification organizations. In general, there is a willingness to outsource functions–such as credentialing–where there are established outsourcing vendors; there is little competitive advantage associated with proprietary solutions.

THE FUTURE

The most important technology developments that will affect managed behavioral health care over the next decade are described in the following sections. Some of the developments involve new technologies–such as wireless handheld computing devices–that will ease provider adoption of computer-based technologies. Some involve technology improvements that are just coming of age; for example, voice recognition, which enables direct voice-to-computer entry with interactive components for obtaining complex data from consumers and providers. Some are new uses of existing technologies such as Web-enabled practice-management systems, telemedicine, and data warehousing. For all these types of technological applications, the challenge is to develop the care-management and -delivery processes that will take advantage of developing technologies to achieve new levels of efficiency and effective care. An overarching issue relating to electronic transmission and storage of patient information is that of protecting patients' privacy and the confidentiality of information—a topic that will be addressed after the discussion of the new technology applications themselves.

New Technology Applications

Data Warehouses for Decision Support

Reporting requirements to purchasers, accreditation organizations, and regulators will continue to increase. The type of data required will change, and with it the data-collection methods and the problems that need to be addressed. MBHOs can expect to find it increasingly challenging to achieve and maintain both the *decentralized* reporting from components of their companies to external organizations, and the *centralized* reporting of aggregated data from all of these components. This challenge will be further intensified by the emerging demands— from general health care organizations (whether in managed care or representing providers), from child welfare agencies, and from the criminal justice system—to integrate MBHO data with selected and appropriate consumer data. In order to respond quickly to new reporting requests, and also to gain the most value from the data they have collected, managed care firms are turning to decision-support systems (DSS). The core of every DSS is a data warehouse.

The purpose of a DSS is to provide management with the tools they need to transform raw data into useful information to support the decision process. The most common data warehouses or data marts (several smaller, single-purpose data warehouses) incorporate data extracted from other modules in the managed care system. These other modules, such as the claims module and the authorization module, are typically online transaction-processing systems (OLTP). These systems are designed to manage the transactions required to *conduct* business but are not optimized to *report* on that business. By extracting the data from these modules or systems and by then storing it in a data warehouse, the data can be aggregated in a manner that is optimal for data mining and reporting. Data from many systems modules (and other external sources) can be stored in the same database so that the data are more accessible to the decision support and reporting tools. Queries and reports that use the data from a variety of sources can then be easily defined, and can be run on the warehouse without affecting the performance of the rest of the managed care system. Often, the data will be stored in a different format than that of the transaction systems. They may be denormalized (stored in formats using longer records, which enables users of the DSS to formulate and run queries), or stored in a schema that will facilitate multidimensional analysis.

A complete DSS can include data-mining tools, an executive information system, online analytical reporting (OLAP) tools, and the data warehouse itself. MBHOs will choose a configuration of tools that serve their specific needs. Regardless of the exact configuration, the goal of the DSS is to provide the information that will best support decision making. Because the data are available in one location, and because the reporting tools allow users easily to add and change elements on reports, the DSS provides MBHOs with the flexibility to meet the numerous reporting requests they receive.

The most recent advances in DSS technology include: multidimensional reporting tools that allow users to examine information quickly along several dimensions; drill-down capabilities that allow users to examine the layers of data underlying each summary statistic; and data-mining tools that decipher trends in the data that are not intuitive or apparent to the user. Health care data that have been extracted from transaction systems can also be amended and adjusted in ways that are not feasible within the OLTP modules. For example, the service and claims information can be risk adjusted, and claims can be grouped into episodes of care. Processes like these can provide users with a deeper understanding not only of the trends in the data, but of the quality and cost of health care.

Telemedicine/Telemental Health

Technology and technology applications for telemedicine and its subspecialty of telemental health have expanded very rapidly. This expansion has been aided by the growth of the Internet and by the increased bandwidth available from telecommunications companies. The expansion also been aided by the introduction of improved telecommunication devices. Although the era of very inexpensive, high quality, real-time, two-way telecommunications has not quite arrived, the progress made in recent years indicates that that era is very close at hand.

Previously, video teleconferencing required high-bandwidth leased lines, dedicated rooms, and expensive, proprietary equipment. Today, at the very low end, it is possible to send an electronic image of reasonable quality over the Internet with a $150 digital camera attached to a PC. Although this type of very low end system is not recommended for real-time videoconferencing, it is possible to build a system that would provide "true" videoconferencing by using standard, commercially available products that cost less than $1,000 per user in hardware costs. The charge for a high-bandwidth cable or phone-line connection is now well under $1,000 per year. What this means is that telemedicine is about to become commonplace. As an outgrowth of this new technology, many telemental health sites arc emerging throughout the United States, particularly to improve behavioral health access in rural areas. Some of these sites, such as RODEO Net in Oregon, have formed business alliances with MBHOs.

Voice/Speech Recognition

Another technology that, though not quite mature, has made enormous strides just prior to this writing is voice recognition. Just a few years ago, in order to use speech-recognition software, it was necessary to pause between each word to give the computer a fighting chance at parsing the communication. Today, due to improvements both in the software and in the processing power of computers, continuous speech is possible with these programs. Further, the software has become much better at recognizing homonyms from their context. For example, the sentence "I went to the store to buy two balls, too" can be correctly deciphered by the newest products.

Despite such obvious progress, the products still need to be trained in order to recognize the speech patterns of each particular speaker. This training process can take many hours over many weeks before any of the speech-recognition products now available reaches a level where the product is not taking more time (including the correcting process, which must also be performed audibly) than typing for many people. Although a well-trained product may produce text that is up to 98% correct, this percentage is still not quite high enough: correcting the last 2% requires proofreading the entire document.

Speech recognition is extremely important because it removes typing as a barrier to entering information into the computer. The need to enter data manually (by whatever method) has been a significant issue in the effective use of computers in the clinical process. Now, dictation can be entered directly into computer-based records, or into a recorder that reads it into the computer later.

The one major caveat with the use of this technology is that it may increase the amount of less useful data in the computer system. One of the current problems with medical records—and with clinical notes, in particular—is that they are too loosely structured and do not preclude the inconsistent use and definitions of terms. These problems make it impossible to summarize groups of records and also make it difficult to search for information or trends in the data. Speech-recognition applications will need to enforce standard charting structures, levels-of-severity definitions, treatment definitions, and other conventions. Otherwise, the end result will only be an increase in the amount of less-than-useful free text in the system, and the only real gain may be the money saved on dictation services.

One area where speech recognition has already proven itself is in applications where single words or short, well-defined phrases can be used to record information or to direct electronic devices. Speech recognition is also especially helpful in fields, such as dentistry or radiology, where the practitioner's hands are busy.

Although speech recognition has thus made significant headway in some clinical areas, it has yet to make substantial advances in clinical behavioral health. Speech recognition is nevertheless proving its usefulness in behavioral health as an administrative tool. Client companies and providers now use speech-recognition software (in the form of IVR systems) to check on the status of claims or on the eligibility of consumers. Providers use IVR systems to enter and receive authorization requests. Consumers use IVR to respond to satisfaction and outcome questionnaires. These systems all have the advantage of not being dependent on a PC.

The Public Internet and Other Internet Protocol (IP) Networks

The Internet is a wonderful example of the enormous gains in access, content, and ease of use that are possible when the world converges on a single set of common, nonproprietary standards: at its core, the Internet and the World Wide Web constitute an agreement to communicate using a common set of electronic protocols. It is the computer equivalent of all the world's people agreeing to speak English. When we use a browser based upon these shared communications conventions, we have access to all the information on all of the connected networks. This is the power of the Internet.

The Internet has already transformed many industries and is rapidly transforming many aspects of health care. Indeed, the information systems for managed behavioral health care will eventually move to the Internet, which is opening the possibilities of universal provider connectivity, of accessible electronic health profiles and medical records, of more efficient markets for medical supplies, and of completely restructuring the health care claims process. For example, in the case of the adjudication rules for behavioral health companies, the rules will be, in essence, "objects" of programming code. Their precise location on the Internet will be irrelevant. When practitioners have claims for services provided to eligible members, they will place that claim via the Internet. The claims will be routed to the appropriate adjudication rules for the appropriate health plan, and the result of applying those rules will be returned to providers. The system will then automatically transfer the appropriate funds to the providers' accounts (or, if requested by the provider, the system will stop prior to the funds transfers in order to enable providers to check the claims payments). There will be no claims backlogs. There will be no claims delayed for missing or inaccurate information. A claim that is missing information will be returned to the provider within seconds, along with a message describing each of the problems with the submission. In essence, providers will not be able to submit incomplete or nonpayable claims. There will be no claims submitted and then denied for lack of an authorization; the adjudication rules will be examined by the provider's system prior to the delivery of the service so that any required billing procedures, authorizations, or ineligible services are discovered and remedied. In fact, there will be no "claim" as we know it today; the process will be reduced to a series of electronic messages on the network.

While we have used behavioral health claims as an example of how IP networks like the Internet will affect future transactions and the connectivity between behavioral health entities, these technologies will obviously affect any type of message or transaction. Regulations to be published under the Health Insurance Portability and Accountability Act (HIPAA) of 1996, for example, will lead to the standardization of many types of electronic transactions, including claims and attachments, referrals and authorizations, payments and remittance advice, COB, claims-status inquiries, first report of injury, plan enrollment, and premium payments. All of these transactions are, indeed, already being conducted over computer networks such as the Internet.

IP networks other than the public Internet will also be used for health care transactions. Although such services cost more than the public Internet, they have all of the advantages of the Internet without some of the negatives. For example, a value-added network (VAN) Internet site can guarantee service availability, provide an additional level of security, and perform many of the network's administrative functions. These services are popular because they allow clients to use all of the technologies developed for the Internet (browsers and so on) in a network that looks and behaves like the Internet, while not actually using the Internet. Therefore, the behavioral health records and transactions are never exposed to the public Internet, and variations in utilization and traffic on the Internet do not affect communication speed and reliability.

The intranets that many organizations have developed are another example of a secure network. Like the VAN described above, they use all of the same tools and protocols, but are not the Internet. Many intranets do have connections to the Internet, but ones that are protected by firewalls to prevent external users from accessing the system. Since intranets are confined to a company, they are useful only for communications within the organization. It is possible, however, to extend the secure network onto the Internet through tunneling protocols and other means of encrypting messages so that they cannot be deciphered. This advance has led to another recent Internet-related trend, the development of "extranets." An extranet is an extension of an intranet out onto the Internet. Extranets are used, for example, to connect trading partners. Although the messages that travel between the companies leave their respective intranets and cross the Internet, the encryption process renders them unreadable to third parties.

As dramatically beneficial as Internet technologies may be with claims transmissions and other business transactions, their impact upon clinical care is likely to be even more profound. The World Wide Web is rapidly becoming a source of clinical information used widely by both consumers and providers. The ease with which information can be accessed through this medium makes it possible for clinical care to be guided more readily and consistently by best practices, and also makes more feasible the efforts of MBHOs to obtain providers' compliance with the companies' recommended practice guidelines, outcome measurements, and other quality and accountability initiatives. The primary beneficiaries of this increased access to clinical information will be consumers, who are likely to experience an overall improvement in the quality of treatment services they receive.

Several software and technology companies are emerging as Application Service Providers (ASPs) that offer practice-management software leased over the Internet. Many clinicians will experience less of a financial hurdle by being able to access practice-management products and services in this way; clinicians can rent ASP products for a modest but predictably constant monthly rate rather than purchase them outright and upgrade them regularly. Clinicians are also likely to experience less of a technological adjustment hurdle since ASP products are directly accessible through the Internet, which they have already learned to use, and therefore do not require the potentially new skills associated with downloading, installing, and periodically upgrading software. This increased ease of adoption is likely to induce many clinicians–ones who are in independent practice and contract with managed care networks–to computerize their clinical and business operations. As a result, managed care companies will find it easier to use electronic communication as the primary mode of exchanging information with their network providers. The eventual cost savings to be realized by all parties through this new development are likely to be substantial.

New Computer Devices

Wireless, handheld devices are the new frontier for computer hardware manufacturers. These devices are very quickly becoming smaller, more mobile, and more powerful. The current medical handhelds are the first ones that physicians have begun to endorse as compatible with care-delivery workflow. The speed and size of the newest machines, coupled with improvements in the speed of wireless transmissions, have made them practical for the first time. Simultaneously, the logic and presentation of the user interfaces have improved to the point that most functions performed by the physician can be achieved with one to three clicks or taps of a pointing device. One particularly promising application is the handheld prescription pad. This pad is the missing link in what is otherwise completely electronic prescription-benefit management. The latest devices contain not only the updated drug formularies for all of the major managed care organizations, but also drug-drug interaction algorithms and access to the each patient's claims history.

At the time of this writing, one behavioral health software company has announced the integration of a handheld device into its product suite. The application downloads appointments, a to-do list, client records, assessment forms, and treatment-plan information directly to clinicians with handheld devices. Clinicians can then record new appointments, completed forms, client-record updates, and progress notes. The forms are definable by the client organization. The application uses a Palm Pilot, so the usefulness is somewhat constrained by the small screen size, but all of the standard Palm entry methods are available, including graffiti, shortcuts, and the virtual keyboard. The Palm Pilots can be shared by several clinicians through the use of separate security codes.

Although this initial behavioral health software application is focused on clinicians and practice management, several of the functions described above could also be useful for MBHOs. Additions specific to managed care are easy to imagine—for example, the transmittal of authorizations directly to clinicians who have handhelds. As of this writing, however, no MBHO-specific software is commercially available for handheld devices.

Within the next 10 years, several of the technology trends described in this section will converge to create much more useful handheld devices. The combination of wireless technology, voice-recognition software, and handheld computing devices will combine to create a device that is useful, easy to operate, and not an intrusion in the therapy process.

Securing the Privacy of Patient Data
and Safeguarding Data Privacy

Consumers and their treatment providers share a common perception that their control over confidential patient information is compromised severely due to managed care relationships. Because of this heightened sensitivity to data privacy, most consumers and providers have given a cold reception to computerized patient records and to the electronic communication of patient information. Consumer and (particularly) provider reluctance remains a major obstacle to moving ahead with increased adoption of information systems technologies and electronic communication between providers and managed care.

Several major efforts are under way to develop and promote standards for electronic storage and exchange of patient information. Some of the best-known national efforts include those by the Institute of Medicine (Donaldson & Lohr, 1994), the Computer-Based Patient Record Institute, and the American Health Information Management Association. Standards specific to behavioral health lag behind, but efforts to develop such standards are under way through the American Psychiatric Association, American Psychological Association, and Workgroup for the Computerization of Behavioral Health and Human Services.

The most influential new standards are likely to come from the public sector. The U.S. Department of Health and Human Services has been spearheading an effort through the Committee for Vital and Health Statistics—an effort that is now, after several years, nearing completion. In addition, the new administrative regulations formulated under HIPAA will address confidentiality and data-privacy concerns in relation to the electronic transmission of patient data within a managed care environment. The regulations will try to balance the protection of data privacy against the need for rapid transmission and easy sharing of appropriate and necessary clinical information. One likely new regulation will require that a record be made of all persons who accessed a consumer's record, along with the date and reason. This record will be available to consumers and will thereby institute a greater degree of accountability for patient-record access by persons other than the treating provider.

Another government-driven initiative in this area is that of the U.S. Center for Mental Health Services: the project on "Analyses for

Improve Information in Managed Care" (Abt Associates, in press). This project, spanning several years of work with many national experts, proposes the data elements and electronic-interchange policies for a complete managed care information system that satisfies all functional requirements. The project also proposes how the data produced through this information system should and should not be shared.

The electronic storage of confidential client information and the use of the Internet have raised many new concerns regarding the security of behavioral health information (Gellman & Frawley, 1997). These developments do, to be sure, introduce new areas of security risk, but many security issues are present regardless of the means of storage and transmission, and apply equally to paper-based record systems (Barrows, Tracy, & Wald, 1996). All of these concerns, taken together, create the need to take appropriate steps to protect behavioral health data.

Security Procedures

Formal, well-documented administrative procedures must be in place to protect and manage confidential data. These procedures should include specific policies regarding the oversight of staff, access to information, appropriate use of confidential information, sanctions and termination procedures, security training, and contingency plans.

Physical Access

Measures to physically safeguard the data should be in place. These measures should protect the data and facilities from both physical intrusion and from natural or other disasters that may potentially damage or destroy data. Examples of such measures include secured access to the computer and to medical-record facilities, and backup procedures to insure that data can be recovered in an emergency.

Electronic-Transmission Security

Transmission-security measures need to be established to prevent unauthorized access to data as they are transmitted over a communications network. These measures include firewalls and proxy servers, digital signatures, encryption, public/private keys, virtual private networks, and VAN Internet solutions. The last uses the same tools and protocols as the Internet, but on a network that is not the public Internet and is therefore more protected from unauthorized access. Security solutions for data transmission are improving rapidly. The best solutions will include a combination of these various techniques to assure both the integrity of the data and their security. MBHOs have been especially sensitive to security issues because of the confidential nature of the information they are transmitting, and all of the techniques described above have been used in behavioral health. The most common are firewalls, proxy servers, and encryption. Some of the largest MBHOs have access to their own VAN solutions. (One behavioral health firm even attempted, albeit unsuccessfully, to create a nationwide behavioral health VAN for the use of all providers and MBHOs.) MBHOs will not be a leader in this area but will continue to adopt successful strategies developed in the broader health care field.

Passwords and Other Logical Security Measures

Logical security measures are those that are programmed into the software code itself. Such software includes security applications that can group users into various role categories and grant them permission to certain screens or even fields based on their designated role. Since the user must be identified by the system in order for the system to grant the privileges associated with his or her role, passwords (or some other form of identification, such as biometric identification, automatic log-offs, call-back systems, and physical tokens) are necessary for these controls to work. The goal is to permit access to confidential data only for users with the correct authorization on the computer system. These measures should be based on users' positions in the organization and on their need to access the information to perform their jobs. As described above, the system will assign different levels of access to each role type. Consequently, the medical director, for example, might have access to some types of records that a case manager or human resources representative might not have.

In order to protect sensitive information and systems, each organization should implement all four of the above types of security measures. If any of the four is missing, the opportunity for security problems is greatly increased. Again, although some of these measures are specific to electronic systems, many are not. Little is gained if an organization goes to the trouble and expense to encrypt data for transmission over the Internet, but leaves the printed records in an unlocked room where any of the organization's employees might access them.

COLLABORATION

MBHOs will have to depend upon providers and consumers to supply a substantial amount of the data that they need to meet increasing reporting requirements, and will have to develop user-friendly means of collecting the data: the process of data gathering must appear clinically useful and administratively feasible to both consumers and providers. MBHOs will also have to depend upon other organizations (for example, managed general health care organizations, child welfare organizations, criminal justice agencies, and so on) in order to obtain data on their covered members who may have used services in these other organizations. To some extent, this data sharing will be facilitated through purchaser requirements and through clearer state and federal regulations regarding data privacy and data exchange. Good will and a spirit of collaboration will be essential, however, to enable this data exchange to proceed efficiently.

In the somewhat longer term, behavioral health information from providers' practice-management information systems and from MBHOs' information systems will be linked to each other electronically and, in a more automated fashion, directly to the therapy process. Eventually, symptoms, treatment plans, outcomes, and other measures captured electronically during the therapy process will be matched in real time to the treatment guidelines and benefits covered in the patient's benefit plan. Both therapist and patient will know more readily the extent to which insurance will cover the course of treatment as it is being planned and delivered. Similarly, outcome information collected using standardized measures can be compared to normative information in order to determine the effectiveness of the intervention and to compare the patient's progress to others with similar symptoms. In this scenario, information technology will provide the therapist with direct assistance in the therapeutic process, while at the same time handling most of the time-consuming administrative tasks inherent in managed care. Patients will benefit through enhanced quality of care and through faster communication between caregivers and third-party payers.

MBHOs will benefit greatly from electronic communication with their clinical providers through greater efficiencies and reduced costs. The quality and timeliness of MBHOs' communications with providers will also improve, thus enabling MBHOs to influence more quickly the direction of care and with it, the quality of care itself. For this dramatic transition to occur, however, there must be a sufficiently large provider adoption of these various new technologies. Provider reluctance to go in this direction must be overcome with workable incentives, such as: giving providers the necessary software, downloadable through the Internet; working with other MBHOs to standardize forms, or at least the content within forms, to address providers' concerns about the growing set of data elements they must collect; and working with staff and providers to train them in the use of computers, the Internet, and data-collection methods.

Public interest in improved knowledge regarding the capacity, efficiency, and effectiveness of treatment and of system interventions has created yet another reason for collaboration. MBHOs are receiving increased requests for data from many stakeholders. It is essential that MBHOs work with government agencies, professional and trade associations, accreditation organizations, and consumer groups to develop common standards for performance and outcome measurements, practice guidelines, data structures and terminology, the structure of forms and the associated data elements, and electronic information exchange.

Managed behavioral health care has influenced the shape of organized care systems throughout the country. It has accomplished this feat through the leadership of visionary, entrepreneurial, and independent-minded people, and through the extensive use of computer-based technologies. The next steps appear to be ones that will take technology applications even further but that will require the collaboration of MBHOs, providers, consumers, standards-setting organizations, accreditors, regulators, and public and private sector purchasers. The goals are within reach, and MBHOs are in a position to lead the way.

REFERENCES

Abt Associates. (in press). *Analyses for improved information in managed care* (conducted under Center for Mental Health Services grant No. CMHS-DSC-280-97-8009).

American Managed Behavioral Healthcare Association. (1998). *Performance measures for managed behavioral healthcare programs (PERMS 2.0)*. Washington, DC: Author.

American College of Mental Health Administration. (1997). *Preserving quality and value in the managed care equation*. Pittsburgh, PA: Author.

Anderson, S., & Van Eik, G. (1999). Recruitment: Is anyone out there? *Behavioral Healthcare Tomorrow, 8* (1), 47–49.

Barrows, R., Tracy, N., & Wald, J. (1996). Privacy protection: Paper or computers? *Behavioral Healthcare Tomorrow, 5* (1), 38–44.

Brown, G.S., & Kornmayer, K. (1996). Expert systems restructure managed care practices: Implementation and ethics. *Behavioral Healthcare Tomorrow, 5* (1), 31–34.

Coke, J. (1996). Integrating behavioral and medical/surgical data. *Behavioral Healthcare Tomorrow, 5* (5), 73–76.

Docherty, J. (1996). Disease management strategy: Initiative links pharmaceutical and mental health data. *Behavioral Healthcare Tomorrow, 5* (1), 51–53.

Donaldson, M., & Lohr, K. (Eds.). (1994). *Health data in the information age: Use, disclosure, and privacy*. Washington, DC: National Academy Press (Institute of Medicine).

Gellman, R., & Frawley, K. (1997). The need to know versus the right to privacy. In T. Trabin (Ed.), *The computerization of behavioral healthcare: How to enhance clinical practice, management and communications* (pp. 191–212). San Francisco: Jossey-Bass.

Goldman, W., Sturm, R., & McCulloch, J. (1997, September). *New research alliances in the era of managed care*. Paper presented at the National Institute of Mental Health Conference on Improving the Condition of People with Mental Illness: The Role of Services Research.

Guptill, B., Stewart, B., Marcoccio, L., Potter, K., & Claps, C. (1999, April). *GartnerGroup strategic analysis report: 1998 IT spending and staffing survey results*. Lowell, MA: GartnerGroup.

HayGroup. (1999, April). *Health care plan design and cost trends–1988–1998*. Washington, DC: National Association of Psychiatric Health Systems and the Association of Behavioral Group Practices.

Joint Commission on Accreditation of Health Care Organizations. (1997). *ORYX: The next evolution in health care*. Oakbrook Terrace, IL: Author.

Kramer, T., Trabin, T., Daniels, A., Theriot, R., Freeman, M.A., & Williams, C. (1997). *Performance indicator measurement in behavioral healthcare: Data capture methods, cost-effectiveness and emerging standards*. Portola Valley, CA: Institute for Behavioral Healthcare.

Maloney, W., & Hill, G. (1997). Computerization in managed behavioral health care companies. In T. Trabin (Ed.), *The computerization of behavioral healthcare: How to enhance clinical practice, management and communications* (pp. 172–190). San Francisco: Jossey-Bass.

Mental Health Statistics Improvement Program Task Force on a Consumer-Oriented Mental Health Report Card. (1996). *The MHSIP consumer-oriented mental health report card.* Rockville, MD: Center for Mental Health Services.

Moran, M. (1998). Managing care with outcome data: New hopes, new responsibilities. *Behavioral Healthcare Tomorrow, 7* (3), 21–24, 40.

National Committee for Quality Assurance. (1997). *1997 Standards for accreditation of managed behavioral healthcare organizations.* Washington, DC: Author.

National Committee for Quality Assurance. (1999). *Health plan employer data and information set (HEDIS) 2000* (Vols. 1 & 2). Washington, DC: Author.

Oehm, M. (1991). Information systems. In S. Feldman (Ed.), *Managed Mental Health Services* (pp. 143–164). Springfield, IL: Charles C Thomas.

Sperry, L., Brill, P., Howard, K., & Grissom, G. (1996). *Treatment outcomes in psychotherapy and psychiatric interventions.* New York: Bruner/Mazel.

Strosahl, K. (1998). Selecting a clinical outcomes system. *Behavioral Healthcare Tomorrow, 8* (3), 48–51.

Trabin, T., & Maloney, W. (1999). Structured interviews with IS executives regarding IS trends and challenges in their managed care organizations: Homer Chin, M.D., Portland Oregon Kaiser Permanente; Chuck Clabots, United Behavioral Health; Robert Esposito, ValueOptions; Elizabeth Ferris, CNR Health; Robert Glas, M.A., Managed Health Network; Catherine Gross, Magellan Health Services; Sidney Hegseth, United Behavioral Health; and Rick Jackson, Integra.

Trabin, T. (1998, June). Industry consolidation and quality of care: Ambivalent partners? *Behavioral Healthcare Tomorrow, 7* (3), 8, 39.

Trabin, T., & Freeman, M. (1995). *Managed behavioral healthcare: History, models, strategic challenges, and future course* (revised and expanded from report for Center for Mental Health Services, U.S. Department of Health and Human Services, 1994). Tiburon, CA: CentraLink Publications.

Waller, A., & Darrah, J. (1996). Legal requirements for computer security: Electronic medical records and data interchange. *Behavioral Healthcare Tomorrow, 5* (3), 45–47.

Workgroup for the Computerization of Behavioral Health and Human Services, Inc. (1995). *The state of computerization among managed behavioral healthcare companies: A national survey.* Rockville, MD: U.S. Center for Mental Health Services.

Chapter 14

SERVICES RESEARCH

Brian J. Cuffel

Discourse on managed behavioral health care has been character-ized as polarized, confused, and uninformed by empirical research (Feldman, 1999; Mechanic, 1994, 1996). Confusion exists about basic concepts such as what constitutes managed care, and lead-ers of managed behavioral health organizations–even when they attend to existing research–consider much of it irrelevant (Feldman). In the absence of basic information about managed care organizations and their practices, there remain numerous controversies about the intended and unintended consequences of managed care. This uncer-tainty has eroded public trust in health care systems, both medical and behavioral, resulting in unprecedented interest in legislation to regu-late them (Mechanic, 1997). Despite these controversies, managed behavioral health organizations (MBHOs) have sustained consider-able growth over the past 15 years, and 176.8 million Americans (78% of the publicly or privately insured) now receive their behavioral health care through a managed system (Findlay, 1999).

The empirical research literature on managed behavioral health care may best be characterized as a loose collection of a little more than one hundred, largely unrelated studies that have little cumulative value (Feldman, Cuffel, & Hausman, 1999). The studies are so dis-parate in their populations, in the managed care arrangements being examined, and in their research methods that contradictory findings in the literature are easily attributable to these differences. Just as psy-chotherapy researchers in the 1960s produced study after study of the effects of what were, in fact, loosely characterized and poorly measured treatments, researchers in the 1990s have tended to study managed behavioral health systems as if they were singular interventions whose mechanisms are well understood and well isolated. Nothing could be further from reality. To borrow a phrase from a critical crossroads in psychotherapy research, studies are needed to determine "what managed behavioral health care practices, by whom, are most effective for this set of individuals with that set of specific problems, and under which set of circumstances" (adapted from Paul, 1967).

Shortcomings notwithstanding, the empirical literature has grown considerably in the 1990s, with important accomplishments evident in some areas. Initially driven by the interests of public payers, academic researchers, and the availability of funding from public and private research-granting agencies, early research focused on the effects of various managed behavioral health care arrangements on public care systems. The confluence of stakeholder interests in this research resulted in a literature that encompassed the effects of managed behavioral health care on cost, utilization, and treatment outcomes. More recently, as a reflection of growing policy interest in national and state parity legislation, research on privately insured populations has accelerated. Although the resulting literature on the effects of managed behavioral health care in the private sector has been quite sophisticated in its examination of cost and utilization, it has failed to include research on how treatment outcomes are affected by different managed care practices.

This chapter provides an overview of (1) early research on managed behavioral health care involving public sector studies of prospective payment, (2) more recent studies of the effects of MBHOs, (3) new and innovative research on outcomes and quality of care, and (4) the research that remains to be done.

EARLY RESEARCH LITERATURE ON MANAGED BEHAVIORAL HEALTH CARE: PREPAYMENT OF PUBLIC BEHAVIORAL HEALTH CARE

The early research literature equated managed behavioral health care with services that were paid for on a prospective basis. Demonstrations of various forms of prepaid care took place in collaboration with state and local mental health authorities and often involved high cost, severely mentally ill, or Medicaid populations. State and local governments attempted to encourage behavioral health providers to deliver services more cost-effectively by placing providers at financial risk for the services required by these populations.

Early demonstrations of prepaid care were simply labeled "capitation" or "managed care" programs, thereby obscuring important differences and making results difficult to generalize. A widely cited but overly broad definition of "capitation" published in the late 1980s stated that capitated systems pay providers "a fixed price per person served for a defined range of services and for a specified time period" (Mechanic & Aiken, 1989, p. 6). This definition failed to anticipate capitation arrangements with intermediary organizations other than providers, and it confused prospective payment systems that were little more than case rates from those in which providers were paid for enrolled populations on a risk basis. Managed behavioral health care demonstrations in the public sector have involved case rates, capitation rates paid to providers, and capitation rates paid to intermediary organizations such as HMOs or MBHOs.

Demonstrations of Prospective Payments to Providers

Three controlled studies have evaluated the effects of making prospective payments directly to behavioral health providers. Although labeled a "capitation experiment," a study in Rochester, New York, evaluated a group of severely mentally ill individuals randomly assigned to providers, who were paid either a case rate or a fee-for-service rate. Groups were comparable in psychiatric symptoms and global ratings of functioning at two-year follow-up, but the case-rate group experienced fewer hospital days than the fee-for-service group (Cole, Reed, Babigian, Brown, & Fray, 1994). Prospective payment appeared to result in a favorable cost-benefit ratio with no deleterious outcomes (Reed, Hennessy, Mitchell, & Babigian, 1994). Another controlled study in New York found that prospective payment for intensive case management reduced face-to-face contact between case managers and consumers, increased the provision of ancillary services, and reduced the amount of unmet service needs (Shern, Donahue, Felton, Joseph, & Brier, 1995).

In a demonstration program that has received sustained attention in the academic research literature, Utah capitated behavioral health providers in geographic areas serving approximately one-half of the state's Medicaid population. Results through the first two years showed that inpatient mental health admissions and expenditures were significantly reduced in the capitated areas (Christianson et al., 1995; Stoner, Manning, Christianson, Gray, & Marriot, 1997). Providers were not at risk for outpatient expenditures, which were not affected over the two-year study period (Stoner et al.). A recent report suggests that clinical outcomes under the Utah program were poorer for persons with schizophrenia as measured by the Brief Psychiatric Rating Scale and the Global Assessment Scale (Manning et al., 1999).

The limited number of studies of prospective payments made directly to providers prevents firm conclusions. Although studies tended to agree that prospective payment allows public payers to maintain more stable and predictable budgets, studies are mixed regarding the outcomes associated with such financial arrangements.

Demonstrations of Prospective Payments to Intermediaries

Three controlled studies have examined the effects of paying capitated Medicaid dollars to an intermediary MBHO or HMO. In Massachusetts, an MBHO (Value/Options) accepted capitated payments to manage Medicaid mental health and substance abuse services. The MBHO did not subcapitate its providers but used concurrent review, case management, and a provider network to control costs. Because Massachusetts's demonstration program was implemented statewide, evaluation was limited to pre/post comparisons of expenditures and to interviews with administrators, providers, and clients regarding qualitative changes to the system (Beinecke, Shepard, Goodman, & Rivera, 1997; Callahan, Shepard, Beinecke, Larson, & Cavanaugh, 1995; Dickey, Normand, Azeni, Fisher, & Altaffer, 1996; Frank & McGuire, 1997). Medicaid expenditures were lowered by 27% compared to levels expected based on prior trends. Providers reported that access to services was unchanged relative to the precapitation period but that administrative problems related to utilization review increased with the implementation of managed care.

In Hennepin County, Minnesota, severely mentally ill individuals were randomized to either "mainstream" HMOs or fee-for-service

Medicaid. No consistent differences in utilization, symptoms, functioning, and health status were evident in the first seven months of this demonstration program (Christianson, Lurie, Finch, Moscovice, & Hartley, 1992; Lurie, Moscovie, Finch, Christianson, & Popkin, 1992). Unfortunately, the demonstration was terminated in the seventh month when the largest capitated health plan withdrew because of problems with adverse selection of beneficiaries into health care plans. Nevertheless, results suggested that at least short-term outcomes for the severely mentally ill treated in HMO-model care are not different than outcomes in traditional fee-for-service Medicaid systems.

Finally, research on Colorado's Medicaid capitation demonstration is of interest because it compared two forms of prepaid care—direct capitation of behavioral health provider agencies and capitation of an intermediary organization—to fee-for-service care. The cost, utilization, and treatment outcomes of severely mentally ill individuals under each form of prepaid care were evaluated at baseline and followed for a two-year period. Results suggested that both forms of prepaid care were less costly than fee-for-service care, with no evidence that treatment outcomes were compromised. Where outcome differences were observed, they tended to favor the prepaid sectors of Colorado's mental health system (Bloom et al., 1998; Cuffel, Bloom, Wallace, Hu, & Hausman, 1999).

The six controlled studies of managed behavioral health care in the public sector encompass a range of prepaid care and a broad range of clinical and economic outcomes. Results have been relatively consistent in showing savings through large reductions in inpatient expenditures but have been mixed with regard to compromised outcomes or quality of care. Published studies have tended to focus on demonstration programs that have been successfully implemented. Studies of poor implementations have not received much attention in the literature, although research on such demonstrations may have yielded a more negative set of findings (Chang et al., 1998).

STUDIES OF MANAGED BEHAVIORAL
HEALTH CARE IN THE PRIVATE SECTOR

Although the origins of managed behavioral health care are in the private sector—where large, self-insured employers began to require specialized management of mental health and substance abuse benefits–research grew more slowly than in the public sector. In contrast to the coalescence of stakeholder interest in public-sector demonstrations of prepaid care, only recently have research-funding agencies, private payers, consumer groups, and academic researchers turned their attention to the activities of private-sector MBHOs. This emergence of empirical research on managed behavioral health care in the private sector is attributable to several factors, including (1) the development of relationships between MBHOs and academic groups (Goldman, Sturm, & McCulloch, 1999), (2) the maturation of data systems within MBHOs, and (3) the resurgence of national health care policy issues such as national health care reform and mental health parity that made plain the lack of data on managed behavioral health care (Frank & McGuire, 1995). As a result of these forces, early research on privately insured populations has focused almost exclusively on the economics of managed behavioral health care. Significant work has been accomplished on (1) risk sharing in MBHOs, (2) the effects of expanded benefits under managed behavioral health care, and (3) questions related to how MBHOs reduce costs. (In addition, a small group of innovative studies that have examined MBHO practices and their impact on the process and outcomes of care will be discussed in the section after this.)

Studies of Risk Sharing in MBHOs

Analagous to studies of prospective payment in the public sector, four private-sector studies have examined the influence of risk sharing either with either providers or an MBHO. The findings suggest that managed behavioral health care results in dramatic changes in cost and utilization even when financial incentives for MBHOs are relatively weak (Huskamp, 1998; Ma & McGuire, 1998). This phenomenon was most directly examined in a study of Massachusetts state employees: an MBHO reduced behavioral health payments by 30 to 40% after adjusting for trends, an amount that exceeded the direct contractual incentives for the MBHO. Economists Ma and McGuire hypothesized that indirect incentives, such as the MBHO's reputation, may have had a more dramatic impact on performance than the financial incentives written into the contract between the payer and MBHO. As an alternative hypothesis, they noted that managed behavioral health care practices are relatively constant across contracts and thus may be insensitive to differences in financial incentives placed on MBHOs by health care purchasers.

Support for this latter conjecture comes from two sources. First, Sturm (1997a) directly studied the influence of contract incentives and noted that they had a relatively weak effect on behavioral health care utilization in 63 health plans of a large MBHO. Capitation of the MBHO was associated with no significant changes in access rates, cost per user, cost per member, or referral rates to psychiatrists. There was some evidence that capitation lowered the cost per inpatient user although it did not lower the likelihood of an inpatient admission. Second, in a large California-based employer that paid a large MBHO an administrative fee for care-management services rather than being placed at financial risk, access to services increased over a six-year period, inpatient costs declined, and outpatient behavioral health service use remained stable (Goldman, McCulloch, Cuffel, & Kozma, 1999).

The results were strikingly different in the one study that analyzed risk sharing with providers in a privately insured population. The study examined an MBHO responsible for approximately 2 million covered lives in its conversion from a negotiated fee-for-service schedule to a risk-sharing case-rate arrangement with providers. In the pre-case-rate period, the MBHO used a preferred provider network and utilization-management strategies to control costs. After the case rate was introduced, the MBHO dropped utilization management and allowed providers to manage episode length. The result was a 25% reduction in the number of sessions per episode. Provider groups with internal utilization-review procedures showed much greater reductions in episode length than those without such procedures. Provider groups having a lower percentage of their total revenue coming from case rates evidenced smaller reductions in episode length.

Taken together, these four studies suggest that risk sharing may have a larger effect on providers than risk sharing with intermediary organizations such as MBHOs. It is interesting to note that where providers have been given control of utilization-management decisions and have been placed under financial incentives to control costs, their decision making regarding clinical care becomes more fiscally conservative and results in greater rationing of care. None of this research examines, however, the impact that various financial arrangements with MBHOs and providers have on the quality of care and the outcomes associated with that care.

Benefit Studies

An important field of research on MBHOs in the private sector took shape as researchers began to reexamine long-held beliefs about the relationship between behavioral health benefit design and the cost of behavioral health care. Studies conducted by Sturm, Goldman, and colleagues show that generous behavioral health benefits do not appreciably increase the cost of care and do not promote inflationary cost trends in managed behavioral health systems (Goldman, McCulloch, et al., 1999; Sturm, 1997b; Sturm, 1999). In plans covered by an MBHO, the estimated costs of removing annual and lifetime limits were dramatically smaller than the projections by the Congressional Research Service (CRS) and Hay/Huggins, which were largely based on assumptions drawn from pre-managed-care analyses of mental health service use (Sturm, 1997b). The MBHO's removing even low annual limits of $10,000 was estimated to cost approximately $4 per enrollee per year, and removing day and visit limits on inpatient and outpatient care was estimated to raise costs only $7 per enrollee per year. In contrast, the CRS-Hay/Huggins projection was that removing these limits would cost over $100 per enrollee per year. Sturm's findings have been replicated in analyses of 46 benefit plans managed by another MBHO (Peele, Lave, & Xu, 1999).

Ohio's expansion of benefits for state employees provided an opportunity for an empirical test of the effects of parity benefits in a managed behavioral health care setting (Sturm, Goldman, & McCulloch, 1998). Removal of discriminatory dollar, day, and visit limits, coupled with the adoption of managed behavioral health care, was associated with lower rather than higher behavioral health care costs.

Other longitudinal studies suggest that MBHOs have been able to sustain cost savings in the long run for generous employer-sponsored plans (Goldman, McCulloch, et al., 1999). These crucial studies of managed behavioral health care in the private sector have influenced the development both of more generous benefit plans for federal employees and of state parity legislation around the country.

Although these results are encouraging, some critics correctly point out that benefit parity does not assure equitable administration of services, particularly if the MBHO criteria for access to, and use of, services are different from those for other types of medical care (Burnam & Escarce, 1999; Frank & McGuire, 1998; Mechanic & McAlpine, 1999). If managed behavioral health care has simply replaced benefit restrictions with other barriers to care, then the effects of parity will be illusory. Rather than facing benefit limitations, patients may face other kinds of barriers to seeking care, such as those induced by utilization management or by the financial incentives on providers to restrict care. Whether benefit expansion in a managed setting achieves a more equitable system for persons with behavioral health disorders cannot be determined with any certainty from available data because of insufficient research on how MBHOs have achieved cost savings.

Studies on How MBHOs Reduce Costs

The literature on how MBHOs effect change in service delivery is sparse. A literature search identified eight studies in which the introduction of MBHOs was determined to have affected one or more of the following cost components: (1) the probability of using any behavioral health services, (2) the probability of using inpatient care, (3) the probability of using outpatient care, (4) the amount of outpatient care used, (5) the amount of inpatient care used, (6) the cost per inpatient bed day, and (7) the cost per outpatient visit. Findings from the eight studies are summarized in Table 1. Studies were included in the table if they tested the intervention of an MBHO covering a publicly or privately insured population. Studies were excluded if the only intervention they took into account was prepayment of care.

The studies in Table 1 showed spending reductions ranging from 25% to 60%. Other than the studies by Goldman, McCulloch, and Sturm (1998) and Ma and McGuire (1998), researchers have not comprehensively analyzed how savings have been achieved, and these two studies yielded somewhat contradictory findings. Ma and McGuire found that reductions in costs by the MBHO were partly achieved by reducing average outpatient visits and the likelihood of outpatient use. Access to outpatient services declined from 12.3% before managed care was introduced to 9.3% thereafter. In contrast, Goldman and colleagues found that cost reductions were associated with increased

Table 1

SUMMARY OF MANAGED CARE STUDIES

Study	*Cost component*						
	Any use	Any inpatient	Any outpatient	Days per user	Visits per user	Cost per day	Cost per visit
Ma & McGuire, 1998			↓	↓	↓	↓	↓
Goldman et al., 1998	↑	↓	↑	↓	↑	↓	
Goldman, McCulloch et al., 1999	NC			↓	↓		
Sturm, Goldman et al., 1998				↓a	↓a		
Cuffel et al., 1999	↑						
Brisson et al., 1997	NC			↓	↓		
Callahan et al., 1995	NC	↓	↑			↓	
Grazier et al., 1999	↑		↑		↓		

Note: (indicates an increase, and (a decrease, found by the study. NC indicates no change. A blank entry in a cell indicates that the study did not report that cost component.
a Per 1,000.

access to, and use of, outpatient care.

Of the seven studies examining access to care, the Ma and McGuire (1998) study was the only one to find reductions in access to care. Three studies found that managed behavioral health care actually increased the probability of using any behavioral health services. It therefore appears, based on this limited number of studies, that savings from MBHOs are not attributable to reductions in initial access to care.

In terms of amount of inpatient and outpatient care, the studies in Table 1 consistently show reductions in average length of stay for inpatient care but conflict with regard to average outpatient visits per user. Four of five studies found decreases in outpatient visits per user, whereas one study showed steady increases in the six years following implementation of managed behavioral health care (Goldman et al., 1998). A sixth study reported decreases (on a per thousand basis) suggesting either access to outpatient care or length of outpatient treatment had declined (Sturm et al., 1998).

Two studies clearly suggest that MBHOs have been able to negotiate more favorable rates with inpatient providers and that changes in the cost per unit of care have had a significant impact on overall cost savings in these systems. One study found reductions in the average amount paid to outpatient providers per visit–which might derive either from lower negotiated rates with outpatient providers or from the MBHO's use of lower-cost providers.

The literature also contains some research examining another possible mechanism of behavioral health care cost reduction, namely, the shifting of behavioral health care costs to general medical settings. Little research has examined this question in large controlled studies. The only test of cost shifting in the public sector occurred in a study of the effects of Massachusetts's Medicaid Program (Dickey et al., 1995; Dickey, Norton, Normand, Azeni, & Fisher, 1998; Norton, Lindrooth, & Dickey, 1997). Analyses suggested that the use of an MBHO decreased behavioral health care costs in the short run but also led to increases in other components of Medicaid costs, namely, medical and pharmacy costs.

A comparable study of a privately insured population evaluated the effects of Alcan Aluminum's behavioral health carve-out on its spending for general medical care (Cuffel, Goldman, & Schlesinger, 1999). Using data for two years prior to the introduction of the MBHO and three years thereafter, the study examined the use and cost of behavioral health and general medical services. Controlling for prior trends, the probability of any behavioral health service use increased, though total spending for behavioral health services declined on both a per member and per user basis. Total spending for general medical care also declined selectively for behavioral health care users–a pattern not indicative of cost shifting.

Although managed behavioral health care research in the 1990s has clearly established that cost savings have been achieved, it has failed to produce a coherent body of literature explaining how that has happened. Development of research on the "how" rather than the "how much" of managed behavioral health care will require a shift in mind-set for investigators–away from studying the effects brought about by MBHOs, and toward studying the principles and practices of effective care management. Recognition that managed systems of care are likely to be the de facto system of care used in the United States may encourage clinical and policy researchers to take a more differentiated look at what MBHOs do and how they do it.

STUDIES OF QUALITY AND OUTCOMES

Whether and to what extent the savings produced by MBHOs have come at the expense of poorer outcomes and reduced quality of care is not clear. Central questions are whether MBHOs disrupt the normal course of help seeking and result in poor coordination of care; whether they refer patients to the lowest-cost providers; and whether they use the lowest-cost, rather than most cost-effective, treatments. Data are inadequate to draw conclusions about these concerns, but a few innovative studies have provided glimpses by looking more closely at the activities of MBHOs and how they affect the quality and outcomes of care.

One study examined MBHO referral patterns and found that rather than systematically referring to lower-cost providers such as master's-level therapists and social workers, one MBHO increased the rate at which persons with major depression, schizophrenia, and bipolar disorder were seen by psychiatrists. For persons diagnosed with depression, 78% in MBHOs received some psychiatric care for their depression—versus an estimated 29% in HMO settings and 66% in unmanaged settings. Less severe cases within the MBHO, such as those with adjustment disorder and V-code diagnoses, tended to be seen by nonphysician, doctoral, and master's-level providers rather than by psychiatrists (Sturm & Klap, 1998).

Some evidence is emerging that MBHOs improve coordination of care following a hospitalization. Research on Massachusetts's state employee carve-out found that reductions in inpatient admissions and length of stay were accompanied by increases in aftercare follow-up rates, which went from 67% of admissions before the carve-out to 84% following it (Merrick, 1998). Readmission rates remained constant over this same time period (Merrick). Findings in this area are conflicting, however; other research shows that treatment restrictions imposed through managed care have reduced hospital stays but have increased hospital readmission rates (Wickizer & Lessler, 1998).

Other studies have looked at the effect of MBHOs on length of outpatient treatment episodes. Two independent studies (of separate MBHOs) have identified an unintended consequence of the common practice of prior authorization (Howard, 1998; Liu, Sturm, & Cuffel, 2000). In the case of outpatient treatment, prior authorization involves referral to a particular provider for a specified number of sessions, at the end of which the provider can obtain authorization for further treatment by submitting a written or electronic request. In one study, providers contracting with one small MBHO were guaranteed approval for requests for sessions beyond those initially authorized (Howard). Providers were then randomly divided into three groups with prior authorizations of 5, 10, or 19 sessions. Even though approval for ongoing treatment was guaranteed, the modal number of sessions in each group corresponded to the number of sessions initially authorized. Evidence also suggested that master's-level therapists were more likely to terminate treatment at the end of the prior-authorization interval than doctoral-level psychologists.

The influence of the prior-authorization level was replicated in a study of another large MBHO, United Behavioral Health (Liu, Sturm, & Cuffel, 2000). Although ongoing approval was not guaranteed (unlike the study discussed above), the MBHO approves the vast majority of requests for additional outpatient care (Koike, Unutzer, & Klap, 1999). Again, treatment terminations peaked at the end of the prior-authorization interval (Liu et al.).

The data from the two above studies of prior authorization provide little insight into the explanation for the findings. Providers may terminate treatment because they believe that further sessions will not be authorized, because they prefer to avoid the administrative hassles of requesting additional sessions, or because they seek to gain favor from an important referral source. Whatever the ultimate reason, findings regarding the unintended effects of prior authorization suggest that the managed behavioral health care practices introduce complex dynamics into decision making by providers and perhaps also by patients.

The complexity of patient-provider-MBHO interactions is underscored by a recent survey of reasons for terminating outpatient treatment episodes in a large MBHO (Cuffel, McCulloch, et al., 2000). The survey involved pairs of providers and patients (n = 190) recently completing outpatient treatment in a large MBHO. Across most reasons for termination, patients and providers showed little agreement. Agreement was high, however, when the reason for termination was "the MBHO denied care because of lack of medical necessity" (kappa = .48). Of these cases, only 1 of the 10 providers had even submitted a request for additional sessions (and received a denial). In the remainder of the cases, no request for ongoing treatment had even been submitted. An interesting twist is that patient-rated satisfaction with therapy and the therapist was significantly higher when the reason for termination was denial by the MBHO than when treatment terminated for any other reason. What providers understand about the utilization-review process of MBHOs and what they communicate to patients about the termination of treatment under managed behavioral health care is an important area of future research.

More comprehensive schemes for evaluating the quality of care are under development and have received some attention in the literature. One method, which arose from Oregon's conversion from fee-for-service to prepaid behavioral health care for its Medicaid beneficiaries, focuses on detecting underutilization on a population basis (McFarland et al., 1998). As part of the conversion, "service packages" were developed by expert panels of clinicians in order to estimate the cost of treating people with different disorders. These service packages cover 55 behavioral disorders of adults and children, and address the service needs for typical, outlying, and extreme-outlying patients. McFarland used the service packages to develop expectations about the amount of service to be delivered on a population basis. Measures included the number of outpatient visits per year, the proportion of the population that would require more than outpatient treatment, and the average length of inpatient stay (McFarland et al.).

The method was piloted in Oregon both in an HMO and in a large MBHO (United Behavioral Health) for attention deficit hyperactivity disorder (ADHD) and major depression, respectively. Analyses showed a close correspondence between the expected and observed utilization patterns for ADHD within the HMO on percentage of patients receiving outpatient treatment, the amount of outpatient treatment, and the percentage of cases receiving some inpatient treatment. HMO utilization was somewhat lower than expected on percentage of persons receiving day treatment. Utilization rates for major depression in the MBHO also showed a close correspondence with the guidelines in all areas (McFarland et al., 1998).

McFarland and colleagues' (1998) proposed method for detecting underutilization, as described above, appears to hold great promise for evaluating MBHOs in that it (1) integrates diagnosis-specific clinical standards derived from expert opinion in the detection of underutilization, (2) provides empirical benchmarks for detecting underutilization, and (3) is low cost and relies upon readily available data within MBHOs. The potential that these population guidelines have for detecting underutilization has apparently not been recognized by agencies attempting to monitor MBHOs.

Other methodological approaches with potential for measuring the performance of MBHOs have been proposed by Frank and colleagues, who define a measure they refer to as "system cost-effectiveness" (Frank, McGuire, Normand, Sharon-Lise, & Goldman, 1999). The measure is a ratio of costs and outcomes, and integrates data on effectiveness of different treatment modalities with data on how behavioral health systems distribute patients to these modalities. Such system cost-effectiveness measures would allow policymakers, health care purchasers, and system administrators to examine the value of the health care dollar in an MBHO or in any other system. Using data on the effectiveness of psychotherapy and medication management in the treatment of depression, Frank calculated system cost-effectiveness over a six-year period (1991–96) in a national database of privately insured individuals, and found generally increasing system cost-effectiveness. Results suggested that systems were improving the extent to which patients received the most cost-effective treatments for depression. It is interesting to note that the lowest-cost treatment modalities were associated with the worst system cost-effectiveness.

More common but lacking in empirical research are "performance measurement" schemes that have been proposed by various private organizations, including the National Committee for Quality Assurance, the Foundation for Accountability, and the American Managed Behavioral Health Association (Merrick et al., 1999). These performance-measurement systems have included relatively few indicators specific to mental health and substance abuse services, and have not generated research on the validity of their behavioral health indicators. Surveys suggest that employers do not attend to these indicators in selecting among managed care health plans (Hibbard, Jewett, Legnini, & Tusler, 1999).

WHAT REMAINS TO BE DONE

Research has not yet accumulated on important questions raised by the wide array of interventions and strategies employed by MBHOs. Existing research has served to confirm easily observable and large-scale changes that had been noted long before the published studies in the 1990s (England & Vaccaro, 1991). At present, the research literature is so sparse and so poorly understood that any changes observed in behavioral health spending are attributed to "managed care," with little attention to the forces operating within and outside MBHOs that contribute to those changes (Leslie & Rosenheck, 1999). Improving our knowledge of managed behavioral health care will require research tied to better conceptual models of how financial, organizational, and administrative aspects of managed behavioral health systems interact with the behavioral health needs of populations to affect societal costs and benefits.

Ideally, future research will examine a number of topics that are only now beginning to receive attention in the literature. There is an overwhelming need for research that relates managed behavioral health care practices to the type of treatment that is delivered and to the outcomes that are achieved by providers. Outcome data is relatively scarce for public care systems and virtually nonexistent for private systems. No studies have examined whether managed behavioral health interventions can increase the use of "best practices"–even though MBHOs are in a pivotal position to affect the nature of care that is delivered (just as they have affected its cost). Linking managed care practices to outcomes will involve learning a great deal more about the internal workings of MBHOs, including their utilization-management techniques, intake and referral processes, methods of paying providers, and methods of developing and maintaining their provider networks.

Additional research needs to expand our understanding of the effects of care management on how people function at work and, more generally, contribute to society. Behavioral health advocates argue that large-scale changes in access, amount, or quality of behavioral health care has implications for a host of workplace costs and benefits. At least one large-scale study supports this notion (Rosenheck, Druss, Stolar, Leslie, & Sledge, 1999). The next generation of research will need to move beyond studies focused narrowly on behavioral health care cost and utilization.

Finally, managed behavioral health care will need to understand the effects of managed care practices on different subpopulations. Unknown are the managed behavioral health arrangements that are best suited to various special populations such as women, minorities, and disabled workers.

The next generation of managed behavioral health research cannot proceed by having researchers and managed behavioral health organizations working at a distance. At present, university-based researchers may lack sufficient opportunity to learn about the internal workings of MBHOs and about how MBHOs influence the delivery of behavioral health care. Saul Feldman, CEO of United Behavioral Health, has written about the factors that contribute to stasis in the development of research in managed behavioral health care, and has organized a series of meetings devoted to promoting a research agenda for the industry (Feldman, 1999). Clearly, the next generation of research on managed behavioral health care will be more difficult and will depend on the development of complex relationships among stakeholders in the behavioral health system, on the willingness of MBHOs to share data with outside parties, and on the willingness of MBHOs to examine and measure what they do and to share this information with the outside world. The success of this research effort will depend upon the degree to which funding becomes available for collaborative research with MBHOs and also upon the degree to which the "market" for MBHOs rewards organizational cultures that foster self-study.

As research evolves from its current state to more complex analyses of how organized-care systems can promote access to high quality, cost-effective behavioral health care, the field will learn much about the general principles of effective care management. Given that it is unlikely that one of these principles will be to "not manage care," research in the next decade will link specific activities of MBHOs with specific economic and clinical outcomes. Understanding these linkages will have several kinds of benefits for the field. Findings considered conflictual or ambiguous in the 1990s will be clarified, which will lead to a better understanding of the system, population, and MBHO differences that contributed to such findings. And as more credible data become available, discourse on managed behavioral health care will become grounded in an evolving empirical base. Such research should place a premium on the quality of behavioral health care and broaden our myopic focus on the cost of care. Perhaps most importantly, the organizations responsible for managing behavioral health care can begin to ground their practices in an empirical base relating managed care activities and interventions to their effects on clinical practice and outcomes.

REFERENCES

Beinecke, R. H., Shepard, D. S., Goodman, M., & Rivera, M. (1997). Assessment of the Massachusetts Medicaid managed behavioral health program: Year three. *Administration and Policy in Mental Health, 24,* 205–220.

Bloom, J. R., Hu, T., Wallace, N., Cuffel, B., Hausman, J., & Scheffler, R. (1998). Mental health costs and outcomes under alternative capitation systems in Colorado: Early results. *Journal of Mental Health Policy and Economics, 1* (1), 3–13.

Brisson, A. E., Frank, R. G., Notman, E. S., & Gazmararian, J. A. (1997). Impact of a managed behavioral health care carve-out: A case study of one HMO (NBER working paper). Cambridge, MA: National Bureau of Economic Research.

Burnam, M. A., & Escarce, J. J. (1999). Equity in managed care for mental disorders. *Health Affairs, 18* (5), 22–31.

Callahan, J. J., Shepard, D. S., Beinecke, R. H., Larson, M. J., & Cavanaugh, D. (1995). Mental health/substance abuse treatment in managed care: The Massachusetts Medicaid experience. *Health Affairs, 14* (3), 173–184.

Chang, C. F., Kiser, L. J., Bailey, J. E., Martins, M., Gibson, W.C., Schaberg, K. A., Mirvis, D. M., & Applegate, W. B. (1998). Tennessee's failed managed care program for mental health and substance abuse services. *Journal of the American Medical Association, 279,* 864–869.

Christianson, J. B., Lurie, N., Finch, M., Moscovice, I. S., & Hartley, D. (1992). Use of community-based mental health programs by HMOs: Evidence from a Medicaid demonstration. *American Journal of Public Health, 82,* 790–796.

Christianson, J. B., Manning, W., Lurie, N., Stoner, T. J., Gray, D. Z., Popkin, M., & Marriot, S. (1995). Utah's prepaid mental health plan: The first year. *Health Affairs, 14* (3), 161–172.

Cole, R. E., Reed, S. K., Babigian, H. M., Brown, S. W., & Fray, J. (1994). A mental health capitation program: I. Patient outcomes. *Hospital and Community Psychiatry, 45,* 1090–1096.

Cuffel, B. J., Goldman, W., & Schlesinger, H. (1999). Does managing behavioral health care services increase the cost of providing medical care? *Journal of Behavioral Health Services & Research, 26,* 371–379.

Cuffel, B., McCulloch, J., Wade, R., Tam, L., Brown-Mitchell, R., & Goldman, W. (2000). Patient and provider perceptions of outpatient treatment termination in a managed behavioral health organization. *Psychiatric Services, 51* (4), 469–473.

Cuffel, B. J., Bloom, J. R., Wallace, N., Hu, T., & Hausman, J. A. (2000). Two-year outcomes of fee-for-service and capitated Medicaid programs for the severely mentally ill. *Health Services Research, 37,* 341–359.

Dickey, B., Normand, S. T., Azeni, H., Fisher, W. H., & Altaffer, F. (1996). Managing the care of schizophrenia: Lessons from a 4-year Massachusetts Medicaid study. *Archives of General Psychiatry, 53,* 945–952.

Dickey, B., Norton, E. C., Normand, S. L., Azeni, H., Fisher, W., & Altaffer, F. (1995). Massachusetts Medicaid managed health care reform: Treatment for the psychiatrically disabled. *Advances in Health Economics and Health Services Research, 15,* 99–116.

Dickey, B., Norton, E. C., Normand, S. T., Azeni, H., & Fisher, W. H. (1998). Managed mental health experience in Massachusetts. *New Directions for Mental Health Services, 78,* 115–124.

England, M. J., & Vaccaro, V. A. (1991). New systems to manage mental health care. *Health Affairs, 10* (4), 129–137.

Feldman, S. (1999). Strangers in the night: Research and managed mental health care. *Health Affairs, 18* (5), 48–51.

Feldman, S., Cuffel, B., & Hausman, J. (1999). Managed behavioral health services: A bibliography of empirical studies, articles of interest, and books. *Administration and Policy in Mental Health, 27* (1/2), 5–88.

Findlay, S. (1999). Managed behavioral health care in 1999: An industry at a crossroads. *Health Affairs, 18* (5), 116–124.

Frank, R. G., & McGuire, T. G. (1995). Estimating costs of mental health and substance abuse coverage. *Health Affairs, 14* (3), 102–115.

Frank, R. G., & McGuire, T. G. (1997). Savings from a Medicaid carve-out for mental health and substance abuse services in Massachusetts. *Psychiatric Services, 48,* 1147–1152.

Frank, R. G., & McGuire, T. G. (1998). Parity for mental health and substance abuse care under managed care. *The Journal of Mental Health Policy and Economics, 1,* 153–159.

Frank, R. G., McGuire, T. G., Normand, S. T., & Goldman, H. H. (1999). The value of mental health care at the system level: *The case of treating depression. Health Affairs, 18* (5), 71–88.

Goldman, W., McCulloch, J., Cuffel, B. J., & Kozma, D. (1999). More evidence for the insurability of managed behavioral health care. *Health Affairs, 18* (5), 172–181.

Goldman, W., McCulloch, J., & Sturm, R. (1998). Costs and use of mental health services before and after managed care. *Health Affairs, 17* (2), 40–52.

Goldman, W., Sturm, R., & McCulloch, J. (1999). New research alliances in the era of managed care. *Journal of Mental Health Policy and Economics, 2,* 107–110.

Grazier, K. L., Eselius, L. L., Hu, T., Shore, K. K., G'Sell, W. A. (1999). Effects of a mental health carve-out on use, costs, and payers: A four-year study. *Journal of Behavioral Health Services & Research, 26,* 381–389.

Hibbard, J. H., Jewett, J. J., Legnini, M. W., & Tusler, M. (1999). Choosing a health plan: Do large employers use the data? *Health Affairs, 16* (6), 172–180.

Howard, R. C. (1998). The sentinel effect in an outpatient managed care setting. *Professional Psychology: Research & Practice, 29,* 262–268.

Huskamp, H. A. (1998). How a managed behavioral health care carve-out plan affected spending for episodes of treatment. *Psychiatric Services, 49,* 1559–1562.

Koike, A., Unutzer, J., & Klap, R. (1999). Utilization management in a large managed behavioral health organization (RAND Working Paper No. 165).

Leslie, D. L., & Rosenheck, R. (1999). Shifting to outpatient care? Mental health care use and cost under private insurance. *American Journal of Psychiatry, 156,* 1250–1257.

Liu, X., Sturm, R., & Cuffel, B. J. (2000). The impact of prior authorization on out-patient utilization in managed behavioral health plans. *Medical Care Research and Review, 57,* 182–195.

Lurie, N., Moscovie, I. S., Finch, M., Christianson, J. B., & Popkin, M. K. (1992). Does capitation affect the health of the chronically mentally ill? *Journal of the American Medical Association, 267,* 3300–3304.

Ma, C. A., & McGuire, T. G. (1998). Costs and incentives in a behavioral health carve-out. *Health Affairs, 17* (2), 53–69.

Manning, W. G., Liu, C. F., Stoner, T. J., Gray, D. Z., Lurie, N., Popkin, M., & Christianson, J. B. (1999). Outcomes for Medicaid beneficiaries with schizophrenia under a prepaid mental health carve-out. *The Journal of Behavioral Health Services & Research, 26,* 442–450.

McFarland, B. H., George, R. A., Goldman, W., Pollack, D. A., McCulloch, J., Penner, S., & Angell, R. H. (1998). Population-based guidelines for performance measurement: A preliminary report. *Harvard Review of Psychiatry, 6,* 23–37.

Mechanic, D. (1994). Managed care: Rhetoric and realities. *Inquiry, 31,* 124–128.

Mechanic, D. (1996). Can research on managed care inform practice and policy decisions? In A. Lazarus (Ed.), *Controversies in managed mental health care* (pp. 197–211). Washington, DC: American Psychiatric Press.

Mechanic, D. (1997). Managed care as a target of distrust. *Journal of the American Medical Association, 277,* 1810–1811.

Mechanic, D., & Aiken, L. H. (1989). Capitation in mental health: Potentials and cautions. In D. Mechanic & L. H. Aiken (Eds.), *Paying for services: Promises and pitfalls of capitation* (pp. 5–18). San Francisco: Jossey-Bass.

Mechanic, D., & McAlpine, D. (1999). Mission unfulfilled: Potholes on the road to mental health parity. *Health Affairs, 18* (5), 7–21.

Merrick, E. L. (1998). Treatment of major depression before and after implementation of a behavioral health carve-out plan. *Psychiatric Services, 49,* 1563–1567.

Merrick, E. L., Garnick, D., Horgan, C. M., Goldin, D., Hodgkin, D., & Sciegaj, M. (1999). Use of performance standards in behavioral health carve-out contracts among Fortune 500 firms. *American Journal of Managed Care, 5,* SP81–SP90.

Norton, E. C., Lindrooth, R. C., & Dickey, B. (1997). Cost shifting in a mental health carve-out for the AFDC population. *Health Care Financing Review, 18,* 95–108.

Paul, G. L. (1967). Strategy of outcome therapy in psychotherapy. *Journal of Consultative Psychology, 31,* 109–118.

Peele, P. B., Lave, J. R., & Xu, Y. (1999). Benefit limits in managed behavioral healthcare: Do they matter? *Journal of Behavioral Health Services & Research, 26,* 430–441.

Reed, S. K., Hennessy, K. D., Mitchell, O. S., & Babigian, H. M. (1994). A mental health capitation program: II. Cost-benefit analysis. *Hospital and Community Psychiatry, 45,* 1097–1103.

Rosenheck, R., Druss, B., Stolar, M., Leslie, D., & Sledge, W. H. (1999). Effect of declining mental health service use on employees of a large corporation. *Health Affairs, 18* (5), 193–203.

Shern, D. L., Donahue, S. A., Felton, C., Joseph, G. R., & Brier, N. (1995). Partial capitation versus fee-for-service in mental health care. *Health Affairs, 14* (3), 208–219.

Stoner, T. J., Manning, W., Christianson, J., Gray, D. Z., & Marriot, S. (1997). Expenditures for mental health services in the Utah prepaid mental health plan. *Health Care Financing Review, 18,* 73–93.

Sturm, R. (1997a). How does risk sharing between employers and managed behavioral health organizations affect mental health care? (RAND Working Paper No. 113).

Sturm, R. (1997b). How expensive is unlimited mental health care coverage under managed care? *Journal of the American Medical Association, 278,* 1533–1537.

Sturm, R. (1999). Cost and quality trends under managed care: Is there a learning curve in behavioral health carve-out plans? *Journal of Health Economics, 18,* 593–604.

Sturm, R., Goldman, W., & McCulloch, J. (1998). Mental health and substance abuse parity: A case study of Ohio's state employees program. *The Journal of Mental Health and Economics, 1,* 129–134.

Sturm, R., & Klap, R. (1998). Use of psychiatrists, psychologists and master's-level therapists in managed behavioral health care carve-out plans. *Psychiatric Services, 50,* 504–508.

Wickizer, T., & Lessler, D. (1998). Do treatment restrictions imposed by utilization management increase the likelihood of readmission for psychiatric patients? *Medical Care, 36,* 844–850.

Chapter 15

EMPLOYEE ASSISTANCE PROGRAMS

Tamara Cagney

Managed care has had a major effect on the definition, design, and delivery of employee assistance programs (EAPs). Historically, EAPs were employer based and known as internal EAPs. The last 20 years has seen a rapid increase in EAP services provided by external firms under contract with employers, frequently as part of managed behavioral health organizations (MBHOs). There are now over 60 million people with EAP benefits covered by MBHOs. This increase–130% since 1994 (EAP Digest, 2000)–is a manifestation of how dramatically the EAP field has changed.

EAPs were originally focused on alcohol and drug problems in the workplace, and were staffed by employees who had themselves struggled with these issues. Later, in the 1970s, EAPs became more comprehensive, offering help with a wide variety of mental health and emotional issues. These programs came to be staffed by individuals with professional clinical training such as social workers, family therapists, and psychologists. In the 1980s a core technology was delineated, which helped define the field. The Employee Assistance Professional Association (EAPA) defined EAPs as follows:

> EAP is a work-site-based program designed to assist: (1) work organizations in addressing productivity issues, and (2) employee clients in identifying and resolving personal concerns including, but not limited to, health, marital, family, financial, alcohol, drug, legal, emotional, stress, or other personal issues that may affect job performance. (Employee Assistance Professional Association, 1997)

As delineated by EAPA, the core technology spells out the components that create a unique approach to addressing work/organization productivity issues and personal issues that affect employees' job performance. EAP core technology includes:

1. Consultation with, training of, and assistance to work organization leadership (managers, supervisors, and union stewards) seeking to manage the troubled employee, enhance the work environment, and improve employee job performance; and, outreach to and education of employees and their family members about the availability of EAP services;
2. Confidential and timely problem identification/assessment services for employee clients with personal concerns that may affect job performance;
3. Use of constructive confrontation, motivation, and short-term intervention with employee clients to address problems that affect job performance;
4. Referral of employee clients for diagnosis, treatment, and assistance, plus case monitoring and follow-up services;
5. Consultation to work organizations in establishing and maintaining effective relations with treatment and other service providers, and in managing provider contracts;
6. Consultation to work organizations to encourage availability of and employee access to health benefits covering medical and behavioral problems, including but not limited to, alcoholism, drug abuse and mental and emotional disorders; and
7. Identification of the effects of EAP services on the work organization and individual job performance. (Employee Assistance Professional Association, 1997)

EAP client target groups include both (1) employees who are aware of personal difficulties that may be affecting, or may start to affect, their work lives, and (2) employees whose performance shows a pattern of decline that is not readily explained by supervisory observation of their job circumstances.

This focus on performance problems and early identification allows the EAP to intervene at an early stage and to deal with non–DSM IV Axis I diagnoses. Approximately 80% of employees receive the assistance that they need at this level and do not go on to access their health insurance. Throughout the early developmental years of EAPs, the employee assistance (EA) professional's relationship with benefit providers and insurance providers was distant, at best. The EA professional was often struggling with limited chemical-dependency treatment benefits, level-of-care limitations, and access barriers. Insurers and employee-benefits staff had little understanding of EAPs and, in some cases, saw them as a substitute for behavioral health insurance benefits (Cagney, 1999).

The EAP approach to case finding (that is, problem identification) and early intervention differs from the focus of traditional insurers. EAPs work to develop proactive case finding. High utilization is seen as a positive. This approach continued to dominate EAPs at the same time that the insurance industry came to be focused on lower utilization and lower costs. EAPs encourage intervention at early stages when a disorder may be a "V Code" and not qualify as a clinical or DSM IV diagnosis covered by insurance. EAPs use constructive confrontation to motivate employees–ones having little insight or external motivation to address their problems–to seek treatment for chemical dependency. Since these employees tend to minimize their symptoms, they often do not meet traditional criteria of medical necessity (Cagney, 1999).

Into this atmosphere of poor communication and divergent goals came managed care and a reorganization of the behavioral health care benefit. Some MBHOs saw EAPs as duplicative, as not performing any function that their panel of clinicians could not provide. Some did not share the EAP focus on aggressive case finding and early intervention. In the 1990s there were people in MBHOs who predicted the demise of EAPs and only reluctantly offered EAP services. In many cases the fit between managed care organizations and EAPs was awkward, at best.

EAPS AND THE EMERGENCE OF MBHOS

MBHOs brought with them new organizational patterns of care and a changing scenario of economic incentives. Major payers were looking to the MBHO to contain health care costs that had risen at an alarming level over the previous two decades. Close to $200 billion of the total health care bill could be attributed to chemical dependency, and in the late 1980s, 75% of that amount could be attributed to inpatient treatment (Mark, 2000).

The initial response to contain costs by a number of insurers and self-insured employers was to form access barriers–for example, by increased copayments and deductibles, and by placing restrictions on benefits. Utilization management was implemented, including criteria for admission and level of care. EAP referrals were channeled into these new designs. The focus shifted to medical necessity and to the lowest appropriate intensity and level of care.

This one egg, one basket approach led to an erosion of EAPs' traditional services. Managed behavioral health care brought about significant cost savings; EAPs, seen more as a "soft" service and undistinguished in providing cost savings to customers, began to assume an inferior position, viewed by some as a loss leader.

Case finding, a major focus of EAPs, became more of a secondary process as treatment of substance abuse and mental health disorders became primary. Less attention was paid to early intervention and workplace support, since their only demonstration of "success" was anecdotal. Some MBHOs decreased their number of EAP-focused activities and began downsizing their EAP programming. Ancillary services, formerly under the umbrella of the EAP, were segregated—for example, dependent care and financial and legal services.

In an attempt to be more competitive, some MBHOs subscribed to the same or similar speed-to-answer and telephone-abandonment rates as their health plan counterparts. EAP phone counselors were therefore held to similar standards as in health care, where the primary job was exclusively to assess and determine medical necessity. Experienced EAP frontline staff, accustomed to comprehensively dealing with presenting problems through additional inquiries about the caller's ecosystem, felt pressed to take more and more calls, and to omit nonclinical questions. Already plagued by competing demands for time and attention, many frontline EAP counselors left managed care altogether or switched to MBHOs that were more compatible with what the counselors perceived as their own professional roots.

Employers' Responses

Those employers who were already familiar with EAP services were able to differentiate MBHO and EAP services. Those who previously had internal EAPs or had contracted with external specialty vendors had come to recognize the EAP as a valuable resource for managers. Supervisors could trigger a referral based on declining job performance without dealing with "medical necessity." Employers also knew that the use of the EAP both provided an alternative to discharging valuable trained employees and facilitated the return to effective performance levels of employees in whom the employer had a financial investment.

Although the clinical skills possessed by EA professionals mirror those of MBHO network clinicians, the EA professional must also be well versed in work and organizational dynamics, human resource management, and legal and legislative workplace issues. In addition, EA professionals need to become skilled at working with multiple constituencies. They recognize that the employer, the union, the safety manager, security, and the employee all have legitimate interests in EAP cases.

As more employers began to contract with MBHOs, EAP services were often bundled with other health care benefits (including those for behavioral health care). MBHOs began to receive calls from employers regarding supervisors wanting to refer employees seeking care for nonclinical issues that did not yet qualify for a clinical DSM IV diagnosis, and there was an obvious demand to treat employees who had tested positive on drug tests but had no insight into their problems. Some MBHOs, particularly those generated by insurers and benefit managers, did not have a system in place to deal with these nontraditional service demands coming from employers.

A Changing Role for EA Professionals

Non-MBHO EA professionals viewed the splitting up of EAP services by MBHOs–that is, with EA providers/professionals covering V codes, outside vendors covering ancillary services such as legal and dependent care, and licensed clinicians covering remediation and rehabilitation–as a further dilution of the EA professional's role. They criticized their fellow EA professionals who were working within particular MBHOs for compromising their work-site-based skills because of the pressure to focus exclusively on clinical issues. They considered such professionals and others as having "sold out" to a direct service/pathology mentality that has obviated the focus on workplace counseling and education.

Some MBHOs, when looking for clinical staff, viewed workplace skills as an asset, but not as a criterion for hire. The assumption was that clinicians with good clinical skills would make good EA professionals. The staff answering the phones for MBHOs were being hired for their clinical skills, with the workplace expertise as secondary.

Clearly, these staff had to be clinically competent to look for and discern clinical problems, but they were also called on to address a plethora of ancillary issues such as installment debt, child custody, divorce, and mediation. Since these issues were not clinical in character, some behavioral health staff perceived them as less significant rather than as being forerunners of potential clinical problems such as substance abuse. Some staff even believed that as behavioral health professionals, they should not address or ask questions about such issues. Consequently, frontline staff often ferreted out the next clinical steps but frequently forgot to provide education and information about ancillary/wrap services. When employees called for continuing or post-hospitalization care, frontline staff looked for additional clinical services instead of taking the more traditional EAP approach—bringing community supports into play and recognizing that solving one clinical problem may disclose another.

The EAP approach would be for frontline staff both to listen with their "third" ears in order to discern workplace issues, and to mobilize callers to take the next steps to address their concerns. Many callers need to be directed toward community resources (for example, self-help groups) and recovery-maintenance programs for additional assistance in dealing with chronic and persistent problems such as alcoholism.

Frontline managed care EAP staff, as well as managed care provider panels of clinical professionals, needed to increase their understanding of EAP technology. Many of these clinicians were unfamiliar with the role and goals of EAP. Some dealt with EAP referrals exactly like all other managed care referrals. In fact, some clinicians felt that the only difference between a clinical referral and an EAP referral was that EAP clients did not have a copayment for the first several sessions when they accessed their EAP benefit.

EA clinicians in MBHO panels differ from traditional EA professionals in yet another very significant way. EA professionals with the goal of assessment and referral often do not establish a therapeutic relationship with their employee clients. Understanding the limits of engagement and the limits of confidentiality are critical for traditional clinicians to make the transition to providing EAP services. When the scope of EAPs expanded to include short-term problem resolution, this relationship was, by necessity, changed. The MBHO model takes this even further. Often the clinician who receives the initial EAP referral will also be asked to continue to provide psychological care under the managed care benefit. This role of the EAP staff is thereby complicated, with varying and sometimes contradictory performance expectations for the clinician that are not present in traditional EAPs. Consider, for example, the dynamic tension between the rights of EAP clients and the safety of persons in the referring organization.

Some MBHOs worked with consultants in order to design national training programs to address core EAP issues. Some MBHOs also assigned geographical overseers to review EAP case documentation and to provide case support as appropriate. These initiatives were driven both by the managed care companies' recognition that contracted EAPs were not consistently addressing workplace issues and by consumers or customers who were beginning to take a more active interest in determining objectives for their EAP programs.

The training programs for clinicians who were now dealing with EAP cases attempted to communicate the unique neutral role that is played by EA professionals. EA professionals recognize the organization, the supervisor, and the employee as clients. The EAP assessment asks questions that may not be part of a clinician's standard intake—for example, concerning work and disciplinary history, and whether there any such problems currently unresolved. An EAP assessment also reflects the roots of EAPs, with alcohol and drug use always being assessed. A large part of the EA professional's intervention is to provide decathexis, clarification, and short-term problem solving. If the employee presents with a problem that is not amenable to short-term counseling, the EA professional needs to have highly developed skills to motivate the employee to transfer to an appropriate level of care. Knowledge of community resources is critical.

THE CONSOLIDATION AND SUBSEQUENT DEVELOPMENT OF EAPS WITHIN MBHOS

MBHOs, like all developing organizations, have come to recognize that EAP staff need to have some control over their work, to feel honored and dignified in their work setting, and to experience a sense of reward and accomplishment no different than the consumers or customers that they serve. MBHOs, with their internal EAP advocates leading the charge, consequently began more concerted efforts to redirect or retrain staff, and established internal training programs to focus on workplace assessment, return-to-work coordination, follow-up, and aftercare.

Enlightenment was also driven by the consumer/customer's need to respond to more extensive federal regulations, such as Department of Transportation (DOT) drug-testing requirements, the Family and Medical Leave Act, and Americans with Disabilities Act (ADA). EA staff and professionals within MBHOs–aided by customers dealing with violence in the workplace and by those in regulated industries–assisted the MBHOs' internal programs to gain clout and recognition. Likewise, the 1996 changes in the ADA, which made mental impairment a recognizable disability, enabled internal EAPs to gain recognition within their own organizations. Customers knew that they needed workplace support to develop appropriate interventions both on a macro- and a microlevel. They were even more deliberate about their needs as they began outsourcing human resources services.

MBHOs were directly affected by the federal regulations mentioned above, particularly the DOT drug testing, which covers more than seven million employees. Employers looked to their MBHOs to help them with compliance issues and to provide the required specialty assessments. MBHOs learned that EA professionals were themselves directly affected by the Omnibus Transportation Testing Act of 1991 because it included them (as certified EA professionals, or CEAPs) as one of the five groups of credentialed professionals to evaluate employees who fall under the DOT. In order to practice within the requirements of the DOT guidelines, MBHOs beefed up their efforts to include in their networks EA providers with expertise in the assessment and treatment of substance abuse/dependence.

MBHOs had long pushed the argument that greater numbers of providers made them more competitive. In the new regulatory environment, however, the focus had to change. There was not a large number of behavioral health professionals who both understood substance abuse/dependence assessment and level-of-care determinations. In the mid to late 1990s, MBHOs were compelled to play catch up–focusing on core EAP services, rather than clinical rehabilitation and remediation, because their constituencies had changed. The stakes were high for regulated companies that had entrusted their mental health/substance abuse services to MBHOs and were subject to litigation on safety issues.

Because MBHOs had to be responsive to both the clinical and the workplace issues, staff began receiving additional in-house training on these issues, as well as encouragement to use external training hours to augment their "legal awareness/learning." While there are now fewer fatalities in the workplace, due in large measure to the Occupational Safety and Health Act of 1970, consumers/customers continue to need assistance following the occurrence traumatic workplace incidents. Since companies are also increasingly concerned that the off-hand, hostile remarks or the aberrant behaviors of their employees might result in legal or financial reprisals, they are looking to MBHOs for guidance and assistance.

The MBHOs began to realize that they needed to develop systems to deal with EAP issues. The major MBHOs began to look for existing national and regional EAP firms that could be purchased. What followed was a flurry of acquisitions and mergers. The 2000–01 Open Minds survey of managed behavioral health market share disclosed 675 surveyed companies–a record number–mainly as a result of the EAP-specific concentration (Oss, 2000). Summarizing that same survey, the *EAP Digest* noted that "EAP enrollment climbed to a record 62.1 million lives in 2000, a 7.8% climb since 1999 and a jump of 130% since '94." It is estimated that approximately 49.4 million people are covered in stand-alone EAPs, with the remaining 12.7 million covered by integrated EAP/managed behavioral health programs. "While enrollment in stand-alone EAPs grew by almost 6 million since 1999, enrollment in an integrated product actually dropped 1 million following a downward trend" (*EAP Digest*, 2000, p. 10).

EAPs Broaden Their View and Their Services

The traditional EAP field has been in an intense struggle over whether the core functions of EAP can be preserved–those workplace-oriented services that make EAPs unique for the employer–and at the same time adopt the principles of managed care and be integrated with other products. While this discussion continues in many sectors, it is clear that the purchasers have embraced integration and managed care concepts. The EAP's historic function of helping employees receive behavioral health treatment and return to full productivity has become just one component in a broad array of services.

Traditional EA professionals have been slow to recognize that their colleagues who are delivering EAP services through MBHOs are, indeed, their colleagues and are ideally situated to help expand employee access to EAP services. EAPs housed in MBHOs rarely have to struggle with being inappropriately seen as benefit replacement for employers offering few or no behavioral health benefits. Similarly, these EAPS have the financial resources to respond, without raising their rates, to purchaser pressures to diversify their menu of services and to offer a wider range of work/life and other activities.

EAPs and Managed-Care Best Practices

Now that our nation, via managed care, has forced our health care delivery system through a cost-cutting revolution, consumers, payers, and providers are participating in a second, quality-oriented revolution. As the market place and mergers settled down in the late 1990s, the immense job of establishing best practices began. The focus has shifted from controlling costs to maximizing value. EAPs within MBHOs are adopting a customer-friendly stance, showing a willingness to be accountable for services provided and finding ways to demonstrate value and effectiveness.

Effectiveness in the area of EAP is often in the eye of the beholder. Clinicians generally look at clinical measures; EAPs look at return to satisfactory job performance; and clients focus on how they feel and how they perceive their quality of life. For family members the central concern is the impact on the family, while payers and managed care organizations view outcomes in terms of cost. This focus on performance data is new to traditional EAPs and is a positive contribution by managed care to the integrated EAP.

A critical factor in positioning EAPs within these large MBHOs was to educate the decision makers from traditional backgrounds about the unique role played by EAPs. Encompassed within these educational efforts were the individuals responsible for selling products to employers. The EA professionals working within MBHOs delivered this education; those with a traditional EAP orientation were often viewed as strident—pushing their organizations to provide a more well rounded experience base for EAP phone counselors. Several organizations established national EAP certification (CEAP designation) as a desired objective, and allocated resources to encourage experienced and interested internal staff to become CEAPs. Most organizations established a similar objective for their network of contracted providers. They developed specific interview guides for those providing EA services, and published EAP handbooks to accentuate their commitment to workplace support. EA providers practicing within the MBHOs' contracted networks were offered additional coaching and oversight to ensure both a common body of knowledge and a commitment to focusing on the workplace.

Continuing Challenges

In the mid to late 1990s, MBHOs came to appreciate that pressures to control costs in an extremely competitive environment, compounded by pressures to operate within regulatory constraints, required a change from "business as usual." Some MBHOs chose to separate EAP phone counselors into two units. Consequently, EAP counselors who have more extensive workplace experience focus specifically on management-support services and direct their efforts to the rigors of the regulatory requirements. The remaining EAP phone counselors focus on general assessment and referrals, linking callers to local providers or community resources through zip-code matching.

For EAPs functioning within MBHOs, the reality that they had to deal with was the segregation of services. Because of this separation of basic tasks, EAP phone counselors have to be very adaptive and able to quickly assess the immediacy of callers' needs so that callers could be routed to appropriate resources. Similarly, EAP workplace-support counterparts have to quickly assess the workplace needs of managers and supervisors in order to assist them in determining specific interventions.

One of the newer challenges to complicate the multiple facets of EAPs within MBHOs is that dependent-care companies are offering counseling for emotional issues and presenting themselves to consumer/customers as having a work/life focus. Like the early MBHOs before them, these work/life firms are presenting themselves as capable of addressing the employee's and employer's full range of needs without understanding the importance of being able to intervene when employees are referred on a basis of declining performance. MBHOs have begun to include dependent-care resources both as a coordination service, or vendor relationship, and as an embedded service. In the case of MBHOs that have in-house dependent-care programs, frontline EAP staff who answer phones focus on work/life integration. In the case of MBHOs with a vendor relationship, EAP staff "warm transfer" callers. In the case of MBHOs with neither of the above, EAP staff perform their traditional tasks of determining community resources appropriate to the caller's dependent-care needs. Today's business world includes planning for pet sitting, assistance with trades people, purchasing/concierge services—all stretching the historical role of MBHOs and EAPs alike. (Likewise, most MBHOs have either folded legal services into their other programs or joined with a vendor.)

There are still areas of service in which traditional EA professionals view MBHOs as the enemy. One of these areas is the payment for substance abuse services, which is near and dear to the hearts of EAPs. The practice of some MBHOs to sell a benefit plan that purports to include a substance abuse benefit but offers only a set of inadequate options managed by individuals having a limited understanding of chemical dependency continues to erode the collegiality between EAPs and MBHOs (Rawson, 2000). Many EAPs feel that managed care has forced a return to the days when there were few third-party benefits for managed care, as a consequence of which employees are being shifted to the public sector and forced to pay out of pocket for treatment. Administrative demands, coupled with minimal reimbursement, are leading to the closure of many independent outpatient treatment programs and residential treatment facilities, especially medical-model treatment units (Bacon, 1990).

Access-to-care issues pose problems for EAPs, both outside and inside MBHOs. EAPs in some MBHOs have served as "gatekeepers"; customers prefer to "use" the EAP in an attempt to control access to benefits. When managed mental health/substance abuse services are discontinued, and if a caller's presenting problem is not one that is appropriate for an EA provider/professional to address—for example, medication evaluations, comorbidity, or complicated psychiatric and substance abuse problems—telephone EA clinicians who have been accustomed to "warm transferring" their callers to their managed care colleagues must now spend additional time with the caller in order to determine what benefits or public services are available to address the problem. Complicating this determination is that many publicly funded community mental health resources have had their funding reduced or eliminated.

Another concern is that some MBHOs continue to staff their EAP products with licensed clinicians who have limited chemical-dependency background or workplace experience. The underlying fear is that EAPs will continue to shift to a clinical focus that deals with self-referred employees who have some insight and motivation, and that EAPs will not bother to struggle with identifying the more reluctant troubled employees who are motivated only by the threat of job loss. Since the latter group comprises many employees who have chemical dependency problems and are quite challenging to work with, the fear is that these employees will drop through the cracks of these clinically focused EAPs.

Yet another concern is the vision of "virtual" managed care organizations in which more and more service delivery is geared, as it were, to high tech, not high touch. Experienced EA professionals, as well as many clinicians, recognize the limitations in dealing with chemical dependency without direct contact and labor-intensive case management. The very nature of the disease—characterized by denial and resistance—makes many of these "virtual visions" inappropriate.

To further compound the issue for EAPs practicing within MBHOs, the nation's current full or near-full employment means that every employee is needed in the workplace. Time spent attending to physical or emotional problems is lost time, which affects productivity and ultimately the financial bottom line. Employers want and expect their employees to function with optimal health and well-being, and are often demanding not only quicker turnaround times for re-entry, but the assumption of risk by the EAP.

CONCLUSION

As we move into the twenty-first century, EAPs have become an integral part of managed behavioral health care. The emerging EAP models within MBHOs are now designed to provide ongoing access to highly qualified providers, to use gatekeepers to help control costs, and to provide additional focus on workplace issues. Employers continue to carve out their behavioral health services to specialty vendors. Integrated care today refers to the integration of mental health benefits, chemical dependency benefits, the EAP, and work/life services.

Employers must compete with a dwindling and not-so-loyal labor force, and their focus is on retention. MBHOs that adopt a business solution or that build programs to address customer objectives will be the ones to become major players in this new century. Consumers/customers need consultative expertise and behavioral health or "good-sense" experience and direction. Their employees are driving them to provide effectiveness training and job coaching. Their managers and supervisors are challenged to keep focused on the bottom line and to adapt creatively to the changing needs and demands of their employees. MBHOs with "good ears" and imagination are able to see beyond the expressed needs of the employers they serve and to focus on all-around effectiveness. MBHOs–and not just employers–need to move from an environment focused on productivity to one focused on effectiveness.

REFERENCES

Bacon, K. H. (1990, July 23). Private drug abuse treatment centers try to adjust to life in slow lane. *Wall Street Journal*, p. B1.

Cagney, T. (1999). Models of service delivery. In J. M. Oher, *The employee assistance handbook* (pp. 59–69). New York: John Wiley.

EAP Digest. (2000). News update–Survey: EAP enrollment jumps 130% since 1994. *EAP Digest, 20* (4), 10.

Employee Assistance Professional Association. (1997). *Standards of Practice* (3rd ed.). Arlington, VA: Author.

Mark, T., Coffey, R. M., King, E., Harwood, H., McKusick, D., Genuardi, J., Dilonardo, J., & Buck, J. A. (2000). Spending on mental health and substance abuse treatment, 1987–1997. *Health Affairs, 19* (4), 108–120.

Oss, M. (2000). Yearbook of managed behavioral health market share in the United States 2000–2001. Gettysburg, PA: Open Minds.

Rawson, R. A. (2000). Substance abuse treatment under managed care: The emperor's new clothes. *EAP Digest, 20* (4), 121–134.

AUTHOR INDEX

SUBJECT INDEX